AF248897

Louis Gifford
Aches and Pains

Book Three

Graded Exposure 1-4

Case Histories 1-4

Curriculum Vitae

CNS Press, Aches and Pains Ltd., Kestrel, Swanpool,
Falmouth, Cornwall, TR11 5BD, UK

Email:info@achesandpainsonline.com
www.giffordsachesandpains.com

Copyright @ Louis Gifford, Philippa Tindle, Ralph Gifford and Jake Gifford 2014

Louis Gifford has asserted his right under the Copyright, Design and Patents Act
1988 to be identified as the author of this book.

A CIP catalogue record for the book is available from the British Library.

First published 2014
Reprinted 2015, 2016 (thrice), 2017 (twice), 2018 (thrice), 2019 (twice), 2020 (thrice),
2021 (twice)

ISBN 978 1 7399486 2 7

Louis Gifford Aches and Pains

Book 1 Aches and Pains Sections 1-14. Book 2 Aches and Pains Sections 15-20.
Nerve Root 1-5. Book 3 Graded Exposure 1-4. Case Histories 1-4.

Louis Gifford MApplSc FCSP

All rights reserved. Except for the quotation of short passages for the purposes
of criticism and review, no part of this publication may be reproduced, stored
in a retrieval system, or transmitted in any form or by any means, electronic,
mechanical, photocopying, recording or otherwise, without the proper permission
of the author and publisher CNS Press, Aches and Pains Ltd., Kestrel, Swanpool,
Falmouth, Cornwall TR11 5BD, UK.

Editing   Philippa Tindle, Mick Thacker and Paula Ross

Typesetting and

Figures redrawn by   Harriet Gendall and Julian Tredinnick

Printed and bound by   TJ Books Limited, Padstow, Cornwall, UK.

Contents

LOUIS GIFFORD ACHES AND PAINS

INTRODUCTION TO GRADED EXPOSURE AND PATIENT MANAGEMENT

Chapter GE 1.1
Graded Exposure/patient management

'the art of medicine consists in amusing the patient while nature cures the disease'

Voltaire

Setting the scene...

This is the story I mentioned briefly in chapter 14.1 but elaborate a little here.

It must have been round about 1997 or 1998, I can't remember exactly but I woke up with the most ghastly right shoulder pain. I couldn't believe it. I was totally unable to move. Abduction five degrees... arghhh... flexion, same... arghhh... hand behind back... arghhh, same. I could hardly shrug my shoulder. Philippa had to help me to dress. I struggled at work. This went on for two days and didn't improve. Now like I may have said before I'm not a wimp with pain, I don't have the anaesthetic at the dentist, so here I am thinking, 'Come on Louis you must be able to move the bloody thing, push through the pain.' But you know I couldn't and it made me get shitty with myself. All the static tests with elbow by my side were fine. There was no pain with the arm down by my side. But even trying to passively lift it was agony.

Two days later I was in the clinic with a low back pain patient, doing and observing standard back movements.

'Ruby, I'm going to show you a movement and then I'd like you to have a go and see what you can do – remember you can do as much or as little as you like, you can even refuse if you want.'

We both smiled, like we were thinking 'The Horse of the Year Show', and then I quietly bent forward and with a bit of a bounce at it touched my toes and came back up again.

I stopped, thought a second, ignored Ruby and repeated the movement... down I went and stayed there. My arm was dangling, comfy in more or less full flexion. I paused, and said,

'Ruby, I'll be with you in moment.' She must have thought I was mad.

I now put my hand on my head and came slowly back up to face Ruby.

Full flexion with my hand on my head standing! The next bit was foolish. I tried to actively lower it, bang the searing sharp pain and me going... arghhh, right in front of my patient.

'You alright dear...?' she puzzled.

Well, I'd found something out that was really quite simple, but when I'd finished treating Ruby and had some free time I started to play with what I'd found

Down I went again. I could stay down and by gyrating my trunk a bit and staying really relaxed it would move, but as soon as any muscle tension came in to help the pain shot back. I put my hand on my head and came up like before – what's now called 'hand on head elevation'! This time I grabbed the arm by the elbow and tried to stay as relaxed as I could to lower it passively... eeeyow! No go! I then lent forward slightly and lowered my head so as to lower the arm a little. I tried to let go again, this time taking a deep breath and letting my hand slide off my head to let the arm fall like a dead weight – no pain! It swung back then forward again and with my lowered head at the ready I managed to grab my head and return to the upright position again. That was all in one neat smooth action. Repeat all together now... lean forward, head down, let hand go, drop arm, arm swing down and back, catch back of head with hand, lift head and rise up... tee hee! I'm smiling now.

So next, I'm standing there upright with my hand on my head. The opposite hand is on my raised elbow; I push against it making a strengthening static contraction, good – no pain. I keep that up and then, while pushing hard, I slowly bring the arm down against the resistance – no pain! I relax and try and move the arm normally... arghhh again. Dang!

The story goes on. I was soon able to get good range of big, floppy, pendular movement by leaning forward hand on head, letting go, swinging back up to catch the head, but almost immediately letting it go back down again, loose and floppy. I gradually used the head-grabbing less and less until I could start the swinging-off standing up! I also found I could also lower the arm with resistance and bring it back up with resistance—with no pain—so long as I didn't relax before going back up again.

This was my little shoulder experience that created an 'ah-ha' moment in that it linked 'fear-avoidance' and 'graded exposure' theory and management methods, normally reserved for 'phobic' behaviours – like fear of heights or spiders or water, to that of movement abnormality or loss of movement.

What am I on about? It's simply that a great many patients come to see physiotherapists with a painful loss of movement. Now the loss of range may be wholly like mine, in that the pain was just too bad to allow me to move it even though I wanted to move it and wasn't fearful of it. By messing around with different starting positions and different ways of doing the movement – it is usually possible to find a way of producing it. Another example similar to my shoulder is lumbar flexion in standing, a pain limited movement of many back pains, but in 'all fours curl up' full flexion is often quite possible. Now, some patient's range limitations may also relate to fear of pain or even fear of doing damage, here again the same 'approach' applies – mess around with different starting positions until the patient can do the movement with confidence. The patient who tells me they avoid standing bending forward because of fear of making their back pain worse, will often quite willingly bend well from different starting positions—all fours as above—even simply bending forward sitting.

Not only that, graded exposure is all about starting easy and moving to more difficult and more challenging tasks. As I showed with my shoulder there are a great many options to try and to choose from. The end result is a simple and gradual return of normal movement and function, or should be!

It sounds simple, but the key is the way it's set up with the patient and that's not necessarily that easy.

Let's have a very brief look at how phobias can be overcome (while you're reading this think of a patient with on-going pain).

There are some vital ingredients:

- the sufferer has got to see that they have a problem and that it's impacting their life, that it's stopping them doing normal things and is almost a constant issue – it's 'consuming'

- the sufferer has to be prepared to have a go at confronting it and trying to overcome it

- the sufferer may need kind and expert help – they need to trust the person who is helping

- they need to be gradually exposed to the thing they fear, starting at an easy level and slowly working to harder and more challenging levels and situations

- the therapist needs to be a bit of a genius at finding/inventing ways of bringing or 'transitioning' the sufferer from one level to the next.

Here's a very simple example:

You the sufferer won't go into a room unless your husband/wife/partner has thoroughly checked everywhere for spiders/cockroaches/geckos/ scorpions/ moths/ daddy-longlegs etc. Let's say your thing is 'spiders'.

Start by thinking about and understanding a 'graded hierarchy', for example, by learning a bit more about the common spiders etc., like where they live and how they go about their lives. Look at a few simple pictures of them and learn that they mostly can't harm you, and even if there are ones that can it's very rare for them to be a problem. Maybe even learn about the 'good' that they may do. Learn that the worse that can happen is rarely much more than a tiny bite.

The next level might be looking at real but dead or preserved spiders, say in a display cabinet, which is a simple way to start observing them. Start with the least nasty looking one for you – that might be very small ones. Gradually 'approach' them. Do this every day until it gets easier and you feel you can move on to say bigger ones.

(Note the 'you' choose part of this – not the therapist dictating your choice.)

Next... when you're ready...

Start approaching and touching the dead spiders...

Gradually increase the size/nastiness looking...

Observe live spiders... in an enclosure...

Take the lid off...

Put your hand in...

Let them wander over your hand...

Try a bigger one...

Start going into rooms by yourself, and start with ones you know that have recently been cleaned. Later you can move onto less visited places like the garden shed, the cellar and so forth.

I think most of us have a 'shudder' point somewhere along that hierarchy – the key thing is to get the fear down to a level where it's not intruding detrimentally on your life – like the example above where it becomes possible for the sufferer to enter any room without someone checking for spiders first.

You could do the same with fear of heights – starting with a mere small step and moving onto a low chair – then lower rungs of a ladder and up and up – to low walkways, to higher walkways, to edges of low cliffs then to higher and so forth.

The point is that any easy starting task can always be found, hence our phrase with pain patients '**START EASY BUILD SLOWLY**'. We use this term explicitly with our patients because we want their help in finding a starting point from which to start and begin moving up in a graded hierarchy. All exercises need to be related to a graded hierarchy.

It is important to realise that a great many patients with straightforward musculoskeletal pain problems don't have anything like true 'phobias'. Most patients will have a simple reluctance to do certain movements 'in case it hurts' or 'in case it does more damage and makes the situation worse'. All these patients require is adequate guidance into appropriate movement and lots of practice. However, there's still always some kind of 'hierarchy' and still the need for a 'start easy build slowly' approach in most cases.

I'm sure many of you have seen TV reality shows where volunteers with phobias have been 'cured' of their fears by being thrown right in the deep end – psychologists call it 'flooding'. You'll find splattered all over YouTube the miracles of hypnotism and 'NLP' based 'instant cures' for all sorts of phobias, often pedalled by 'celebrity' hypnotists and the like. Headline: 'cured of spider fear in seven minutes, after having problems for a lifetime' etc.

I'm afraid I'm deeply suspicious of quick cures for long well-entrenched problems – especially when done in front of the TV cameras, where pressure for and expectations of a good outcome are very high. Those who fail, or don't do what they're supposed to, are likely to get binned and never screened. We, the public, never see them and what we're left with is the very powerful impression that the video-star fixes everybody in an instant! If you look you'll quickly find 'back pain instant cures' too! What you won't see though are chronic pain sufferers, who can hardly walk, suddenly running because they've been put in an enclosure with a pile of hungry lions! That's the equivalent of 'flooding' for pain disability as far as I can see.

So, as far as 'graded exposure' and my pain patients are concerned it's all about '**RETURN OF PHYSICAL CONFIDENCE**' – whether the problem is acute or chronic. The fundamental thing is a process of gradual physical challenge. The patient starts off with movements they find achievable and safe and then gradually increases the quality, quantity and difficulty of movement in a slow and progressive way. As I said before, I help do the 'inventing' with the patient and the patient makes the choices of how and where they'd be happy to go.

As mentioned earlier, patients often have concerns or fears about movement and activity – a problem that's termed 'fear-avoidance' and relates to various beliefs about the problem and the pain. For example, beliefs about what is wrong with them; how strong they are where it hurts, or where the pain is coming from; they may have concerns about re-damaging and causing further harm, and most importantly about causing more pain. Structure and pain related fear 'beliefs' lead to 'fear-avoidance' behaviours. For example, you wisely limp when you've just twisted your ankle and you cancel the soccer match scheduled for tomorrow. Or, you're a chronic back pain sufferer and you avoid all bending and only sit with a constant lordosis for fear of setting it all off again. Your life is your back and your lumbar roll is your security blanket.

Take a look at figures GE1.1 and GE1.2

On the left is a patient with an 'acute' presentation (that's a problem that has very recently started, say days or at most a few weeks) who comes to you because of some concern about their problem and a wish for help in getting better. In the figure we are saying that they're 'in a position of fear – of pain/further damage'; and they require a confident therapist who can be clear, reassuring and give good information and guidance! I put an exclamation mark because I almost hear a great many of you going – 'I wish my patient's were that simple' and my response is that surprisingly, most are. But there are some you have to work hard with to grasp and embrace the pathway that you're offering. Patient examples later will help if you're sceptical here. I'll also discuss 'locus of control' too – as understanding whether the patient has an 'internal' locus and therefore keen for knowledge, understanding and guidance so 'they' can help themselves. Or, has an 'external' locus, meaning that they want you to take control, do everything and fix them and they're not keen to take responsibility in their recovery – which in itself is a very significant yellow flag.

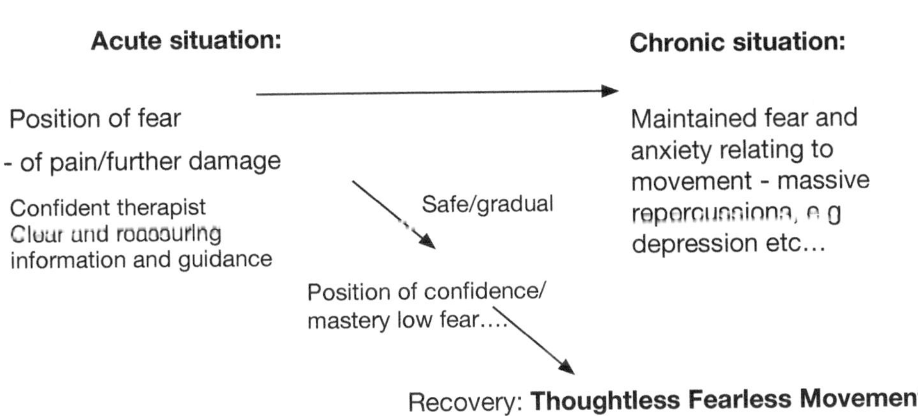

Figure GE 1.1 An 'acute' presentation

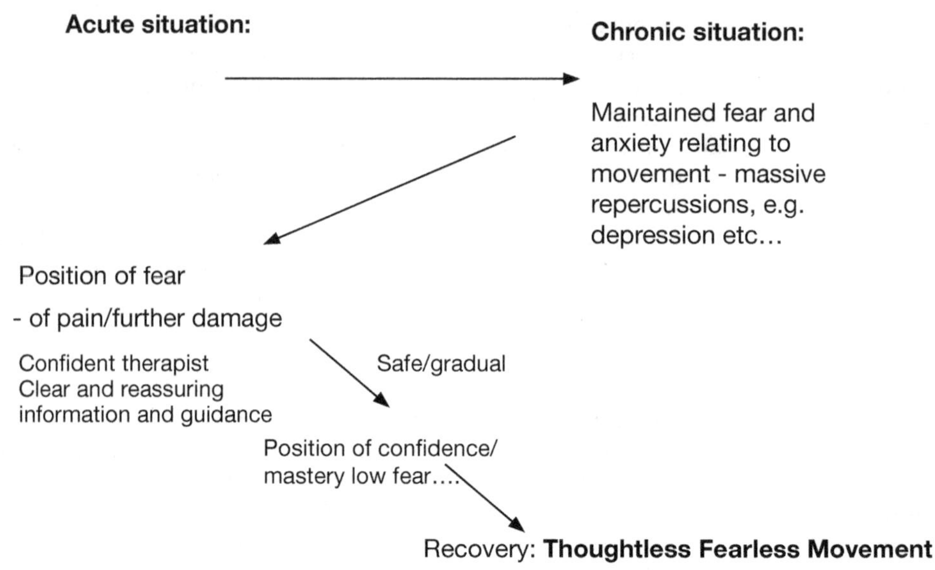

Figure GE 1.2 A 'chronic' presentation

So, as per the diagrams, the process is to take the patient from a position of concern/fear/anxiety about their problem and situation, via gradual and safe stages, to a position of confidence and 'mastery'—what I like to term—the recovery of **THOUGHTLESS-FEARLESS-MOVEMENT**.

I like that phrase and I came up with it after getting fed up with patients coming in who were so 'body' focused. I remember one patient, Veranda, who talked out loud as she moved, it went something like this:

Me: Er, Veranda, I'd like you to show me what you're happy to do when you bend forward.

Ver: Right, ribs out, tummy in, brace the transverse, engage the erectors, curve in, bottom then out a millimetre and forward with slow release 2, 3 and 4 and down don't let go, reverse again and check tummy, bottom tense, curvy in erectors tight and no – here I am again!

She had bent forward, touched her toes and come up again.

Me: Where did you get all that?

Ver: Oh, my physio in Sheen, Naomi. I saw her two years ago with back pain and she was so cross with me and the way I moved. Oh, we spent months getting my core working correctly, but it's paid off I can touch my toes again.

(Sheen is a posh London 'village' for those not familiar with England)

Look, normal movement, normal healthy movement is thoughtless and fearless. 99.999999999% of the world DON'T think like this lady does when they move – yet physios and others into 'muscle imbalance' teach patients to focus on their bodies, on specific muscles and 'correct patterning', like it was super dangerous not to. It makes me mad – hence my goal of thoughtless-fearless-movement. It's my rebuttal of a particularly nauseous physiotherapy fad that's still going on.

My suggestion is you read papers like Eyal Lederman's:

Lederman E (2007). The Myth of Core Stability. CPDO Online Journal, June 1-17

But also go do a half marathon, and/or watch the Paralympics closely and observe hard what you see. Those places are full of people with quite remarkable disabilities and remarkable 'muscle imbalances' achieving the most amazing physical feats using thoughtless-fearless-movement. Please save all that nitty-gritty stuff for the super elite athletes when you can't think of anything else to do and stop teaching normal people to become 'somatisers'!

The second figure (GE1.2) shows the same process for a chronic pain patient with 'maintained' fear and anxiety relating to movement and pain, and of course all those repercussions like helplessness, hopelessness, mood changes and not uncommonly, depression.

So what's the physical approach for chronic? Same as acute! Well, in essence at least!

Here are some important early issues with a 'graded exposure' approach.

1. Alongside a 'graded exposure' process is a strong 'appropriate' educational element, that helps the patient feel confident with what they are doing and lessens any fear of further injury or worry about increased levels of pain. There is no way a patient is going to begin stressing and moving their body if they have no confidence in it and they are fearful of negative consequences. The case histories later will give plenty of examples of how I do this.

2. Patients will only believe what you explain to them if you have listened thoroughly and done a good physical assessment – in their eyes, not yours! They must be confident in you. I sometimes find myself saying to patients' things like: 'Now, I feel I've found out a great deal about your problem and how it's affecting you. I've also done a thorough examination and explained to you what I've found – that's all well and good, but now I want your opinion about it all. For example, have I missed something, is there something you want me to test that you feel is important, or maybe there's something you want to tell me that I haven't asked you about?' The key here is to create an atmosphere with the patient where they can be absolutely honest with you. Remember, you might be thinking you've just done a top notch physical examination but the patient might be thinking that it was all a load of irrelevant fiddling about!

3. Pain as such is not ignored (see shopping basket and all the examples later). However, pain's recovery or lessening generally occurs with improved physical confidence and performance. Check figure GE 1.3, 'The forgotten

pain killer' – movement! The big deal here is that movement helps, but it's movement in the right 'context' as far as the patient's brain is concerned, and that is what makes it all so hard sometimes. Note that this figure was originally produced by Bill Fordyce (1981) one of the great behavioural psychologists who was famous for the following quote:

'Information to behaviour change is like wet noodles are to a brick!'

What he's on about is how difficult it is to change people's behaviour habits by information alone. 'Smoking gives you cancer'. 'Drink drive' campaigns, the preacher in the pulpit, the lecturing politicians, the 'healthy school dinner' campaigns, all wagging their fingers at you telling you what to do – but do people change? Do they heck! For change to occur most people need more than just information, they need their hands holding, they need guidance and some need very close guidance and support. The more ingrained and chronic a problem the more difficult the process becomes.

4. Help with pain relief is very important in the early stages of a disorder. BUT – pain relief and focus on pain response (e.g. manual therapy á la Maitland which I was schooled in) is never the sole form of management. In fact a major feature is to actually de-focus on pain—that means you—the therapist: 'Where's your pain, what's happening to your pain, where's your pain now, what's the pain now? That awful grinding pain chatter that goes on and on

The forgotten pain killer – purposeful function!

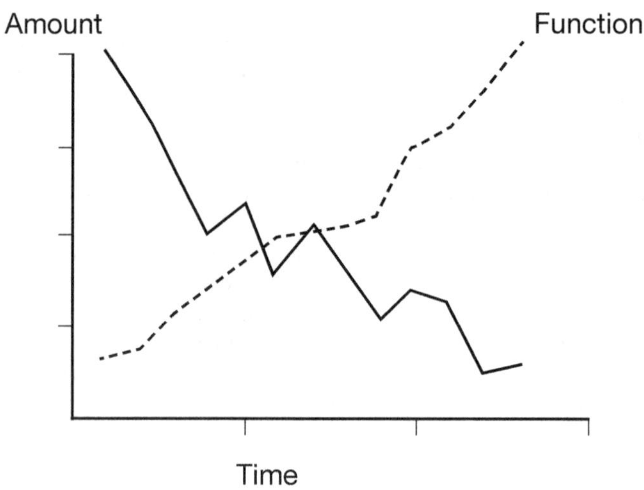

Figure GE 1.3 'The forgotten painkiller' – movement

and on. I have some advice: STOP IT! Stop the habit of constantly asking about the patient's pain! If it's any help, once I realised I was asking too much about pain I reckon it took me a good few months to get out of the habit. If you talk about it the patients will think about it more – you'll train them to maladaptively 'centralise' their pain if you're not careful. Also, get explicit with the patient, quite often I ask the patient if they're finding that their mind is habitually coming back to thinking about, checking on and looking for the pain?   I specifically state that one of my goals for them is to try and get them to dampen that thinking down and recognise when they're doing it.

5. Now a big deal here is to not only reduce patient fear of pain but also to reduce therapist fear of it! If the therapist doesn't understand the pain they're dealing with, hasn't a clue why it fluctuates and isn't confident about its nature and cause, they're hardly going to able to deal confidently with the patient – and the patient will pick that up. Clinicians need to have seen and listened to hundreds of patients and need to know a great many common presentations too. Grumpy old me is getting more and more pissed-off with therapists with a mere three or four years clinical experience labelling themselves as 'experts' or 'specialists' or even 'consultants' (I understand that we can even call ourselves consultants with or without any peer review or exam structure!). Here's me after thirty five plus years of listening, observing and watching pain presentations and recovery and I wouldn't dream to be so arrogant. All I can say is that I've reached a stage in my career where I have no fear of any pain patient who walks in the door. My aim is to help them and I have to work hard with the patient and see how it all unfolds – acute or chronic. Now, after all these years I can usually predict who I will have more success with than others.

6. Leading on from the clinician 'fear' of pain, I also think we need to overcome many irrational fears and fads ourselves; like flexion exercises; 'incorrect' postures and movement patterns; the prescription of lots of 'musts and don'ts'; 'it must be done like this not that' statements. Ghastly things like, 'you mustn't do a sit-up until you've got abdominal control'. If you have firm beliefs like this and refuse to change, then I seriously suggest you take more time to look at normally awful movement habits in the majority of the population who have no pain, and reconsider. The one that really gets me is not allowing the patient to flex until repeated flexion testing stops peripheralising the pain.

7. We must feel comfortable that even the injured musculoskeletal system is strong enough for most everyday movements and activities, even though they may have to be modified a bit for a while. The strained back often likes to be flexed, or flexed and shifted; the injured calf prefers to walk flat-footed and with your foot turned out; the flaring arthritic hip likes a stride with a roll and short extension and so forth. If it's adaptive, do it, but remember one of the goals of good therapy is 'Normal, thoughtless, fearless movement', or 'as far as possible, normal thoughtless, fearless movement!'

Many years ago a local fireman came to see me with acute low back pain. He'd had the problem about three or four days and was desperate as he was doing the London marathon in six days time! Should he cancel or should he carry on were his big concerns. He hobbled in flexed and shifted, he could hardly bend any further, his side flexion towards pain was nil, nor could he come up straight to neutral, all because of nasty, sharp pain. I did a full neuro exam – reflexes, muscle power and sensation – all were fine. This guy was a normally very fit fireman who had never had back pain before, he was 37 years old and the back pain followed a 'lifting drill' at work, basically he'd been carrying a colleague on his shoulders out of a 'burning' building.

That's all we need to know here. I treated him using simple 'hands-on' in side lying and gave him some easy exercises with all the progression details as well as advising him to regularly take some anti-inflammatories. That was on the Monday and the marathon was the following Sunday. When I saw him on the Friday he was a little less shifted and flexed, he said he was about 20% better. What do we do – go for it or not? He had his running kit, I went and put mine on and off we went for a run. After two miles he was going along pretty well and I told him to do a couple more laps of the circuit we were doing and I'd see him back at the clinic. The reality was that I couldn't keep up with him!

He strolled back into the clinic and he felt OK. I told him to go for a five miler that night and to ring me. My words to him were, 'Stu, don't know about you, but I'm feeling increasingly confident you're going to be fine – look forward to the call later and then we'll decide.' He rang later, he'd been fine. He did the marathon in a better time than he'd aimed for and within two weeks was pretty much fully recovered.

Should I have manipulated his back? Should I have done McKenzie stuff? NO! Not for me. You wouldn't 'crunch' a freshly twisted ankle and you wouldn't (or shouldn't) keep pushing 'correcting' movements over and over again and then get the patient do it every hour. Would you? To me that stuff in this situation is just not biology—don't risk it—you could make them one hell of a lot worse. 'Yeah, but you went and let him run a marathon Louis!' Yes I did, but consider running as having been tested, that he was fine when he did it and it loosened him up, plus running does not involve any forceful end range movement (I'm thinking nerve compression and the possibility of neuropathy at worst).

In the next few chapters I discuss some reasoning models that I've found important to have in my head when assessing, treating and managing patients in pain. The last chapter tidies up with a few useful bits and pieces!

Here's the list I'm going to discuss in the following section:

1.   The Biomedical Model.

2.   Evolutionary Reasoning.

3.   The Vulnerable Organism Model.

4.   Johan Vlaeyen and Steven Linton's Model of Fear Avoidance.

5. The Mature Organism Model and Hebb's Rule.

6. Chris Main, Chris Spanswick and Paul Watson's Model of Disability.

7. The Need for an 'In Parallel' Problem and Management Perspective.

8. The Biopsychosocial Model.

Section GE 1
Read what I've read

Fordyce, W. E. (1981) Pain Complaint - Exercise performance relationship in chronic pain. Pain 10: 311-321.

Lederman E (2007) The Myth of Core Stability. CPDO Online Journal, June 1-17.

Section GE 2

MODELS

Chapter 2.1
The Biomedical Model

I have already discussed the 'weaknesses' of the biomedical model when it comes to pain states. One of the main problems with it is that the amount of pain is not necessarily an accurate reflection of the state of the tissues. There can be massive pathology and very little pain at one end of the spectrum, and at the other, massive amounts of pain and very little or no evidence of any pathology.

I will discuss the biomedical model in relation to the 'Shopping Basket Approach' later, it's an essential and natural part of our reasoning once its weaknesses are recognised.

When I used to run my Graded Exposure course I asked the participants to spend a few moments writing down all the key findings relating to typical early sciatica.

I'd get this sort of stuff back:

- limited SLR

- flexed and shifted

- loss of reflex, calf weak, numb little toe...

- pain with movements

- awkward gait

- tenderness to palpation

- 'accessory movements' limited

- the usual 'favourite treatment' related findings, for example, 'muscle imbalance', sacroiliac up/down/side-slip, loss of craniosacral synchronicity etc.

Then I might get a bit of:

- difficulty sleeping...

- constant pain down the leg

- can't get comfortable, restless all the time

- pins and needles and numbness

- hurts to cough or sneeze

- unable to walk far

- can't sit for long

- likes lying curled up on side

- difficulty getting out of a chair or bed

- can't get socks on first thing in the morning

But I didn't get much of this:

- highly distressed with the situation and the pain

- fearful of movement or doing anything, taken to resting

- frightened that something's seriously wrong – and that they might become paralysed

- stopped all hobbies, activities and exercise

- off work and work is getting mad with them

- family are unsympathetic/sympathetic/over sympathetic

- feeling hopeless and fear it may never fully recover

- disillusioned with all the pills and therapy not doing anything to help

- quietly getting more and more wound-up and angry

- stopped socialising

- massive fear of having to have back surgery.

Like it or not, the majority of therapists think in terms of the biomedical model (or they used to) and from what I can see give lip-service to the broader dimensions of pain and illness.

I'm promoting the Shopping Basket Approach here because it integrates this tissue focused/biomedical/impairment based love affair of physiotherapy into a broader perspective – via what can be called 'In-parallel' reasoning[1].

As I will discuss in a later section, 'In-parallel' requires the clinician to absorb material and information from many different 'levels' and bring it all together for best management. It helps us to see that the problem of sciatica, for example, is far more than just 'a disc' extruding and pressing on a nerve.

The biomedical paradigm is responsible for a great deal of useful knowledge however. For example, pain and tissue healing mechanism knowledge is vital. Here's an incomplete list of some of the useful things that biomedical research and knowledge give us:

- knowledge of healing and recovery for a great many recognisable musculoskeletal pain problems

- primary hyperalgesia – tenderness = something is 'wrong' in tender area

- secondary hyperalgesia – tenderness of normal tissues = nothing 'wrong' with them

---

1 - The term 'paralleling' was originally coined by Maitland and he used it to indicate that during your assessment you 'followed' the patients line of thinking and reasoning, and thus asked questions appropriate to it.

- referred pain and referred tenderness

- pain memory

- adaptive and maladaptive pain and sensitivity?

- explains 'crazy' pain's via massive changes in receptive fields and other aberrant processing mechanisms.

The problem is that medicine and physiotherapy are not being schooled in this sort of material well enough – they are still very firmly stuck in the tissues.

To finish off, here are some problems that derive from biomedical model thinking:

- the mechanism/injury that starts a pain problem may not be the same as the mechanism that is currently operating, e.g. a disc extrusion can be an initial cause of sciatica but the sciatic pain that follows is derived from hypersensitivity and reactivity of the sciatic nerve root and other central mechanisms that result

- pain mechanisms move and shift with time

- it focuses on tissues all the time – like most musculoskeletal therapists do!

- it likes single sources of a problem to label and target (dogmatic appraisal/ unidimensional appraisal) for example, 'it's a transverse abdominus sequencing problem', 'it's a disc', 'it's stress'

- it tends to ignore the impact of the problem on the patient and then the patient's impact on their own recovery

- it assumes that pain is an accurate reliable witness of tissue damage – and if the amount of pain is out of proportion to anything found – the patient is a nuisance or exaggerating their pain and therefore isn't to be tolerated.

Think about this sort of thing too:

- so called 'bad' tissues often don't hurt – or if they do they can still stop hurting

- you don't actually need to know exactly where a pain is coming from to effectively treat it! BUT, the patient likes to think you do (good assessment required)

- if you treat a particular 'joint' or tissue and the pain lessens – that doesn't mean that the joint or tissue you treated was the cause of the problem

  The sacroiliac joint is top of the league here I'm sure. A joint that hardly moves (and by the time most of us are past forty is completely seized up) yet for thousands of therapists is blamed for just about everything that hurts from the waist down. My recommendation is to spend some time with some pelvises from fresh cadavers of various ages and look at the real movement – as opposed to the imaginary movement! Sorry, very sceptical here and there's millions of dollars being made out of one of the most stable and strong joints in the human body. The other joints in this category are the cranial sutures. Come on stop believing that garbage; they're mostly fused, period. Look, send a back pain patient to a cranial therapist and they may change the pain, send the same patient to a reflexologist and they'll fiddle with the foot and may too change the pain. What's that about then? Yes, it is a 'processing' change!

Don't hate me I'm making much needed fun of these things. If physiotherapy/ physical therapy is to gain credibility we need to come up with a much better spin than many seem to have so far.

Chapter 2.2
Evolutionary Reasoning

I have already written at length about this in Topical Issues in Pain 4: 'An Introduction to Evolutionary Reasoning: Diets, Discs, Fevers and the Placebo' which can be downloaded for free on my blog: www.giffordsachesandpains.com

Briefly, there are two types of reasoning or two perspectives, that can be applied to the understanding of any presentation:

1. An 'evolutionary' perspective which asks the simple question **'Why?'**

2. And a more traditionally 'scientific' perspective that asks **'What, or how?'** – about structure or mechanism.

The 'what' or 'how' reasoning relates to a *'proximal' or 'near'* explanation of an observation or cause. In medicine proximal explanations address **how** a body works and some people get a disease and others don't for example. On the other hand *'evolutionary' or 'ultimate'* explanations show **why** humans, in general, are susceptible to some diseases and not others.

This type of reasoning can be applied to any observation and in my chapter I used Jared Diamond's amusing example: 'Why do skunks smell bad?'

The proximal answer that a molecular biologist would use might be:

'It's because skunks secrete chemical compounds, with certain particular molecular structures, that result in bad smells.' Molecular biology looks at the mechanism of the bad smell.

The evolutionary biologist would reason:

'It's because skunks would be easy victims of predators if they didn't defend themselves with bad smells. Natural selection made skunks evolve to secrete bad-smelling chemicals; those skunks with the worst smells survived to produce the most baby skunks.'

Applying all this to pain gives rise to two questions; one might be '**How** does tissue injury cause pain?' The other is '**Why** does tissue injury cause pain?'

The proximal answer details how physical and chemical stimulation of sensory nerve endings in the damaged tissue produces impulses that run in various pathways, via the peripheral nerves and spinal cord to the brain, which then, via complex neurochemical processing mechanisms gives rise to pain.

The evolutionary explanation would be that tissue injury causes' pain in order to generate behavioural and physiological responses that are compatible with best recovery, overall function and improved survival chances.

The following example is lifted from my Topical Issues in Pain 4 chapter:

Back and leg pain

When physiotherapists observe patients we seek answers to what we observe. We most often use a proximate style of reasoning, whose very nature is wedded to a biomedical, mechanistic view. We don't often use evolutionary thinking and even less often act on an evolutionary reasoned management strategy. For example, why is the female patient with back and leg pain of one week duration flexed and shifted? How should it be managed?

Many might offer the following 'proximal' style of answer.

'Because she probably has a disc problem and the disc problem has led to irritation of the sciatic nerve.'

Proximal reasoning with regard management might go: reduce disc problem, manipulate its structure in some way, overcome the problem which has mechanical origins and hence relieve patient of the pain. Or, similar thinking involving a different pathway – correct the abnormal posture, get normal movements back and again – fix problem.

An evolutionary perspective considers the following before formulating an answer.

The pain and resultant physical tension produced help her to avoid doing something that might be injurious, or slow adequate healing. The tension and pain are useful for best early physical recovery. Pain demands cautious movements. Pain may 'request' inactivity and stiff fixed postures. If you think about it, pain may also demand regular *activity* of the injured part too; patients are frequently physically restless, often shifting, wriggling and moving with their pain.

Pain helps generate self-care, vigilance and the feeling of vulnerability. The implicit message might run: 'I'd rather not go out gathering food today if you don't mind and I'm not at all keen on having sex.' Pain also generates a need state that requires help and protection. Pain often generates a quick temper, anyone who gets a bit too close, or appears to be clumsy, or in the least bit threatening gets bawled at.

Her posture and movements warn other community members to avoid her – and be very careful when approaching, again helping to provide best healing conditions by not disturbing vulnerable recovering tissues with sudden movements. The fact that an animal that is moving awkwardly or abnormally in some way labels them as weak and hence an easy meal is a problem here! Thus, the buffalo that limps is soon picked out and killed by hunting lions, wild dogs or hyenas. In some circumstances therefore, pain and the behaviours and postures it can produce are worth concealing. No wonder we have evolved a very powerful 'pain-off' system!

The posture and the behaviours generated by pain help her to gain favourable attention and receive protection from those who know her, are close to her and value her. Feeling protected and cared for may be important for best healing, for example, it reduces stress and as argued earlier, stress can slow or even put healing on 'hold'. It also means that the individual can direct all their resources towards recovery.

Having pain can be associated with rewards, more especially if you have some status in the group in which you live. If you are deemed to be important and useful by your peers, you get a lot of attention and protection, you get out of working and doing chores that you dislike doing – 'you' are given more time to heal – which may be a good deal more than that given to others of low ranking. High ranking individuals in a hunter-gatherer community may have vital knowledge and skills in relation to things like security and wellbeing of the group. Without that skilled and/or knowledgeable individual the community is potentially more vulnerable (see Diamond 1991). Evolution (continued species survival) often demands cruel efficiency and thus endows some higher social mammals with behaviours and emotions that says, 'Look after those who are valuable, take less time and care with those who are not or are a burden.' Think about it and it becomes quite obvious that even though we try to suppress them, these deep rooted sentiments and prejudices persist in the humans of today. They are not necessarily nice, but they are acts of evolutionary wisdom that have to be applauded because they have contributed to our being here today. In the reality of our day to day clinical practice, one has to be a very strong willed therapist not to give 101% of our skills and time to a client who is well known or a celebrity of some kind. I'll bet you don't think twice about running well over time here!

Postures, gestures, words and actions that indicate suffering, foster acts of kindness within the immediate family and social group. If you are in a hunter-gatherer community you may get a few days off from hunting and gathering. In our modern society you can get paid by the social services and drinks bought for you by sympathetic friends down at the pub. Recall the innate laziness rule: *'get as much as you can for the least amount of effort'* discussed earlier. The fact that having more than a few days off is being shown to be detrimental to recovery seems hardly surprising. What use are you if you are unproductive? No wonder that our sympathy for those in our midst who are unwell and don't get going in a reasonable time, or are disabled for more than a few days, soon wears thin.

Some uncomfortable words perhaps, but if you're thinking from an evolutionary perspective it starts to help explain and make sense of a great many issues that can often 'leave a lot to be desired' when viewed from more cultural, civilised and social perspectives. Our animal instincts were once valuable; if we appreciate them and accept them for their remarkable usefulness in times gone by, we are far more likely to be able to bear better judgement and understanding and have greater insight on them in the present.

Before addressing management, and bearing the above points in mind, the next important part of reasoning like this is to ask if the presentation (the pain, the postures and the observed behaviour in its context) can be considered to be useful to survival, or '**adaptive**' – therefore to be respected or, of no use whatsoever, hence, **maladaptive**. Or, finally whether the observation is some kind of **imperfection** or **defect**?

We tend to think that we are in a healing profession and the pressure is on us to provide a cure. Evolutionary reasoning invites a shift of thinking to consider that this flexed and deviated posture might be a very adaptive response and one not to be meddled with?

Would you ever consider saying to a patient something like this?

'Don't worry about your flexed and shifted posture. It's very useful and protective at the present time – it will get better as your problem gets better and at the appropriate time I will help you to gradually overcome it. If we attempt to correct the way you stand and move too quickly we may actually prolong your problem...'

In other words if the pain and posture are adaptive—they're an evolved smart response to the situation—what right have we to get try and instantly get rid of them?

If we do deem such a posture and pain to be adaptive, evolutionary reasoning would predict that too early a resolution of the pain, or too rapid a correction of the posture may not be a good thing. For example, it may prolong recovery, lead to further injury (like nerve root) and leave the back in a more vulnerable state than it otherwise would be. This is a very useful type of research question –that is a challenge to many treatment methods and needs answering.

Clearly, whenever we examine a patient it is important to reason whether what we observe can be viewed as <u>adaptive</u>, <u>maladaptive</u> or an <u>imperfection/defect</u>. On the one hand, we need to consider millions of years of success, yet on the other we ought to consider that the phenomenon we are observing and deeming 'abnormal' in some way may not have been at all obstructive to success. The pain and posture adopted by our patient may be of little consequence to the passage of genes from one generation to the next. Eventually, especially if you are ignored, shift or no shift, pain or no pain, you have to get on with life, fend for yourself and your community or you get (adaptively) ignored, ostracised and even eventually die!

The opinion here is that a great deal of acute pain may not be useful pain – in the sense that it should be deemed adaptive and therefore command respect. For example, the early severe pain that is often the result of minor nerve injury (see Nerve Root section), the pain is often out of all proportion to the injury sustained. While pain levels can be incredibly high, continuous, extremely distressing and debilitating, the actual injury to the nerve may be minimal, with the nerve's ability to conduct hardly affected if at all. It could be argued then that most neurogenic or neuropathic pains are maladaptive pain, or an imperfection/defect related pain, even in its acute stages and hence should be subdued as quickly and efficiently as possible without ill effect later on. Maybe? Consider what you'd like to be done if you had acute shingles pain? I think most would agree that to kill the pain in its tracks wouldn't be detrimental. Now think what you'd like to be done if you had acute sciatica? Yes, the same logic applies. The notion that to get rid of the pain would mask the problem and therefore cause more pain is pretty redundant, unless you were to go straight back out on the rugby pitch again? The most important consideration is preservation of nerve function and for me, to this day, it is one of the hardest clinical decisions to consider and think about. My reckoning and observations so far which I'd happily stick with are:

- that further nerve injury/signs of worsening conduction, <u>once it has occurred,</u> is something which I have never witnessed except when there has been serious pathology

- that nerve injury and loss of conducting function can occur **after the onset of 'simple', fairly well localised back or neck pain without pain** radiating into the limb is a far more common observation and invariably follows several things:

  a) the patient 'doing' something that made their problem take a turn for the worse, like an awkward lift, movement or prolonged awkward posture

  b) the patient doing nothing, it simply got worse or was going to get worse anyway

- the patient had been subjected to treatments that may well have compromised/squashed/overstretched the already vulnerable nerve or nerve root, I will cite:

  a) forceful manipulation – clicking and cracking, or therapists trying to click or crack a back/neck

  b) any end-range mobilisation – particularly pressures into extension (like simple postero-anterior pressures done on the prone patient) but end range rotation may be a culprit too

  c) any end-range exercise – in particular extension in standing but also extension in lying – which are often combined with side-gliding manoeuvres that close the facet/foramen down on the side of pain

  (I would like to say flexion too, but I have never come across a patient who has been given regular and strong flexion exercises in the acute stage of their problems. It undoubtedly should be capable of doing the deed given that many patients report that the thing that really caused their sciatica to start related to a bend or awkward lift)

  d) neurodynamic mobilisations – for low back pain, the use of strong SLR or those techniques which combine lumbar rotation with SLR. For neck pain – any upper limb tension tests done strongly. In fact when I was learning these techniques back in the early 1980's I lost sensation in my right thumb for about three weeks following a particularly strong and clumsy procedure by a colleague!

The important thing from this is that none of us want to be responsible for giving a patient a nerve root problem or a nerve injury with neurological deficit. The problem may have been going to happen anyway, but it's best not to be the one who might just have 'pressed the right switches' to bring it on. It is a very hard thing to prove and an area that is in desperate need of unbiased research. The fact that the majority of experienced therapists will have seen a great many 'disasters' from other practitioners is testament to the frequency of the problem.

Let us return to our lady patient with her flexed and shifted posture.

The pain and deformity of this patient may be an unfortunate by-product of the healing chemistry and may also relate to genetic factors (see Nerve Root section). The fact that there are many people who suffer nerve injury or who have squashed, compressed or fibrotic nerves, without ever getting any pain, is in part testament to this 'maladaptive' /imperfection/defect perspective for neurogenic pain.

A major problem for patients **_and clinicians_** is that high levels of pain are often interpreted in terms of seriousness which then generates understandable fear – leading to inappropriate inactivity/rest and/or inappropriate medicalisation. A major factor may well be that the clinician is unable to adequately understand the problem they face. A high level of pain and the distress and suffering witnessed can be scary to clinicians – but recall, the report of a high intensity pain is **_not_** a 'red flag' (for red flags, see Waddell 1998, Roberts 2000) it is a yellow flag and one which appropriate attention and intervention is required in order to prevent the high possibility of chronicity developing.

When clinicians ask themselves whether a problem is adaptive or maladaptive it is important to think beyond just the pain and physical dimensions. Consideration as to whether, psychological, behavioural, social, work and cultural responses are adaptive/maladaptive need reasoning too.

Whatever we decide, whether adaptive or maladaptive, evolutionary perspectives should also be accompanied with thoughts about **'costs'**. This balances the reasoning process, but unfortunately for those who like clear-cut black and white answers – leads to frustration!

In terms of our patient with back and leg pain we need to address the question 'If the patient maintains this posture for some protective or other reason – what are the costs?' Here is a possible list:

1. It might cause more discomfort and pain by straining/loading other structures – which might lead to secondary problems there. Maybe every physiotherapist should adopt a flexed and shifted posture and maintain it for four to five hours – just to get a feel of what happens!

2. On-going poor movement and postural habits may be being set up or 'conditioned' into the organism as 'normal' when they needn't be. On-going and unnoticed movement related 'tension' I think is a culprit of significance!

It's always best to think: restoration of 'thoughtless-fearless-relaxed and floppy-movement'!

3. If they keep going round like this it's pretty obvious they're injured – they'd be an easy target for any predator! If you look vulnerable you are easy prey. Thankfully, nature has endowed us with responses that can extinguish pain and deformity in an instant – 'Set the dogs on the one who's wimping along with the pain will you Jeeves. He'll soon be moving better...!'

4. The sufferer might be unable to fend properly for themselves or their family; they are unable to work effectively; they may suffer financially; they may feel very frustrated and upset and lose their self esteem; they may feel very embarrassed or distressed by it and so forth. The long term consequences of pain and disability are well described (see Chris Main's model later)

5. They are likely to be poor at chasing opposite sex (usually relevant to males) or keeping them off (usually relevant to females!) hence, unsatisfactory reproductive consequences. 'She' may end up being saddled with a child she can ill afford to bring up and 'he' just wallows in the misery of an unfulfilled sex drive, and to a lesser extent, reproductive failure. Or, because they move awkwardly, look weak and unpleasant (hence they're both viewed as poor 'stock', or having poor parental capabilities) they may receive little attention from the opposite sex or only get it from others similarly afflicted!

Having dissected our 'disc' and nerve problem, by raising a few issues on either side of the evolutionary adaptive/maladaptive argument, the reader may well be left thinking – what should I do with the next problem I see like this? Should I tell the patient it's OK to be in pain and be awkwardly immobile, or should I try and correct the problem and lead them back to normal function? The stance advocated here is to provide a balance of both; meaning – avoid the 'fix it/correct it now' style of approach and engender a graded recovery period similar to other strains and sprains, but with the added 'nerve dimension' that it may take a bit longer. And reassure the patient that what they are experiencing is normal and common to all, although annoying it will lessen given some time and an appropriate recovery programme. Also provide and explain that early and effective pain relief is a great advantage for best outcome and the prevention of on-going incapacity (see Linton 1997, Watson 2000). This means that just as drugs should work so should physiotherapy treatments aimed at reducing pain (so long as they don't involve risk to nerve function). If it works, do it. If it doesn't work, for goodness sake keep trying different things until you find something that is effective! A good message here for the patient is that – adequate pain relief may actually speed up healing and recovery; rather than the usual, and more or less opposite line of reasoning that goes 'dull the pain, lose protection and hence promote further injury' – which is how most clinicians and patients react to pain killers. Use some of the examples from chapter 15.4 and tell the patient how helping reduce the pain actually aids and speeds the healing response efficiency.

So far questions have been raised about the value of the back and leg pain and the resultant deformity. Evolutionary reasoning suggests that since this pain and posture are such common occurrences they are likely to have evolved for very good reasons and therefore should be given some respect. After all they evolved and that means they must have helped our ancestors survive. Think of all the common conditions you see every day; think of the associated postures and movement patterns that accompany them. Maybe someone should write a manual of them all or put a DVD out. The classic hip osteoarthritic 'hip roll' gait has come into my head, as well as the less common (in my experience) Trendelenburg gait, which we're taught about as students. By the way, a Trendelenburg gait is due to weak hip abductor muscles and the contra-lateral pelvis tends to drop as the weight is taken on the arthritic leg. The hip 'roll' gait, which to me is far more common, is when the patient throws their trunk/weight over the affected hip as they weight bear on it. If you ever see a marked Trendelenburg I hope you're suspicious of L5 (and possibly L4 or S1 too) root neurological deficit, for these muscles are supplied by these roots.

The point I'm making is yes, there are well established patterns of protection and movement and many may well be 'smart' responses. On the other hand, the hunter-gatherer environment that they all evolved in will only have allowed them to be around for a very short while. In this far less pressured age, and relative luxury we now live in, these responses have the opportunity to hang around for far longer than may be helpful and this factor needs our consideration. So, our clinical question must include, 'Has this pattern of movement or posture been going on for too long?' In my experience the answer is invariably YES!

Anyway, I hope you are willing to embrace a little evolutionary reasoning with your patients?

Chapter GE 2.3
The Vulnerable Organism Model

When you're low you hurt more easily...

For years thoughtful writers on pain have gone out of their way to emphasise that pain **precedes** depression/low mood/emotional changes rather than the other way round. The pain starts with a physical cause and the psychosocial obstacles follow. Let me quote Gordon Waddell (2004 page 153)

'Psychosocial factors influence how patients respond to back pain and they are important in low back disability, but they do not cause the pain. Back pain is not a psychological problem. Back pain starts with a physical problem in the back.'

While I generally agree I would rather like to take this to task a little, because for years I have been listening to patient's stories and very often found it hard to find a reasonable physical cause to explain the amount and on-going nature of the problem they describe. What is evident, if you have time to really listen, is that there is a great deal going on in the patient's life. As we often say in our clinic, 'There's no such thing as a straight-forward patient!' A great many of those with a complicated pain problem have a complicated 'life' story to accompany it. A great many seemingly straight-forward ones do too. Many patients can be described, quite simply, as being 'low' and have been low, on and off for a long time before their problem started. These unfortunate individuals seem pre-sensitised in some way and that's the point I'm trying to make. The Vulnerable Organism is more prone to pain states – when you're low, you hurt more easily!

My exhaustion experience
– how I became 'vulnerable'

During the winter of 2002-2003 I was in training for the Paris marathon on 6th April 2003 (my fiftieth birthday present from Philippa!). During one long training run, about a mile from home, after being out for two and a half hours and feeling weary and extremely tired (I am a plodder) my left hand happened to knock onto my right hand and this gave me an instant cascade of pins and needles in both hands and lower arms. I was rather startled by this and didn't quite pass it off as just one-of-those-things, but thought for a rather mischievous moment – positive 'Tinel's sign'. Neuropathy! For those last few miles I had also become aware of a deep aching pain in my right shoulder – exactly the same as the old shoulder pain I'd had and that had taken three or four months to clear up but had never come back – it was there too!

So there I am in a situation of 'extreme' physical exertion/exhaustion and here are some of the features of me as a 'vulnerable organism' that I started to notice and think about.

1. I've got **increased sensitivity** – my positive Tinel's test plus the emergence of an 'old' pain that had long since gone. Personal evidence for the validity of pain memory perhaps?

2. I'm also generally **more bodily aware** – I can feel every strain in my body, it's all very uncomfortable – it's sending me a tediously repeating but very simple message... 'er, Louis can you give me a rest pretty soon, that'd be really nice... er, Louis can you...' Another part of me is going 'Ignore all that, you're nearly home, you can't stop here and you've done really well!' So, on I plod to get home.

3. I'm also become aware that the whole of my **attention is focused on the possibility of any threat to my goal** and of being constantly on the look-out for anything I can do that would make it all easier and conserve what little energy I have left. So, here I am plodding along at a steady but slow jogging pace, flexed, head down looking at the ground – looking down for anything on the road or path that might catch me out – like tree roots, uneven pavements, puddles, little dips or little mounds that wouldn't normally bother but now might trip me. I'm trying to conserve everything; I'm dragging my feet along low to the ground; I'm not wasting energy standing up with good posture and looking upwards and forwards. I'm doing what 'oldies' do – I'm all bent up and I'm looking down at the ground right in front of me. I'm thinking like an oldie now and starting to feel sorry for them – with all those physios saying, 'Now stand up straight, look ahead and stride out, swing those arms.' Oh yeah, that's **not** wise action when you're weak and knackered and can easily fall over on that little bump in the pavement. I'm with you old guys, keep flexed and your eyes on the floor, there are plenty of hazards out there in front of you. But I notice too that I also take the occasional 'flash' ahead – up comes my head and I give a quick glance, 'Where's the shortest route? That parked car is in the way – there's a corner ahead, best to cut across the road, that'll be easier – can't be bothered to hop up on the pavement, I'll stay on the road until there's any easy gap to follow onto it. Yes? Have you done all that when you're 'cream-crackered[1]'? Bet you have. Remember the rule: 'get as much as you can for the least amount of effort'. Wise action is to conserve energy and more so when your weak, exhausted and in poor shape! Don't just think of 'oldies' though—think of some of your patients—look how they move about, look how slow and cautious they are and they've only got out of their car and walked into your practice/hospital. They've got 'knackered-life-ache-posture-syndrome' without doing anything at all. I had to go running for a silly length of time to catch it. Someone should maybe make a video, 'Hey, this is what you look like, did you know that?'

4. Which nicely brings me to the last thing I noticed, that to conserve energy I was floppy –especially in the face – it's 'knackered-face-floppy-syndrome'! I'd find I was passing people I knew and they'd be shouting 'Alright Louis!' I'd barely look up. I didn't smile – I hardly responded, they got a grunt and a little raise of my hand. I didn't make eye contact. Have you experienced that? Now think of some of your chronic pain patients – long faces, expressionless, mouth all down in the dumps, eyes all saggy and the 'can't-be-bothered life ache' posture – misery and vulnerability are not easily masked.

---

1 - Cream-crackered is rhyming slang for knackered (exhausted)!

It was simple, out of this self-observation came, 'When you are low, weak, out-of-sorts, exhausted (mentally or physically or both) you can hurt more easily.' Plus all the other more subtle features by which we naturally recognise someone who is in a poor 'state' of health. From this grew the 'Vulnerable Organism' idea. I immediately thought of how I was when I had the flu. For example, when you're ill you go quiet and conserve energy, you're grumpy and moody, often expressionless, you 'can't be bothered'—but most of all—you hurt more easily. Your whole body feels sore and stiff, movement isn't nice, joints don't feel like going far out of normal range limits, they want to stay still. The slightest knock makes you groan and hurt, if someone bumps you, or someone sits next to you on the bed and comes down partly on your foot... 'Ohhh, don't do that, just go away, leave me alone, put Leonard Cohen on again can you and when you go out shut the door on the world – I'm not here.'

Let's have a slightly closer look at some issues that lead to someone 'becoming a vulnerable organism[1]'...

The sickness response and becoming vulnerable...

If you enjoy this stuff read Robert Sapolsky's essay: 'Why You Feel Crummy When You're Sick' (see his book of essays, 'The Trouble With Testosterone'). I've used some of his witty spin on this here, so, a big thanks again to a great writer.

The basic components of the sickness response are illustrated in figure GE 2.1.

What's beautiful about the sickness response is, like the stress response and Selye's 'General Adaptation Syndrome', that no matter what the 'illness' (or stressor) is, the reaction or response to it is much the same. We all – whatever mammal we are, whatever culture we come from – feel and look 'crummy'. We get the flu and what happens? In Sapolsky's way of describing things:

> *'We want to sleep at all hours of the day. Our joints ache, and we feel cold and feverish. Sex loses its appeal; we lose interest in food; if the illness persists, we lose weight even if we force ourselves to eat. And we look like hell... we all will get achy and mopey and feel like putting on flannel pyjamas...'*

It's a response we all recognise in each other but also in our pets and any other mammal we might come across. Evolution has been working hard on this one.

Let's start with the answers to the medical mechanism, the 'How?' question and then ponder the evolutionary 'Why?' question afterwards.

---

1 - *Mick Thacker tells me that they have some preliminary evidence that when you are like this you start to raise small immune responses even with no injury, think ME, fibromyalgia etc...?*

Becoming a vulnerable organism

• Illness/ infection - cytokines....illness...hyperalgesia, anti-analgesia....

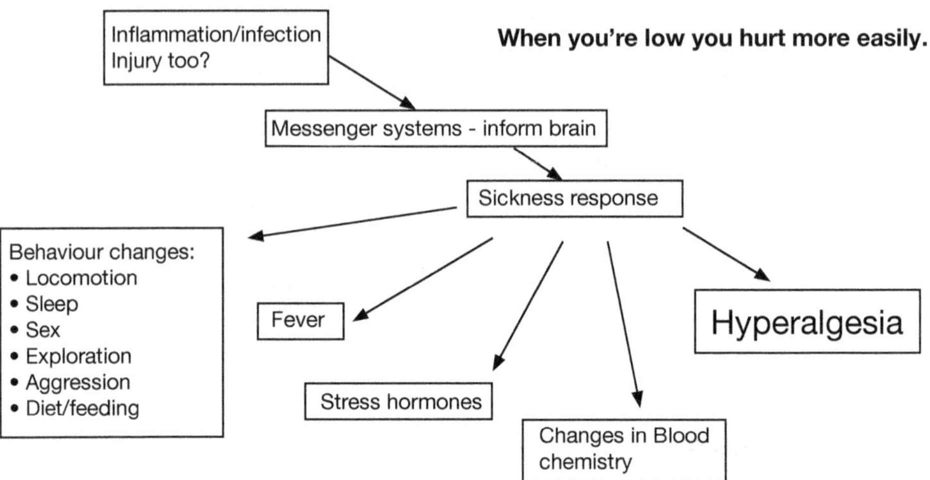

Figure GE 2.1 The Sickness Response.

When a pathogen invades the system the immune system responds – after 'grabbing' the pathogen and scrutinising it – by activating 'killer T cells' that then begin the attack. And because it involves macrophages it's called 'cell mediated immunity'. The second line of defence is called 'humoral' immunity, here white blood cells called 'B' cells start to rapidly divide and differentiate to produce antibodies that again attack the intruder.

The immune system is wonderfully complicated, but a great example of a 'sample-scrutinise-respond' (MOM style) system. After the 'sampling' of the pathogen, one of the main means of communication the immune system uses is via messenger chemicals called cytokines (also called interleukins and interferons). Cytokines travel in the blood and lymph seeking their specific receptor destinations. Interleukin 1 (IL-1) is the most famous one (see section 20) and it principally sends alarm signals from the macrophage to the T cells. But, as we saw in section 20, it also signals via the blood to the brain after crossing the blood-brain barrier. Here, it alters the temperature regulation and causes fever. A while back, when no one had worked out its structure, IL-1 used to be termed a 'pyrogen' (heat generator!)

Now remember the 'preoptic' area of the hypothalamus from section 9? It's here that IL-1 gets sampled and scrutinised when there's a pathogenic invasion, and the response that follows is to reset the body temperature, shifting it upwards a notch or two. You're now running a fever!

So, that's the 'How' question answered for fever. The evolutionary question now is

'Why' run a fever? The point is, that it's not about what the bug is doing to you it's more what you are trying to do to the bug. An increased temperature is wise action because:

a) It makes your immune system work more efficiently. For example, T cells multiply far more rapidly, antibody production is stepped up and key response enzymatic pathways are only operational at high temperatures and...

b) Bugs don't like higher temperatures. Bugs (meaning viruses and bacteria) do best at 98.6 degrees or below, they divide most efficiently here and 98.6 degrees is normal temperature.

What about 'costs?' Well they can be huge, too high a temperature will damage you and keeping the temperature high is a huge metabolic investment, especially when you don't feel like going out and getting supplies in! For example, during malarial fever metabolism increases by nearly 50% and much of this energy goes to producing heat.

Matthew Kluger did a great little study on lizards. Remember lizards are cold blooded but they like a little heat to help get their metabolism up to speed and more efficient, that's why they often bask in the sun first thing in the morning. Anyway, Kluger puts a lizard in a 'terrain' (a fish tank with no water in) and cleverly makes one end of it pretty hot, then 'just-right' in the middle and cold down the other end, so there's a nice smooth temperature gradient. When healthy, a lizard goes for the middle 98.6 degrees but when Kluger infected them with bacterium – they actually chose to become feverish, they moved into the hotter end to raise their temperature above the normal. He then prevented them from doing this and you guessed, they were less likely to survive the infection.

Evolutionary reasoning here makes us think differently and be warned, some Drs are unaware of what's just been discussed, that a raised temperature is a good thing—it's a well evolved survival strategy for infection—that works most of the time. Drs like to cool you down, **which is fine if your temperature is dangerously high** but it could be the worst thing to do! Drs also want to give you drugs to combat the temperature, antipyretics like paracetamol (acetaminophen in the USA) or aspirin, as well as dulling the inflammation or immune response. They may well be blocking our highly evolved defence strategy and putting us at greater risk. Take note parents, when you give Calpol (juvenile paracetamol) to a feverish youngster you may well be prolonging the problem? All this is very easy to say but sometimes it can hard to know where the fine line runs between a dangerous temperature level and a usefully high one?

Recall too from section 20 that IL-1 also stimulates the HPA axis via receptors in the relevant part of the hypothalamus. One of the end results of HPA activation is blocking of energy storage, 'You need all the energy you can get for bug fighting – don't stick any of it in the storage cupboard.' The system also dampens appetite for food, sex and the reproductive process (in the cause of energy efficiency!). As Sapolsky puts it, when there's a stressor about (be it a gang of thugs, a rhino charging at you or a pathogen), 'It's a 'foolish time to waste energy by ovulating or planning lunch!'

IL-1 makes you sleepy and also is a really big deal for us pain clinicians, because it turns up sensitivity and the pain-on system. This aspect of the 'sickness response' has only relatively recently been investigated, focused-on and discussed. It seems likely that there's yet another area in the hypothalamus that networks with the 'physical threat processing/nociceptive processing' areas in the 'interoceptive cortex', to act like a 'dimmer switch' in relation to pain and sensitivity to pain.

That's the metaphor I use when explaining it to patients.

The 'dimmer-switch' of the sickness response winds up our sensitivity to pain, it gives us pain and that pain is quite often a headache, if there's some kind of infection. Why headache? Why pain? Why sleepy? Again, its energy conservation, stay in your burrow/bed, your snug safe place and go quiet. When you're in pain have a fever and feel crummy; the last thing you do is go out exploring, beat up the neighbours or organise a hunting trip! Feeling crummy is smart behaviour for energy conservation and recovery purposes – pain and especially a headache is a great way of forcing the behaviour towards finding somewhere cosy and safe, resting and going quiet while your recovery system goes into overdrive.

But why lose your appetite and why do you lose weight faster than you otherwise would? It doesn't really make sense? One reason mooted for loss of appetite is that it stops you going out looking for food and therefore the danger of getting grabbed by some hungry predator. But, as Sapolsky puts it, 'The trouble with this is that card-carrying carnivores also lose their appetite when they're sick.' My spin on loss of appetite is that it's still good to conserve energy – you might not find any food anyway because you're so grumpy; surely much better to stay in and let your metabolism organise to get the calories it needs by using your energy stores and you for fuel. Getting hungry on top of everything else is only going to make you even more rubbish anyway.

In the book, 'Evolution and Healing' by the famous evolutionary biologists Randolph Nesse and George Williams, they point out that in some bacterial infections we go off food rich in iron – like bacon and eggs and liver! Their point is that dividing bacteria love iron! Good strategy then – don't eat any and any that just might be around and available, quickly hide it somewhere where the bacteria can't get it, like deep inside the liver. It's wonderful to note that when we're infected with bacteria we become anaemic due to this iron hiding strategy. Drs who don't know about this may test you, find you're lacking iron and then force-feed it to you!

Now you'll notice in the flow chart figure GE 2.1 there's a box on the left called 'Behaviour changes'. Interestingly some authorities and Bruce Charlton is a major advocate here, are starting to view the 'Sickness Behaviour' presentation when we're poorly as having a great deal in common with depression. They're basically saying that what they see clinically with their 'Major Depressive Disorder' (MDD) patients is the same as the behavioural presentation in the sickness response.

Let's just revamp the little 'Behaviour' box in the figure and look at it from a psychiatrist's view point. When a psychiatrist sees someone who's fighting the flu or an infection they see (and as you will have experienced):

- <u>anhedonia</u> – the loss of all pleasures in life! eating and sex are not fun anymore – low energy for function, sleepy, tired all the time, dulled out

- <u>impaired cognitive function</u> – the patient can't think straight or be bothered to even try to think; give the patient a crossword or book to read when they're poorly and you'll see what I mean

- <u>a feeling of hopelessness and helplessness</u> – they can't be bothered right now, become very passive, they're lethargic, sleepy and the future's not bright at all. What's the point to life, pass the pills and let's finish it!

- <u>Distress</u> – with all the nasty feelings... ohhh... the body ache, the headache, the grotty guts, the pain, the malaise, ohhh. Unending torment and pain.

What's described here are the basic ingredients of depression and if it goes on for a long while it becomes chronic depression. But when you're poorly, it's acute, it goes away when you recover and you get on with life. The point is that we have all been there when we've been sick, so has your dog and your horse! Think about it though, if we all get it, it has to be an installed, evolved and important **adaptive** pathway. It's simple – we need it in order to adopt the best energy conservation behaviour strategy for the immune system to work at its most efficient. A cost, because the potential for it already resides in our systems, is that it can go on and on, very like the graphs for pain discussed in chapter 13.1.

My viewpoint is this: the early grumpy crummyness is wise and **adaptive** but it can kindle, become more and more complex and become **maladaptive** if it goes on for too long. Yes, but depressions don't always start with some infection and sickness do they? No, but the circuits that produce the mood changes are well installed in all of us and our mammalian relatives too. If a 'programme' for crummy grumpiness is already installed surely it can be triggered by **any stressor** to the system, especially if the stressor goes on for a while?

What about the circuit that triggers the immune response, can that be triggered too when it's not really needed? Maybe, and maybe the pain dimmer switch can be turned up too? Stress and on-going stress in particular might be the key factor, or maybe we should turn our thoughts to 'vulnerability'? It's a simple question to ask yourself about a patient 'Are they in a vulnerability state?' And, if you feel they are the next question follows, 'What is in their story and presentation that indicates this?' The answer is usually some form of on-going stressor that the individual has been struggling to cope with. The stressor may be mental, physical or both of course.

Recall from section 20, that long-term stress can dysregulate the stress system in either of two directions, 'hypo' or 'hyperactive'. If an individual is shifted towards the 'hypoactive' then there's a loss of control of inflammatory and immune response due to low levels of cortisol and other factors. The inflammatory and immune reactions run amok. On the other hand, the 'hyperactive' stress response direction may leave the individual with inadequate immune, inflammation and healing responses.

When we're vulnerable, be it from an infection or any stressor, it challenges our system and our system responds in a stereotypical 'sickness response' way (see figure GE4.1). It's really Selye and the GAS in a different guise or merely coming from a different angle! So, an on-going challenge will often result in depressive type mood states and depressive behaviour accompanied by pain and increased sensitivity – giving that feeling of general malaise.

So why doesn't 'fever' 'maladaptively' crop up when we're under stress but when there's no evidence of infection? Apparently it does and it's called 'FUO' or 'Fever of Unknown Origin'. Most medical papers on it blame lack of a full investigation and demand a fuller work-up to identify the cause. However I did find one paper on the internet that reviewed 'psychogenic fever':

Oka T., Oka K.(2007) Age and gender differences of psychogenic fever: a review of the Japanese literature. BioPsychoSocial Medicine 1:11

Here's a statement from the paper:

'Psychogenic fever is one of the most common psychosomatic diseases. Patients with psychogenic fever have acute or persistent body temperature above normal range in psychologically stressful situations.'

I was actually quite amazed to find this: I'd thought for years that fever is a very stable and reliable indicator of some underlying 'threat' to the system. I shouldn't have been so surprised in retrospect. I had actually reasoned that fever for 'no reason' was unlikely simply because it is so metabolically costly, and because of this, its controlling mechanisms will have evolved a high degree of reliability. They would be above being triggered by 'mere stress'. But hey, it's not according to this one paper. This adds weight again to the potential and likelihood for 'maladaptive' stress and sickness responses to occur out of the blue and for no apparent 'physical or pathological' reason, just like pain. Also, and just like pain, a temperature may start as an adaptive response to say an infection, the body may deal with it quite adequately, but the temperature just like pain or malaise or the positive 'depression' symptoms of the sickness response ,may continue on afterwards when they are no longer of any value. Could I recommend the reader reviews all the graphs for pain that I illustrated in chapter 13.1, and see that fever, depression/feeling low/sickness behaviour and malaise can just as easily be applied and used on those graphs too.

Now a little aside: Bruce Charlton, who's an advocate of this sickness-behaviour-underlies-depression stance, believes that antidepressants work to reduce clinical depression because **they relieve pain and malaise** in these patients. Not only are antidepressants analgesics, they're also anti-inflammatory. The stance runs: alleviate the pain and malaise—which occurs rapidly—and the mood will <u>gradually</u>

lift following this, hence the common statement from Drs and researchers that antidepressants take several weeks before taking effect.

Think about recovering from a bout of sickness or illness; once the pain and discomfort of the malaise goes, the head gradually clears, mood improves and the world seems not so bad again—in that order—and it takes a little time to come about. That's the nub of it! Charlton says:

> *'I suggest that analgesia is not just a fortuitous side-effect of tricyclics, but the primary effect of any specifically antidepressant drugs... So, antidepressants do not 'make people happy' but instead, when effective, they remove a significant obstacle to happiness. It is easy to be happier without malaise, and antidepressants get their effect from being anti-malaise analgesics.'*

What we're looking at here is the possibility that depressive mood or symptoms can be caused by the activation of the immune system. The key little blighters are the interleukins again, IL-1, but also interferons and another called TNF, tumour necrosis factor. Research studies (see Campbell et al 2005 for further refs) comparing depression scores of patients with 'systemic' illness (like flu, fever, sweats, fatigue etc.) and those with physical injury, showed that depressive symptoms were far commoner in the illness group than the injury group. For example, scores of between 5-13 on the Beck Depression Index (BDI) were recorded from 88% of the 'ill' group, but only 11% of the injured group. This score equates to a diagnosis of 'mild depression'. That's a massive difference between the two groups. What's the deal? The argument is that there is far more immune activity and far greater amounts of interleukins and cytokines in the ill folk compared to the injured. Also, it turns out that when macrophages of severely depressed patients are examined they're found to produce IL-1 in significantly greater amounts than normals.

The lack of depressive symptoms from the **injured** subjects is because the 'sickness response' profile of all those cytokines are likely to be at a much lower level. However any review of physical injury, as in previous chapters, reveals plenty of inflammation, local immune activity and plenty of those interleukins too. Further, research into nerve injury is also implicating immune system activity and plenty of cytokine activity. The big thing is that the majority of us don't feel malaise when we're merely injured or have musculoskeletal pain, but being already 'vulnerable' or low prior to the injury for whatever reason, may predispose some to the more global response. So, if you're physically injured when you're low or weak (vulnerable) you not only hurt more easily, you're more likely to get depressed, feel malaise and you may even get a fever!' Think of all your whiplash, road traffic accident, repetitive strain injury, low back—chronic problems—and listen to their stories at the time of onset. My experience is that a great many reveal that they were already under a great deal of pressure before the precipitating 'incident' occurred.

Perhaps depression hits the injured more easily if their system is more predisposed to a high inflammatory/immune response? The prediction would be that these patients already have a stress system shifted towards the 'hypoactive' side of things.

It's all pretty obvious I think. If you're already stressed, you're already 'up' on the vulnerability scale and that makes any further stressor like an injury, even a normally modest injury or strain or an infection, more likely to drive you even lower mentally and physically and be more pain reactive too.

When you're low you not only hurt more easily, you're also likely to get even lower more easily!

I think we are in a strong enough position to say that it is quite within reason to challenge those who emphasise that the pain always comes before any depression/anxiety/mood state. Thinking 'predisposed by a vulnerability state' surely helps to explain a host of presentations that seem to be out of all proportion to the seemingly mild or modest nature of the initiating event that's reported. However, it is still very important to appreciate that on-going unresolved pain is not pleasant and the psychosocial factors that arise are fully understandable.

Overtraining/overuse and becoming a 'vulnerable organism'

We've all heard of athletes and obsessive 'exercisers' ending up with 'overtraining syndrome' and exercise 'burn-out'. These folk tend to lose all energy, get lots of musculoskeletal aches and pains, often get infections that go on for long periods and are generally unwell. They can very rapidly go from being super-active and highly energetic, to becoming super-lethargic.

Here's an abridged list of the various things that can happen:

Physiological

- decrease in white blood cell count – lymphocytopenia, relates to a depressed immune system; hence frequent minor infections and colds going on and on

- weight loss, loss of body fat

- increased resting heart rate and heart palpitations

- decreased muscular strength

- chronic muscle soreness

- tiredness and fatigue

- increased incidence of injury

- constipation or diarrhoea

- absence of menstruation and infertility, especially in females

- insomnia

- lower testosterone and higher cortisol levels...

Psychological

- depression

- loss of appetite

- mood disturbance

- irritability

- loss of motivation

- loss of enthusiasm

- loss of competitive drive.

Performance

- early onset of fatigue

- decreased aerobic capacity

- poor physical performance

- inability to complete workouts

- delayed recovery.

This all looks very familiar to me and much of this list could come from ordinary folk – not just obsessive fitness freaks and athletes. It's got many of the hallmarks of stress and of melancholic and atypical depression that I listed in section 20. If you push yourself too far mentally or physically you end up with a constellation of common features.

In my flow diagram figure GE2.2, looking from top left and going down to bottom right you see the basic issues of overtraining.

In most training and fitness acquisition sessions we push ourselves a bit more than we normally would, which in the context here is called 'training overload'. In the tissues microtrauma results, which when allowed adequate rest soon recovers.

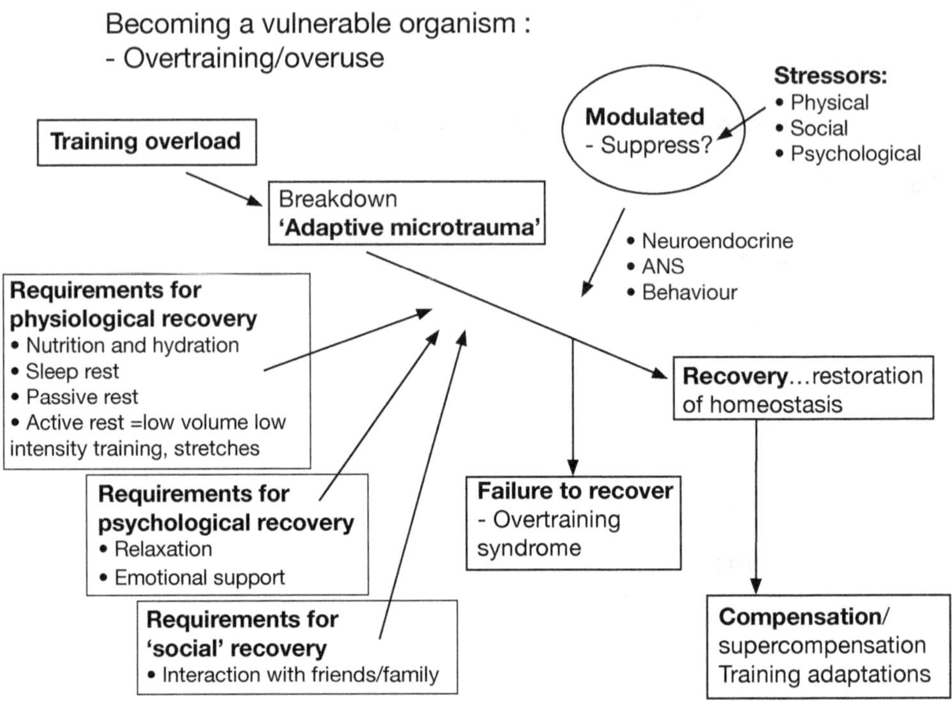

Figures GE 2.2 The basic issues of overtraining.

What's fascinating is that recovery usually occurs to a little stronger level than before the training. This training adaptation is called compensation and if significant is called 'super-compensation'. Simply, the exercise leaves us a little bit fitter than before. As I've already discussed in chapter 13.3 and 13.4 muscles and bone are particularly good at it but ligaments, tendons and other tough collagenous tissues are much more docile and slow to respond. But they all do and, like the brain, they're 'plastic' and can learn and adapt to the conditions they get exposed to.

Now the efficiency of this recovery and compensation process can be 'modulated,' meaning suppressed or enhanced, by various conditions. In the top right of figure GE 2.2, I've got the negative modulators and again, it's all about the multiple dimensions of stress. Think about the obsessed one-track mind athlete, an Andy Murray or a Chris Froome (2013 Tour de France winner from UK) perhaps? But also think of those wannabe athletes too, pushing themselves to the limits every day and who often get to feel anxious a lot of the time about their performance. Many get hung up on their competitors' performance, the inadequacy of their diet, their weight, their technique and probably a whole host of other things real or imaginary. 'I need tight ilio-tibial bands – like Bradley Wiggins has; I need my bike to be 5g lighter; I need an aerodynamic racing helmet.' Rarely are these guys cool, relaxed and satisfied. Those who are or who are able to channel into it easily, end up performing well and making gains. The ones that fall by the wayside may find that their 'stress' (physical overdoing it/plus or minus/psychologically festering/ ruminating over the perceived threatening issues) leads to their downfall and the 'overtraining syndrome' constellation of signs and symptoms above.

Think about the stress response in hyped-up athletes and you'd expect to find increase sympathetic and HPA axis activity levels with the potential for a stress response 'shift' towards the hyperactive side of things.

But, what about positive modulators? On the left of the diagram there's a list of 'needs' for the athlete (think of them for our pain patients too). Physiological equals things like good nutrition and hydration, good sleep, guilt-free relaxing rest and relaxed low grade training too. The overtraining types, like many of our patients, are poor at the rest and relaxation bit. They often say they do it but maybe they're like a great many patients, they're in mental turmoil when they do nothing and physiologically they're really not relaxing at all? Wouldn't biofeedback be so helpful here?

Psychological and social requirements include things like good support and interaction. Look at the entourage that Andy Murray tags along with him! Here's your multidimensional list then: coach, trainer, psychologist, physiotherapist, manager, nutritionist, friends, distractions, your mum and your supportive girlfriend. The bottom line is, when we're in a bit of trouble a bit of support from somewhere comes in handy.

Now aren't many of these things the requirements of all of us who want to keep going, be healthy and recover from injury, pain, infection, sickness or psychological challenge? I think so and I often make it clear to my patients when it's appropriate. I often tell them about some of these basics of overtraining syndrome so they can see what I mean. What I'm after is for them to make a few changes to their life and most often it's a change to the way they're thinking and reacting to the situation they're in. I hope the reader has the 'obsessive wannabe athlete' type chronic pain patient in their mind. These types of patient can be the exact opposite of those that give up, slob-out and need re-activating. These individuals are often the ones who want and try to be constantly on the go, if they're given something to do they'll do ten times as much as they're given; they've no time for stopping, pacing, goal-setting, incrementing, letting go, winding down, socialising, relaxing and so forth. So be it. If we recognise it, it tells us where we may need to try and go with them.

Graphs for explaining to patients

Here's the graph I often use with patients to show them where they are now, figure GE 2.3. I sit with a blank piece of paper and build it up. Vertical axis: capacity to cope or 'batteries charge' level. At the top it's full of life and energy, batteries charged, 'strong organism'. The horizontal axis is time: and the downward graph, which can be drawn wavy/Toblerone, represents how life has gone as the problem has progressed... since the whiplash, the RSI, the back pain...   Thus, the battery gradually drains to leave the individual bumping along the bottom, right on or just above the limits of their 'coping capacity'. I draw the 'dotted line' to indicate the lower limit of their 'capacity to cope' –where their batteries are nearly drained. I use the term 'vulnerable', 'exhaustion' even 'weak' with them if it's appropriate and then explain how small issues, that normally wouldn't be a problem, they find difficult to manage, that small things may easily exacerbate the pain or overwhelm them and make them very tired. The important thing to note is that when in this situation of 'vulnerability,' it doesn't take much 'disturbance' to trigger a problem. When you go through this graph with them most patients are pleased to see you understand their situation and will often nod their heads in agreement.

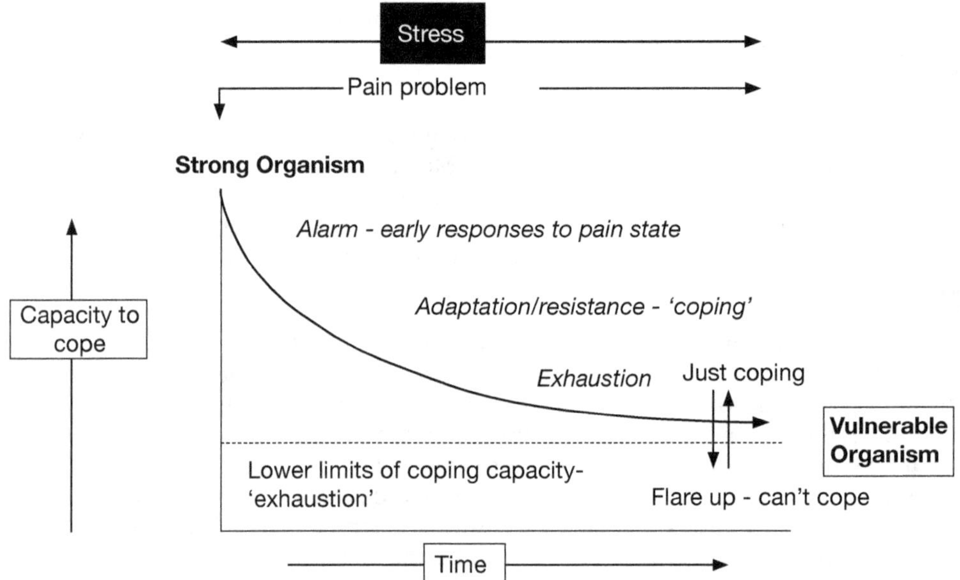

Figure GE 2.3 The coping graph

You'll note that I've put the three 'Selye' stages of the GAS on the diagram Alarm, Adaptation/Resistance and Exhaustion and that I explain this to the patient when appropriate and if it's going to be helpful (I give them an abridged version of Selye and his experiments with rats!).

I then use the recovery graph, which I used with 'Kate' in chapter 17.7 and produce again here for reference (figure GE 2.4). It may be worth returning to the case history in chapters 17.7 to see how I used it. Remember you can put what you like on the graph as you build it with the patient, so long as it's appropriate. The worst thing you can do is just give it as a hand-out. PLEASE DON'T! Find time to go through it and take your time; it's where you show the patient a potential route to a far better place than they are at now. It's a slow and gradual start and quickening improvement as early goals are reached and success builds.

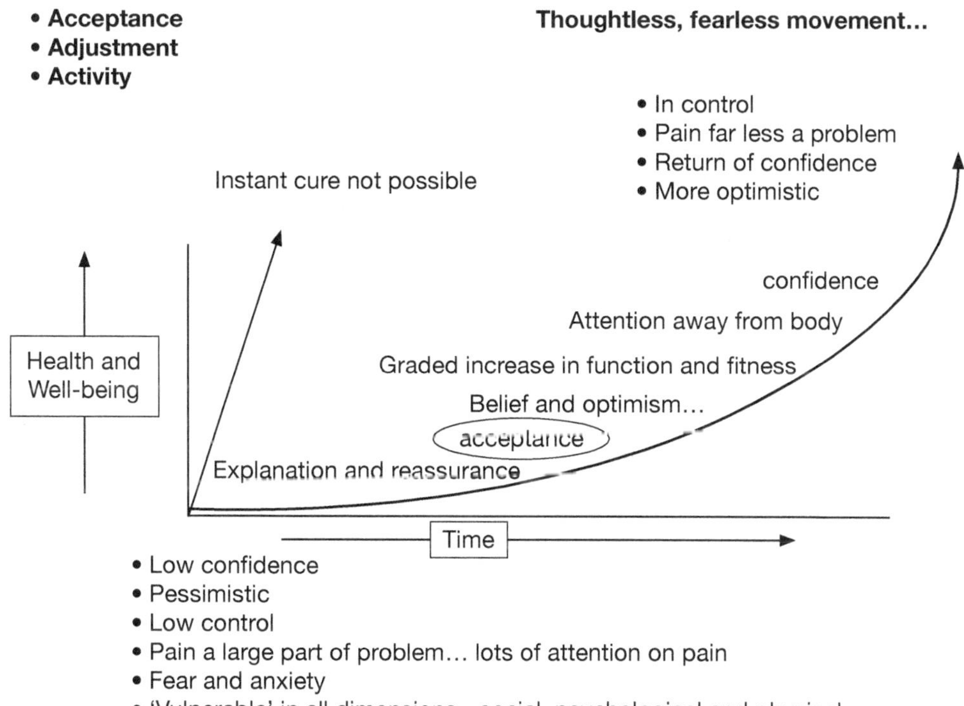

Figure GE 2.4 The recovery graph

Don't forget also that the good old 'Numskulls' can be used here too when you're telling the patient about sensitivity increases and the state of the tissues. Weak and deconditioned tissues in a vulnerable organism are likely to keep the sensitivity dimmer switch on a high setting, get them fitter and the switch can turn it all down. Big point here, it's not necessarily the tissues getting fitter that do the trick – it's **the context in which the tissues get fitter** that is the key. How the individual patient interprets it all can massively help it or massively mess it all up! Giving exercises is one thing but the context in which they are done is another. You need to try to think what the patient might be thinking with the exercises you've given them. If it's, 'I can't see the point of this. How on earth is this pathetic little exercise going to help?' ... then more work needs to be done! If it's 'Louis' given me these five exercises; I know they're not much right now, but if it works out like he said and I get good at them I'll gradually move on and on and it'll be helping me to get fitter and get better again'... then you're certainly on the right track.

So, a little summary of the Vulnerable Organism model to round things off here.

The CNS/brain/individual perceives that 'its body/mind' is weak/not coping and hence vulnerable, and responds by increasing sensitivity to the constant stream of sensory information arriving from the body. Inputs that normally do not reach conscious awareness may now get the opportunity for easier access. It makes evolutionary sense to go carefully if you are physically weak and/or lack confidence. Introducing a hypersensitivity state may be a significant way of achieving this.

It seems likely to me that old injuries (now scar tissue), arthritic joints, wear and tear, age related changes in tissue compliability and strength, old nerve injuries and nerve impairments will be continually bombarding the CNS with their own selfish nociceptive activity. Their constant droning and pestering to the CNS monitoring systems might run 'I'm not so good you know. I'm this bad you know, I need you to be kind to me thank you, don't let your attention wander-off somewhere else. Oi! Back to me, that's it, take notice, keep focusing on me, it's me you want to be thinking of all the time...'

The 'body weak or sick/tissue below par' representational neural circuitry, from the tissues and throughout the body representational-neuromatrix in the CNS, quietly sings its little tune and mostly gets thoroughly ignored by consciousness until the individual enters a vulnerability state – as I did from running and felt my old shoulder pain... (it has never come back by the way).

Some points and thoughts:

> Feeling low, coping poorly or being under stress, may be background mental states that also prime the central hypersensitivity circuitry. Hence spontaneous onset of physical symptoms due to the unmasking of normally muted nociceptive activity or circuitry. Further, psychological factors may be important in triggering pain states or making them more likely. They are also likely to amplify pain above 'usual' levels should the individual sustain some form or strain or injury. That there may not have been an obvious physical incident can be irrelevant if we consider that as most of us age we harbour more and more physical 'abnormalities and imperfections' that are silently signalling their status to the CNS. I think this is one of the major reasons why degenerative changes can be present for a great many years without any symptom manifestation.

> Does the 'interoceptive cortex' also receive inputs from areas of the brain that monitor our mental well-being and vulnerability states? If the vulnerable organism hypothesis is correct this would be expected.

> The notion of a pain 'pre-sensitised' or 'pain vulnerable' individual must include balanced thoughts relating to genetic as well as environmental/developmental factors.

Chapter 2.4
Vlaeyen and Linton's Model of Fear Avoidance

Johan Vlaeyen is a clinical psychologist and expert in fear-avoidance research and treatment. Steven Linton is well known in this area too, but also for his work on prevention of chronic low back pain disability. He is the 'Linton' in the Linton and Halden yellow-flag questionnaire.

Before discussing the fear-avoidance model I'd like to mention Steve Linton's early work on prevention of chronicity. The best way is to simply reproduce here what I wrote in the preface to Topical Issues in Pain 1 (Gifford 2013):

In a very timely editorial to the journal 'Pain' Steven Linton (1998) persuasively argues the case for the instigation of early preventative programmes in the management of acute low back pain:

"...we found that a secondary prevention program in primary care, for first time sufferers, significantly reduced disability and reduced the risk of becoming chronic by 8-fold as compared to 'treatment as usual'. The program included a thorough examination by a doctor and physical therapist, information designed to reduce fear, uncertainty and anxiety, self-care recommendations, and the recommendation to remain active and continue everyday routines"(Linton 1998).

He also makes a plea for the early instigation of adequate pain control since it is well established that intense pain in the acute phase of a disorder is a significant risk factor for chronicity. He bluntly points out that if 'medical' risk factors such as 'pain intensity' are being missed by clinicians, then...

'what kind of job is being done with 'yellow flag' risk factors?'

'Yellow flag' is the term used to represent the psychosocial factors, which have been shown to be powerful and very useful predictors of chronicity and poor outcome for treatment of low back pain (see Kendall et al 1997). They have been shown to have far greater predictive power for a poor outcome than many biologic/structural/anatomic/biomechanical/pathology based findings. These psychosocial yellow flags need our understanding and attention.

Linton (1998) highlights the work of Indahl and colleagues (1995) whose paper title is in itself great food for thought: 'Good prognosis for low back pain when left untampered. A randomized clinical trial'. What they did was provide a straight-forward and low cost intervention for people off work more than 8 weeks because of back pain. Firstly they provided a 'classic clinical examination by a physician', tested physical capacity, and took X-rays. The patients were informed about the findings and advice was provided. Patients were told that 'light activity would not injure the disc, but instead would speed recovery.' This message was given even where discs had verified herniations where surgery was not recommended. They placed great emphasis on removing fear about the back pain and specific recommendations about movements and lifting were provided. In their randomised clinical trial this 'minimal' treatment was shown to significantly reduce sick leave as compared to the control group and the return-to-work rate was more than twice as high in the intervention group.

Linton (1998) notes seven common features of the highly successful programmes for acute or subacute low back pain he reviewed for the editorial:

1. They all appear to take a multidimensional view of the problem. A major emphasis is placed on the psychosocial aspects of the problem e.g. fear and worry involved.

2. A thorough, but 'low tech' examination is provided.

3. After the examination, time is taken to communicate the results to the patient i.e. why it hurts and provision of advice as to how to best manage the problem.

4. There is an emphasis on self-care. 'That the patients' behaviour is an integral part in the recovery process'. But also, the use of effective drug therapy and/ or non-drug therapy to help control the pain is seen as vital. Linton notes that reducing pain appears to lessen fear and other psychological factors that may 'fuel long term problems'.

5. There is an attempt to reduce any unfounded fear or anxiety concerning the pain.

6. The programmes provide crystal clear recommendations concerning activities and in some cases help patients regain function by providing graded exercises.

7. The programmes do not medicalise the pain. By this he means for example: the indiscriminate use of high tech exams, referrals as a starting point, sick certificates of more than a few days, providing extensive prescriptions, or advising the patient to 'take it easy' or bed rest.

The findings from the research are impressive, an eight fold better outcome than standard care is phenomenal and we must take note of these seven features of success. At the time of writing it is now 15 years on since this research but the song remains the same, the words on the hymn sheet haven't changed! I rather feel that the momentum we had back in the late 1990's and early 2000's has vanished into thin air and that my profession has drifted back to 'modality' and tissue based therapies. It is very sad to see. If you look at the list, a recurring issue is dealing with the fear and anxiety involved with back pain.

Let's now review fear and avoidance in relation to everyday pain states.

Von Korff & Moore (2001) looked at the main concerns of acute and subacute back pain patients in a primary care setting. This is what they revealed along with the percentage of people reporting the concern.

1. The wrong movement might cause a serious problem with my back (64%)

2. My body is indicating that something is dangerously wrong (50%)

3. I might become disabled for a long time due to my back pain (47%)

4. My back pain may be due to a serious disease (19%)

I find the figures quite astonishing. The key thing is that we need to openly ask the patients about this sort of stuff, instead, as most therapist do of assuming that the patient wants you to 'fix' them. You absolutely must ASK THEM!

How do you do that?

I sometimes tell the patient the above results and ask them whether they agree or not with the statement, or ask them what they feel about the individual statements. For example:

'Right Sam, I've listened to your problem, I wonder if you'd mind telling me how you feel about the following comments that were taken from a recent piece of research. Patients like you were asked what their main concerns were with their back and these were the top four answers...'

For '1' above: 'Quite a large number of people when asked indicate that any wrong movement of their back might cause a serious problem with it...'

'Well, that's dead right, that sharp pain is telling me not to go there and to be honest it feels like it could snap something...'

For '2' above: 'Right, so do you think something is dangerously wrong with your back... or is it just strained in some way...?'

'I think it's more than strained, as I said the pain is so sharp it makes me feel that if I'm not careful it could be really bad and my disc is out...'

For '3' above: 'How are you feeling about getting better, making a full recovery and getting back to work...? Quite a few people get concerned that they'll end up badly disabled, but others are quite confident they'll be fine...'

'Well, there are two blokes from work who did roughly what I did and they've been off for ages, one's probably coming up to a year now come to think of it...'

For '4' above: ... some people come in here and after a while they tell me that they're worried about some serious kind of disease that might have caused it... what are your thoughts here?'

'Again, the bloke who's been off a year was told he'd got four discs out but they didn't x-ray him until he'd been off work for a couple of months. Then it turns out that he's got arthritis in his back... I spoke to him a week back and he reckons that they might have missed a fracture or something. So, I'm certainly wary of what could have happened.'

All this tells me that a very thorough and well explained examination is going to be important and even then it could be hard to convince this fellow. I'll try and reassure him and make sure I ask him whether or not he actually feels reassured at the end of the session and again when I see him next. I may well have to organise a 'reassuring x-ray' or scan and will have to be very careful with terms like arthritis and discs out, which pathologises or medicalises the situation. The answers he's given are clear 'yellow flags' in the 'Attitudes and Beliefs' category (see GE 4.5 and GE 4.6).

The diligent thinking therapist usually picks up the fearful and avoidant patients during the history taking. For example they're off work, resting a lot, avoiding any normal activity, stopping all bending and pestering their GP over and over again. Even so, questioning like this can be very helpful.

Let's now take a look at the fear-avoidance model. There are two figures (GE 2.5 and 2.6) the first being the older and the second the newer 'amended' model. There's actually a third model that is more complicated and includes anxiety as well as fear. I haven't included it because I've found that the two shown are quite adequate for my day to day clinical needs and reasoning.

This model is key to prevention of 'chronicity'

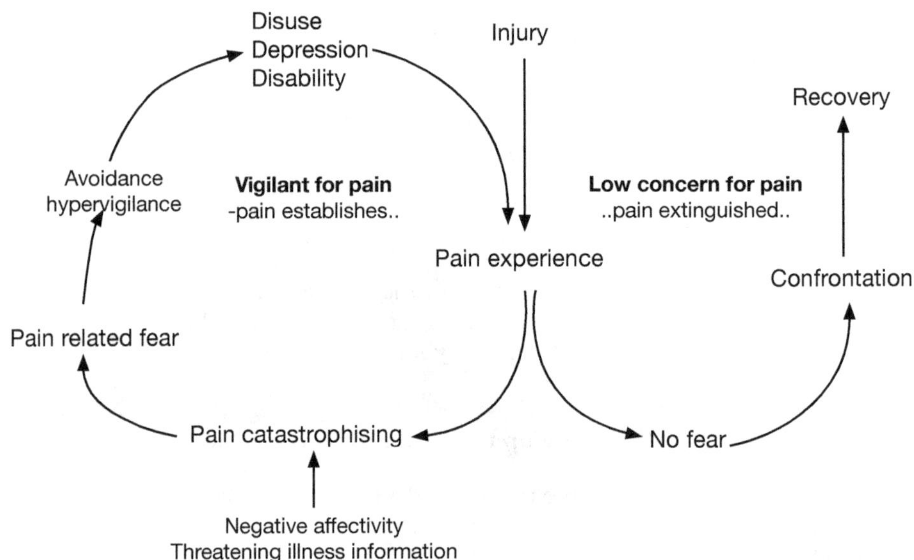

Figure GE 2.5 The Fear Avoidance Model 1

Start in the middle of the figure with the word 'injury' and then 'pain experience' and note that musculoskeletal aches and pains frequently start without specific injury, or a clear precipitating cause. This is an issue of some importance because pain without an obvious reason, though common, should always rouse a little flag for possible concern. Regardless of that the key thing to note is the simple two pronged pathway given—one that leads to chronicity and a self perpetuating pathway—and the other that's open and leads to recovery.

This model is key to prevention of 'chronicity'

Vlaeyen and Linton's amended model of fear-avoidance

Figure GE 2.6 The Fear Avoidance Model 2

When we perceive pain we tend to look for a reason for it and engage in a process of seeking and attributing some kind of cause as well as assessing how serious the situation seems to be. For a skin wound this is quite a straight forward process, it's not particularly nice but it isn't a disaster and we lick it a bit, stick it under the tap, look for a plaster and then carry on our lives but with a bit of modified or restricted movement of the wounded area. As time goes on we start to use it more and more (confrontation) and recover and forget about it. If we do the same with a back strain or pain again think about/assess it, more than likely find it unpleasant and annoying but deal with it the best we can; but keep going and with time gradually we increase activity and recover none the worse.

That's the right side – some might call it a 'confrontational' coping style. The left side is where the situation is assessed by the individual as much more of a problem. I'd use the term 'high threat value' but psychologists like to use the word 'catastrophising' – meaning seeing the problem as a major obstacle and problem for now, the future and no doubt, to infinity and beyond. When a problem is deemed a major issue like this – it's bound to cause emotional upset, hence high levels of distress or 'negative affectivity' and often associated with a great deal of anxiety about the pain or anything else that might exacerbate it or make it worse. There may also be anxieties about the underlying cause too.

The emotional problems and fears can be compounded further by the neighbour, the best friend, the Dr and all the various therapists:

'That Mr Crickbone, you know, the bone what-do-you-call-it-fellow he told me my pelvis was the worst he'd ever seen and that I shouldn't do any exercises or bending or housework for at least a fortnight. And do you know what Milly next door told me...? That her uncle had a back like mine about ten years ago and he never straightened up again; he couldn't move his foot properly and he lost all physical interest in Auntie May. He had to stop work and he never went down the Working Mens club again.'

I dealt with some aspects of 'threatening illness information' in Section 20.

Giving high threat value to a problem, combined with pre-existing high levels of distress, leads to pain related fear and subsequent avoidance of anything that 'just might' stir the pain up. These patients can be in an almost 'frozen' tense state 'just in case' they move wrongly or awkwardly. The term used in the model is 'hypervigilance'. It also means that the attention system is focused on one thing, the pain and being constantly on the lookout for it or anything that might make it worse. In 'brain' terms from sections 16 and 17, the quick and dirty 'low road' and the amygdala and friends are doing all the processing. As time goes on the patient fails to recover, they do less and less and they start to lose fitness and their normal thoughtless-fearless movement patterns. Symptoms relating to disuse and deconditioning start to emerge. For example, lack of energy and muscle strength, further pain, new pains, spreading pains and lack of stamina. Doing nothing, being in pain all the time, being constantly vigilant for the possibility of hurting, getting nowhere with recovery all serve to shift the mood towards depression and the pain cycle revolves relentlessly on.

Note that the second fear-avoidance model (figure GE 2.6) is basically the same as the first but adds a few little bits on. The words 'pain appraisal' in the middle I've already discussed. Over on the left the triangle of arrows indicates some of the top-down and bottom-up relationships. For example, that negative thoughts about the situation – 'I don't want to do that, I know it'll hurt, Oh my God.' This in turn will lead to 'physiological' effects, like increased muscle and sympathetic tone that can feed back into the system, making the feeling even worse and promoting the underlying unhelpful emotions and appraisals (same as the MOM!).

Learning to adequately manage and treat chronic pain sufferers with high levels of fear and avoidance is a very skilful thing. What I've realised over the years is that my job is to take patients and steer them away from the disastrous end of this spectrum – via good examination, good explanation of what I'm finding on examination, physical reassurance; and then getting them going in a fluid, relaxed and graded manner, so that they come to learn that things aren't as bad as they actually thought.

One of the key things about the graded exposure programmes used by Vlaeyen and colleagues is that they work hard at **'disconfirmation'** of patients fears and fear beliefs. They do this by working out feared hierarchies for each individual patient and then get them doing things that they ***think*** they can't do or that might hurt a great deal—but find when they give it a try—that they actually can do them and that they don't hurt as much as they thought it would, hence 'disconfirming' their beliefs. This is a fundamental principle of good pain management.

Kugler et al (Vlaeyen's group) administer an assessment tool called the 'PHODA' – the Photograph Series of Daily Living Activities. The PHODA uses 98 photographs, each one representing a physical daily life activity, like lifting, bending, riding a bike, riding a bike on a bumpy road, twisting, walking, running, being pushed in the back, getting the baby out of the baby seat in the back of the car, hanging out the washing, trampolining, falling over and so forth. The patient is then sat in front of what they call a 'fear thermometer' which is a large sheet of paper that has a vertical line on it, zero at the bottom and marks at 10, 20, 30, all the way to 100 at the top. The patient is then instructed:

'Please look at each photograph carefully, and try to imagine you performing the same movement or activity. Place the photograph on the thermometer according to the extent in which you feel that this movement is harmful to your back.'

Here's a case example... from Johan Vlaeyen and colleagues (2004)

This hierarchy is from a 40 year old female with chronic neck and shoulder pain. The pain followed being hit by a ball while swimming in a pool, from there on it got worse and worse, flare-ups followed 'cracking' noises in her neck. There were all the usual things, Dr diagnosed muscle sprain and told her to rest, she stopped working and never returned—she had various ineffective treatments—the neurologist did nerve blocks which helped for two months but pain returned following another 'crack'. Repeated nerve blocks were ineffective, eventually eight years on she was referred to Johan's rehab programme.

Her PHODA results included these:

100:   Sudden unexpected movements
       Running
       Jumping down
       Falling
       Cycling
       Trampolining

50:   Climbing stairs
      Bending forwards
      Vacuuming
      Lifting light objects

40:   Driving a car

Dressing a child
Washing dishes
Ironing

The brunt of her management consisted of:

- fifteen sessions of sixty minutes over five weeks
comment: that sounds like a lot, but with chronic pain problems the issues
are complicated and a great deal of time is needed. Half an hour slots or less
are really a waste of time –they'll burn you out or, to survive you'll end up just
mindlessly applying some treatment to a virtually lifeless bit of collagen and
that is exactly what you shouldn't be doing here

- measures of pain, pain related fear and difficulties encountered with three
daily life activities were kept in a diary

- she did her PHODA thermometer

- in the first educational session she was provided with a rationale explaining
that painful body sensations can occur without signalling muscle or nerve
damage

- she was also provided with information on how protective behaviours (such
as resting, guarding and vigilance) in the long run can maintain the pain
problem

- this session was followed by the first 'exposure' session starting with activities
with a fear rating of around 40-50 – see above list; she actually started with
picking light objects from floor, followed by some lifting and reaching tasks

- they used 'behavioural experiments' (see below) to challenge the belief that
sudden movements are harmful

- during subsequent sessions, the activities became physically more intense
as the patient 'ascended' the 'fear hierarchy' – meaning they gained in
confidence as they found that they could do the things of which they were
fearful

- **<u>at the end the patient was able to do somersaults and learned to head
a football</u>** – in all my 'manual therapy' days of seeing patients just like this
lady, I never even dreamed that achieving this sort of recovery or level of
confidence would be possible, let alone actually working the patient towards
actually doing it in a treatment session!

- after the exposure therapy the TSK (Tampa Scale of Kinesiophobia) decreased
from a score of 48 at the beginning, to 17 at the end – and the PHODA score
went from 690 to 110

- of interest was that the **pain ratings decreased significantly and in parallel with the pain-related fear ratings**

- daily activities that were chosen as important goals, but avoided because of fear, were gradually resumed.

As you can see from this case study – it's more than just education and telling a patient that they won't 'harm'.

A big part of it is working out an achievable 'fear hierarchy' and then starting easy (around 40 or even lower on the PHODA scale) and then working to harder and harder/more feared or challenging levels. The key thing is that the patients' beliefs and behaviour are being challenged to shift from unproductive ones to more productive. I don't think most physios or other practitioners would be willing or confident enough to take an eight year chronic pain patient and get them doing somersaults and heading a ball by the end. That's the point I've been making about OUR FEAR or CLINICIAN FEAR being just as problematic as the patients' fear.

The big thing is 'disconfirmation' of beliefs. The patient has to actually experience that what they thought about an activity, for example, '...that it was bound to cause worsening of pain and further damage' is actually wrong once they've tried it and repeated it. The key is a carefully designed graded approach to the activity.

Note the 'setting up the brain' part of this, getting the physical challenges in the right context—all the top-down before bottom-up—you can't just take a chronic pain patient and make them suddenly do a somersault, or even bend down and pick a light object off the floor without considerable preparation.

So what does '**Behavioural Experiment**' mean? As Johan Vlaeyen explains it:

'The essence of a behavioural experiment is that the patient performs an activity to challenge the validity of his catastrophic assumptions and misinterpretations.'

What follows is along the lines of what they do plus my own adaptation from about point 3-4 onwards:

1. The patient formulates the dysfunctional belief and rates its credibility. For example, a patient may rate that 'jumping down off a stair will inevitably cause nerve damage in the spine and excruciating pain' as having 75% credibility. That is very high!

2. A realistic alternative belief is also formulated – which is that they'll be able to continue walking without excruciating pain after jumping down from a chair and this will have 25% credibility This is a good thing to do because, like you and I, patients don't often think of the 'opposite' aspect of any given estimate of failure i.e. that it actually just might be OK! When I do this with patients and they think about it some will say 'Oh, hang on a minute I

think I'll make that 90%.' This simply shows how fearful or convinced they are that what you are suggesting will stir their problem up.

3. A 'behavioural experiment' is then designed. For example the patient is asked to give a minimal height that they think will cause a nerve injury and pain exacerbation as well as an 'alternative', which is a height from which they can jump down from and walk away without excruciating pain or nerve damage. Let's say the minimal height to cause injury chosen is around six to seven inches and the height to be OK from is around two inches.

4. Using a variety of boxes or big books, the two heights are set up. The patient is asked to rate what they think will happen and then asked to try and see if it does.

5. Usually the patient finds they're not as bad as they thought and the whole process is discussed. The patient starts to experience that their beliefs may be wrong and that they can do more than they thought.

6. Between us we agree a height that the patient feels OK to do at home and practice. Let's say between you, you agree that two inches for a first time might be the best height to try. The patient may then say that that is so low it seems pointless or ridiculous and that they feel they should try a bit higher. This then leads to the next point.

7. We now discuss what has happened in the past when they try to start doing something again which they 'know' will stir it up, but that they really feel they should start to try and do again because it's being such a source of frustration in their life. The typical thing here for chronic low back pain is simply bending over and picking things up of the floor, or giving a hand lifting the shopping out of the car. The patient quickly gives examples like these and then relates that every time they do it they regret it because it stirs it all up for days on end, the family get mad with them and that they then make an even stronger effort not to do it again. In other words, their efforts to return to doing normal things again are invariably stymied by failure which reinforces their 'avoidance' strategy. This leads to the next point.

8. I now introduce a little saying that I use very frequently in the clinic, it's **'SUCCEED NOT FAIL'**. I tell the patient that what they've just described is very common, that patients want to try and get going again, but it often bites them back and leaves them even more frustrated. As I have noted in other areas of the book, the key is **START EASY BUILD SLOWLY**... that often means, for the patient who has repeatedly failed and been knocked back, that they have to start at an almost ridiculously easy level in order to 'succeed and not fail'.

9. I often take the patient back to the 'Recovery' graph (figure GE 2.3) discussed in the previous chapter and note the very flat and long initial part of the curve of recovery.

10. I also review the 'Toblerone' nature of on-going pain and the fact that they may well find there's an increase in pain some time after the practiced activity, but that they may also find there are occasions when there isn't an increase. In a way, I try to get them to shift their attention towards looking for times when the reaction doesn't go the way they expect – to look for evidence of pain inconsistency, where it has a 'mind of its own' and that it doesn't always follow-on from an activity. The idea is to slowly 'disconfirm' the patients' deeply held beliefs as far as is possible and at the same time increase physical confidence.

The big skill is picking an activity (or quite often an exercise or movement that's relevant) that can easily be done and be easily incorporated into a hierarchy of difficulty. In later chapters there will be plenty of patient examples. The main thing is that as far as possible the activity you use should be functionally relevant.

That's the first skill; the second is picking the right level of difficulty/fear from which to start. When I do this with patients I generally start at very low fear levels, or even no fear at all, just to get the patient going. I also get them to give me their level of 'confidence' about the task on a scale of 0-10 before, sometimes during and again afterwards. If they rate their confidence as 7-8 or above we go for it, if it's 4-5 or below I adjust things until they're more confident.

As you can see the behavioural 'experiment' is an 'exposure' task and the patient is already learning how to break something that is feared down into more manageable steps or components. What's good is that patients soon pick up the 'method' of re-learning how to do something that they've avoided for a long time and frequently show you what they've tried and achieved outside the things that you were focusing on.

A great deal of this is about shifting peoples' catastrophic and anxiety fuelled beliefs about activity, function and exercise, which at a biological level means re-process the whole thing away from the 'quick-and-dirty-threat-processing' low road. Thoughtless-fearless-movement!

Chapter 2.5
The Mature Organism Model. Desensitising and Hebb's rule

See sections 10 and 18 for the MOM. For Hebb's rule see sections 5 and 6; but for discussion and practical use of Hebb's rule, see 'Runner Pete's calf problem', chapter 14.2

The Mature Organism Model

I used to use a modified diagram of the MOM to explain chronic pain to some patients, but its major use was as a teaching tool or vehicle to try to persuade dyed-in-the-wool manual therapists to see a bigger picture. I wanted them to see that the way patients were reacting to their pain, what was in their heads, was an important issue and had a huge impact on how they reacted to their pain problem. After all these years it's rather nice that I'm still getting regular emails from therapists thanking me for it and telling me that it changed their professional lives for the better! That has been very pleasing, but I'd like to slip in here that I wish that the 'Vulnerable Organism Model' and the 'Shopping Basket Approach' were as popular!

Anyway I've included the MOM in this section on 'Models' for pain we need to take on because I firmly believe this way of seeing the whole pain situation is vital for all pain clinicians.

Explaining pain using the MOM worked reasonably well with a few patients, but over the years I found it a bit too cumbersome, complicated and unnecessary for the majority in the chronic pain patient bracket I was seeing. I always wanted to make it as simple as possible and some of the case histories later on show this.

The Desensitising Rule

Have you ever jumped out of an aeroplane and done a bit of sky diving, or off a cliff doing some bungee jumping perhaps, or maybe been swimming with dolphins, or stood at the top of Eiffel Tower? Exciting, thrilling, ghastly, amazing and never to be forgotten! Novelty and excitement often give a great buzz to life but most of us find that if we keep doing that stuff over and over again it loses the buzz, it becomes everyday and eventually we can get bored with it and the thrill is gone. Think about the security man who's at the top of the Eiffel tower every day. I bet he's not that interested in the view or the amazing feeling of height? If he has lost interest, he's habituated or desensitised to it.

We can apply the same to some pain states. Keep repeating a movement or activity that hurts and eventually the pain lessens and you get used to it. Though it's always best to start easy and build slowly, as I've already discussed. Recovery from injury or sprains and strains is a great example. You start walking on the recently twisted ankle and it hurts a bit, keep going and it gets easier and freer. It flares a bit when you rest but as you go on and on every day the flare reaction gets less and less and the pain on walking diminishes too and you do more and more.

With patients when I want them to start moving into the pain with movement or function I tell them about desensitising. The easiest way I've found to do this is (I live near the sea!):

'If you go down to the beach right now, take off your shoes and socks and wade into the water up to your knees, it'll be horribly cold and you'll probably want to get right back out again? Stay there and put up with the pain – wait and after a minute or two the pain will ease down. The water hasn't got warmer—you've got used to it—you've started to desensitise. Now do this for about three or four minutes day one and tomorrow go down and do it again and the next day, keep going every day – build up the time you stay in for and you'll find as the days go by you'll find it easier and easier. You adapt, you desensitise, your pain-off system gets a boost, it gets a bit of excitement, it kicks it out of bed and it gets the endorphins flowing. Now you know we have folk who swim in the sea all the year round, you could do that too. Anyone who's reasonably fit and healthy should be able to. The big thing for success is you've got to want to do it—you've maybe got to even look forward to it— and also see it as a positive challenge.'

'So, we're now going to apply that principle to your hip pain when you walk. Small walks to start with – some pain is more than likely and a bit of a flare afterwards may happen too. You won't be damaging it. Keep repeating it and try and slowly increase the time on your feet... The key to success is that you can cope with it and tolerate it and if at all possible you get to enjoy it and look forward to it.'

The patient gets all the pacing and incrementing rules and our little phrase that accompanies 'start easy build slowly', which is 'succeed not fail', meaning – if you overdo it and it puts you off, it's your fault! It's far better to do less and succeed, than do too much and start to get anxious or fearful of it. 'Tobleroning' may be included!

Hebb's Rule again

Hebb's Rule approach to things is almost the exact opposite because it avoids pain (see chapter 14.2).

Agnes has chronic and awful shoulder pain. I've examined her and she can abduct to about 40 degrees, stopping due to pain. Flexion isn't much better, about 60 degrees. During my examination of her I find that leaning forward dangling is pain free and a good range. She can swing the arm quite freely if she stays relaxed and doesn't swing too far. I also find that using the reciprocal pulley is pain free in flexion too and that she likes it – her good arm helping the bad up. Pulleys are old-fashioned, but for some shoulders they're brilliant. You can get them with simple little wedges that fix them over the top of a door, we have about three or four in our clinic and lend them to patients for a week or so and if they like them they buy one.

The conversation might go like this...

'Right, Agnes here's the principles of getting you going! I'm going to ask you a question and you give me the answer... your car? ... mini ... your phone number? ... 314987 ... your dog? ... Scamp!'

'Right, every time I ask you a question, the question makes a little circuit in your memory start to activate and it then finds the answer, by engaging the circuit in your memory that has the answer. So, 'dog' circuit turns on and that links to the 'Scamp' circuit and you give me the answer. When one circuit makes another circuit activate we say the two have 'wired together'. It's how we learn and remember. Here's an example of mine, when I brush my teeth in the morning I immediately want to have a pee – for no reason whatsoever, maybe it's the running water thing! But somehow the two circuits have wired together. Now, when I go to America skiing I find that this link disappears – it's probably because of the time change, when I'm doing my teeth in the morning there my body thinks it's one or two o'clock in the afternoon so it doesn't happen. What I'm saying is that things seem to get linked up in us but, they can become unlinked, if we go about things differently or we change something. Have you noticed any links like that?'

'Well Louis, yes I have, a bit embarrassing but when I speak to my mother on the phone I soon get desperate to go to the loo – like you!'

We both laugh as you'd expect.

'Your shoulder pain has been going on for ages and it seems to me that some of the pain circuits have become linked to some of the movement circuits; every time you take your arm out to the side or lift it up forwards, you get the pain. But, when I get you to do it differently – leaning forward or using the pulley, there's no pain link to the movement. The circuits stop getting each other to go off – just like when I go to the USA and clean my teeth!'

'We call the rule 'circuits that fire apart depart', it means that the more you do a movement that normally hurts, without hurt, you'll find that the pain and movement circuits will eventually leave each other alone. So, the plan is to get you doing nice big pain-free movements for a bit and see what happens to the usual pain-when-you-lift-your-arm-up pattern.'

Again, it's 'start easy build slowly', but instead of going immediately into pain—we start with no pain—but with the biggest movement possible. If it's not possible to do a big movement we just start with a small movement and then build up to larger ones when it allows. Later, if things are going well Agnes will get on to the desensitising approach (producing and going into pain, repeating and doing it until the reaction gets less, then doing a little more etc.). Again, the key is to try and make the exercise enjoyable, relevant and meaningful. Be explicit about these things, tell the patient that it needs to be enjoyable and that they should feel confident, but that if they're not sure why they're doing it or it doesn't make sense, they must say.

It's 'Top down **before** bottom' up and 'Top down **during** bottom up.'

A key thing in this is to keep a close eye on and deal any with fear and anxiety. Use the confidence rating scale to find out how they're feeling about it when doing it.

Chapter 2.6
Main, Spanswick and Watson's Model of Disability

It's best to read this first hand in their book. It's a great model and broken down, studied and thought about, it brilliantly helps us understand the multitude of factors that cause and determine chronic pain and related disability. It's my belief that if we appreciate the complex factors and the manner in which they interact we cannot fail to become better clinicians.

Start simple with the first flow chart, figure GE 2.7.

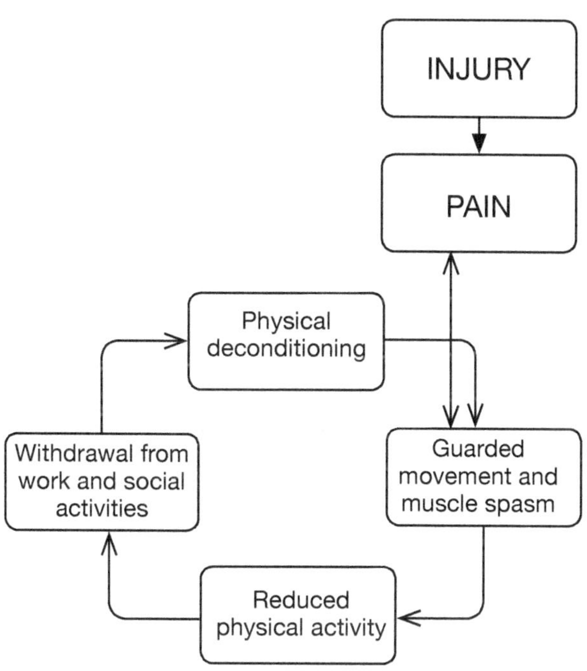

Figure GE 2.7 Development of deconditioning and disuse – model 1

Injury and pain in all of us leads to guarded movements and increased tension and tone. I'm not sure about the label 'muscle spasm' here. I prefer the terms increased tone and 'guarding' especially when it applies to movement and activation. Many acute pain sufferers are able to get their problem comfortable and relax it very well, but when they move it, it's usually very slow, tense (i.e. increased tone) and cautious. I don't see this as 'spasm' clinically. Spasm is a sudden tensing of a muscle and more a part of neurological problems. Clearly there are still many acute pain patients who do have constant increased tone – particularly back pain and are quite unaware of it. If you find it – put it in the shopping basket! (See later). For now, reason whether it's adaptive or maladaptive muscular tension with movement and keep it fairly high on the list of findings that need to be addressed – above range of movement! When there is severe guarding and increased tone it's as if the patient is stuck in the 'freeze' moment of the acute stress response.

When things have just started to hurt we go carefully and stop doing normal activities. This reduction of physical activity goes on for a variable length of time, but as we saw in the fear-avoidance model, most people quietly do their best to get on, confront the problem and gradually get going. On the other hand some will remain in a reduced activity state for too long – it's the adaptive acute response starting to become maladaptive.

When patients with pain reduce activity for a long time they generally stop normal activity, go off-sick from work and may even stop socialising. As anyone who's spent time ill in bed, it doesn't take very long to lose fitness. The term 'physical deconditioning' is an excellent term to use with patients if they need activating. The problem though is that physical deconditioning leaves the sufferer vulnerable, sensitised and also more prone to on-going pain. The tense and guarded movement remain.

What this flow chart is telling us is the importance of easy relaxed movement – if we're using Hebb's Rule approach, then the movements are going to be big and pain free where possible. For example, a low back pain patient who can hardly move standing up, but with standard lying supine tests actually does good crook rotation and 'grab a knee'—plus hip and lumbar spine flexion—is in a good position to start to get going.

On the right of the next figure (GE 2.8) a 'cognitive' component is added on; what the patient thinks is going on, what it means and what they feel might have caused it, their 'attributions' or more correctly for those with chronic pain their 'misattributions'! As discussed in chapter GE 2.4, 'misattributions' relate to a belief that there is bad

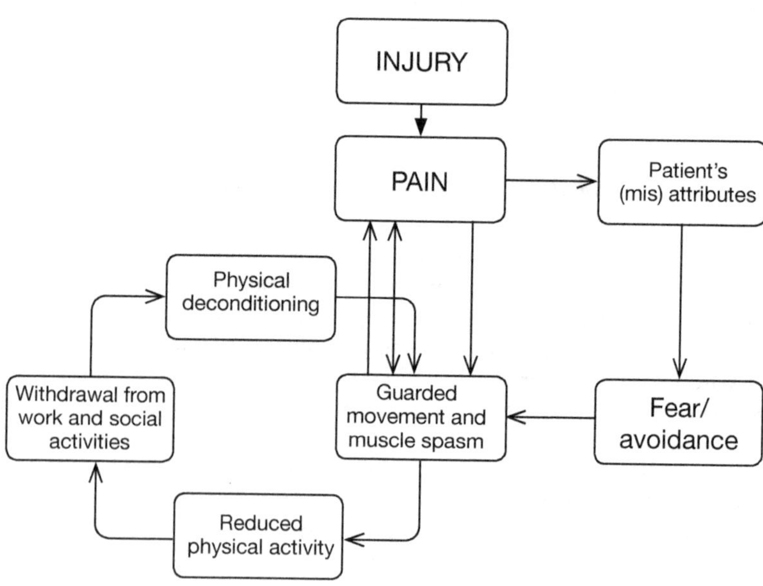

Figure GE 2.8 Influence of fear and avoidance – model 2

damage or something seriously wrong, or that movement and normal activity are likely to make the pain and the problem a lot worse. This way of thinking leads to increased tension and reduced activity levels i.e. Fear-Avoidance!

Clinically, this means that the therapist must always enquire as to what the patient feels is wrong and what their attitude to getting movement going and gradually doing more and more might be. A great many 'acute' pain patients come to me wanting my knowledge and advice here. That's fine, but it's those whose beliefs are very firmly stuck in the 'rest is best and don't move it until the pain goes' corner that are likely to be more problematic. It's no good going in head first with movement and exercises until a patient's beliefs and attributions about their problem have been ascertained. Remember—'top down before bottom up' is essential here—the person with the pain has to understand and go along with the physical recovery and reactivating process.

The third figure (GE 2.9) acknowledges the importance of depression and that it's often associated with this prolonged withdrawal from normal activities, the on-going pain and the feeling of being useless and a burden to others. If you keep stopping a human from doing things, if you stop them from being an important cog in the wheel of the household or their work, they tend to feel annoyed, frustrated and also hopeless and helpless. 'What's the point? I won't even try, it'd just stir it all up, they'd all get cross with me, I'd probably make a mess of it all anyway, I might as well be a picture on the wall.' Feeling like this all the time means that the individual is likely to be doing very little – thus has plenty of time to focus on and get to grips with their pain and on goes the self sustaining cycle continually nourishing itself.

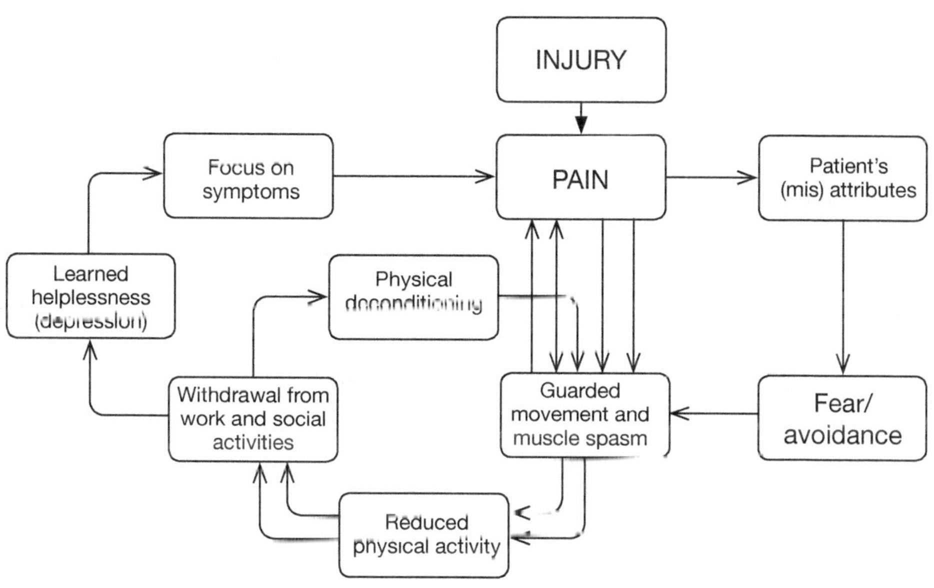

Figure GE 2.9 Influence of depression – model 3

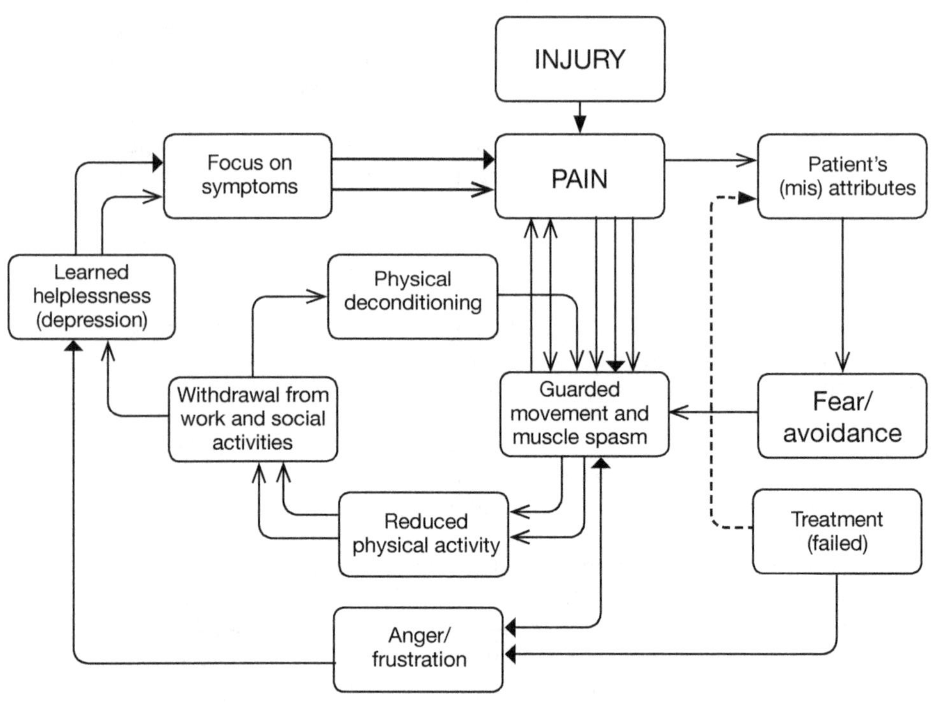

Figure GE 2.10 Influence of anger and frustration – model 4

Figure GE 2.10 brings in all those clinicians who diagnose and/or treat these patients. Clinicians try and help, but a great deal of the time they feed in conflicting and worrying diagnoses with lots of conflicting advice about what to do. Many advise even more rest when the patient reports ghastly flare ups. Some clinicians take great glee in ridiculing other clinicians' diagnoses and treatment attempts, then go on to offer yet another treatment that is bound to end in failure when observed over time. Failed treatments and the confusing and conflicting things that clinicians say to these patients often add to their frustration and anger.

Frequently these types of clinicians feed the patient's misattributions and beliefs about the seriousness of their problem even more. This again confirms and reinforces the patient's beliefs that doing nothing and resting is the only way to go. **Failed treatments**, practitioners unable to help, practitioners even blaming patients for not responding to their treatments (sometimes directly, but often indirectly via body language and tone of voice); or getting annoyed with the patient for not complying with the exercises or tasks they were given to do – all lead to mounting frustration and quite often bitterness and anger. That's yet more stress/distress and not at all helpful. It's yet another layer of useless reinforcing feedback into the pain, but so too the low mood and depression, as denoted by the arrow going from 'anger/ frustration' to the 'learned helplessness/depression' box.

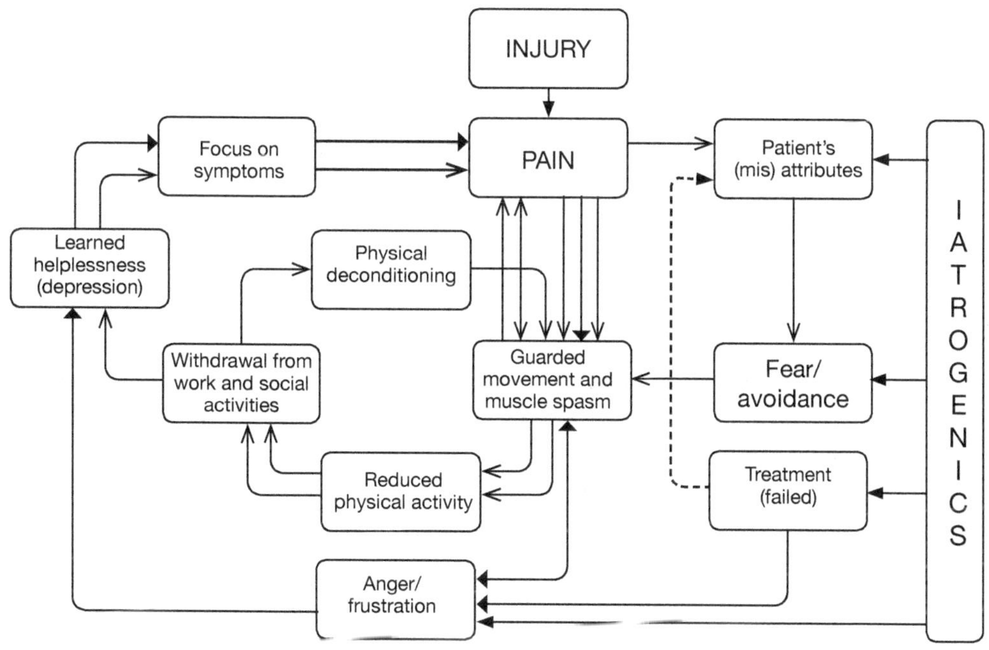

Figure GE 2.11 Influence of iatrogenics – model 5

Figure GE 2.11 adds the beautiful word IATROGENICS on the right hand side, that's medicine and therapists making things worse! For medics iatrogenics is usually associated with the side effects and toxicity of drugs and injections; for surgeons it can be more drastic, like cutting the wrong bit in operations! Rarely is the term used when it actually should be, for the detrimental effects caused by <u>what they have said to or told the patient</u>. Drs almost inadvertently use complicated medical language and diagnostic labels for the patient's problem, that are a cause for great confusion and concern. Physical therapists can be just as culpable. WHAT COMES OUT OF YOUR MOUTH AND THE WAY YOU SAY WHAT COMES OUT OF YOUR MOUTH CAN BE DANGEROUS!

This is what one of my patients told me their Dr had said to them:

'Look, what more do you want me to do? You've got arthritis in your neck, that's cervical spondylosis. It's here on the x-ray report and it's incurable. There's nothing I can do, there's nothing a physiotherapist can do and there's nothing anyone else can do. If I x-ray you today and you come back in a year and I get you x-rayed again I promise you, it will be worse. Now, its painkillers, give up the golf, don't do anything strenuous and learn to live with it.'

The patient was understandably devastated and basically gave up. The patient was 56 when he was told this. I saw him with his wife when he was 60. She said from that day he'd changed out of all recognition from the person she'd known before. She'd persuaded him to come and see me. Six months later he was playing golf again. He's now 70 and he's still playing golf. He still has cervical spondylosis and undoubtedly it would be worse, but he got his life back together, got moving, got fitter and got his physical confidence back – despite the x-ray – despite the diagnosis and despite what the Dr said. I didn't cure him at all, but what I did do was show him how to get to his full physical potential despite the x-rays and the cervical spondylosis.

I have to say that a great deal of my professional life has involved sorting out the mess caused by these sort of words—not just from Drs and consultants—but from physiotherapists, chiropractors, osteopaths and many alternative practitioners too. It used to make me mad but I've come to accept that it is unlikely to ever change, until medicine and clinicians see the sort of picture of pain that I'm trying to get across in these pages... hah!

So my advice is to start thinking about your communication and your normal patter with patients and think what bad it might be doing, as well as what good too. Think about those little frowns those subtle shakes of the head and those under the breath sighs and maybe give some thought to the impact they may be having.

A major problem is that if your approach to the on-going pain patient is to fix; manipulate; unbalance the imbalance and rebalance; re-establish the core stability; to correct the pelvis; lengthen the leg length; tape the glide of the patella; untwist the supinated foot; un-torsion the torsioned tibia; revert the inverted leg; down slip the up-slipped innominate; revive the accessory glide; correct the myofascial plane and its unreleased fibres; smother a cranio-sacral antagonism; make an un-dynamic nerve dynamic; eviscerate the visceral tone; even seeing if you can improve your patient's graded motor image – you're missing the multidimensionality of the problem that this model is crying out to all practitioners to see.

When I was teaching my courses I used to get therapists come up to me in the breaks and tell me about 'their techniques' and how they get fantastic results all the time with all their chronic patients. All I can say is that in the old days, when I was a pure Maitland manual therapist, for a short while I thought I got fantastic results too with all the patients, including the chronic pain ones. But the reality, when I really listened and when I honestly followed them up, was that this was never true. I worked with Geoff Maitland in his practice for two years and the practice was bursting with chronic whiplash, RSI and spinal pain problems and I saw nothing that impressed me (in terms of 'successful' treatments). In fact that experience was one of the main things that made me want to look further and seek better understanding and better answers. There are plenty of myths in the world of pain treatments.

I've listened all my life to stories of chronic pain patients and what treatments they've had and their transient initial improvements but then the later failures and the frustrations that this can cause.

I'd like to quote a passage from Main, Spanswick and Watson's book, page 100:

'Waddell et al (1984a) found that in a large sample of patients with chronic low back pain the amount of treatment received (e.g. bed rest, injections, physiotherapy) was related more to patients' levels of distress and illness behaviour than to the presence of physical indications for such treatment. Patients attending pain management programmes frequently have had a lot of previous treatment, but, of all the sources of anger and frustration evident in patients attending pain management programmes, the influence of failed treatment among chronic pain patients is perhaps the most powerful.'

My advice is to try and tame the arrogance that makes you believe that your treatment technique might be better than those who have gone before and failed. Remember, having multiple treatments and the patients continued use of passive treatments is a yellow flag. Keeping passive treatment going with chronic pain patients, as I witnessed to a marked extent in Geoff Maitland's practice, is contraindicated. To be fair and this is important, back then in the 1980's through to the mid 1990's or later, most of physiotherapy knew nothing about chronic pain mechanisms or pain management approaches. We were all doing our best. The tragedy is now, when there is no excuse. The obligation is for those who teach undergraduates to buck up and get with it. Curriculums for undergraduate

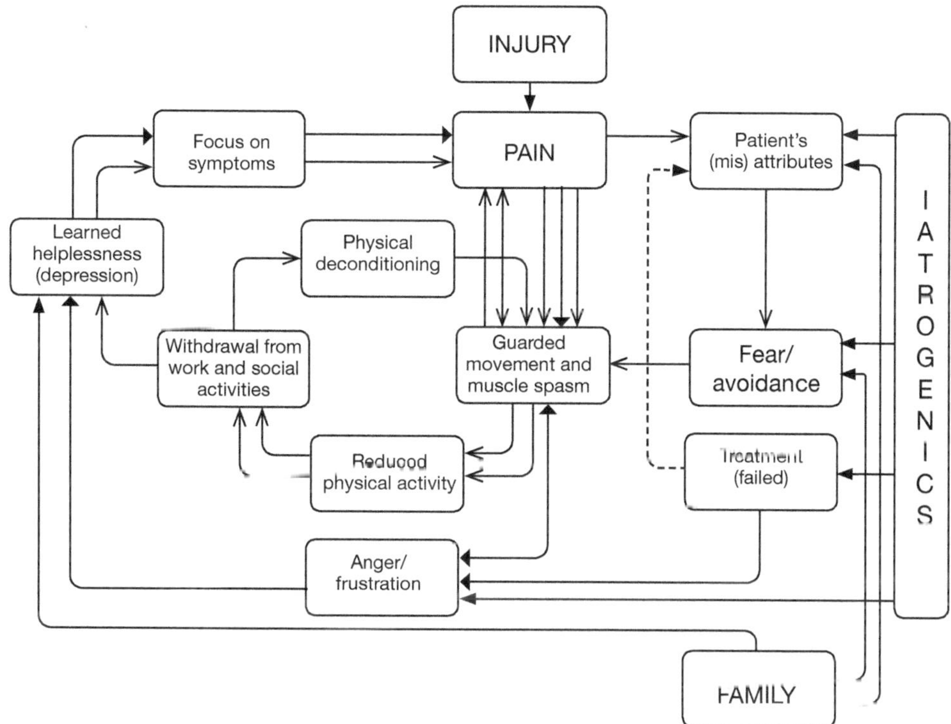

Figure GE 2.12 Influence of the family – model 6

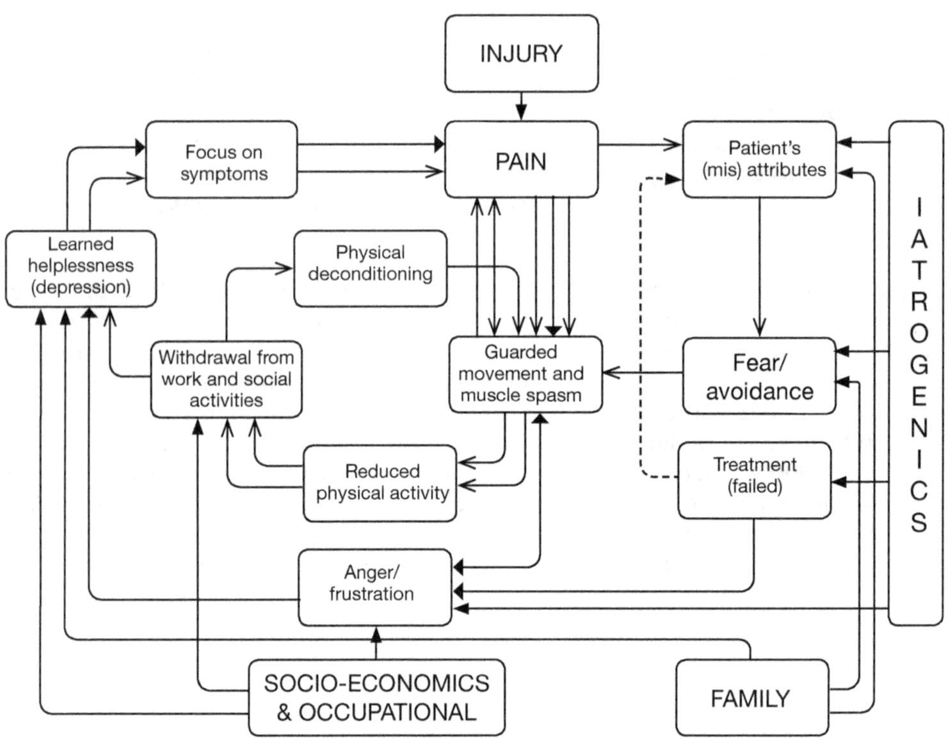

Figure GE 2.13 Influence of socio-economic and occupational factors

physiotherapy must include the teaching of models like this one combined with practical CBT methods relevant to pain. That means the teaching team including practicing pain psychologists or highly trained CBT trained physiotherapists.

Figure GE 2.12 adds the effect of the family into the mix! What does the family do to a pain sufferer? I want you to think about those patients you've had who go, 'Do you mind if my wife/husband/partner come in too?' Sometimes the actual patient can't get a word in edgeways. 'Mr Pecked, what's your problem?' Mr P pauses and then Mrs P pipes in 'He's got it in his back, he's got seven discs out in his lumbago, his sacro-whats-it has never been put back in place properly and now his hips gone; I do my best to not let him do anything that'll put more of his discs out and I've moved the bed downstairs into the lounge so he can watch the telly all day in bed.'

Partners have their own spin on the problem, their own attributes, fears and beliefs as to what should be done or not be done. They can feed into the model – note where the arrows from 'Family' go! The particularly dangerous spouse is one who takes over and doesn't allow the suffering patient to do anything. That's the 'over-solicitous spouse'. There's also the spouse that insists that regardless of all the negative tests that have come back, 'There must be something wrong. There must be something that can be done.' Partners can often stymie the best efforts of pain management and rehabilitation; they may not even seem to want the patient to try and get going or get fitter! At best the spouse, partner or the family can be hugely supportive and encouraging with the rehabilitation and reactivation process—at worst—they can as good as sabotage it.

The last 'stage' of the model, figure GE 2.13 adds on 'socio-economic and occupational factors'. Chapter 4 in Main and Spanswick's book is devoted to this important and complex topic. Also see a great many of the chapters in Topical Issues in Pain 5.

Long term pain disabled people nearly always have gripes with their employers, with the 'Social', with their finances, with benefits and with the Drs and consultants who are employed to assess their fitness to work or not. Here's the example Main, Spanswick and Watson use at the end of chapter 5:

Mr S. had been called for a medical for his disability benefit. The examining Dr hurt him during the assessment. Mr S later learned that the Dr felt there was nothing wrong with him and his benefits were withdrawn. Meanwhile Mr S's trade union was seeking compensation on his behalf. Mr S therefore had to undergo a number of medical examinations from Drs instructed by his union's solicitors and those of his previous employers. Mr S felt insulted when he read some of the reports, which seemed to imply he was putting it all on and malingering. He became very angry and depressed. His wife and family, meanwhile, had to adjust their lifestyle as the family's income had effectively halved.

Hopefully the messages of all these models are clear...

1. Pain is complex, chronic pain even more so. The notion that there's one thing wrong that needs finding and fixing is just not tenable. There are a vast number of interacting factors operating in the present and a great many chiming in from the past. It all adds to the difficult multidimensional mix of factors that go to explain why the patient is so troubled. A great many humans have very fixed and seemingly unshiftable beliefs, attributions and ideas. A great many are unwilling to change and we should not feel we have failed if we can't get anywhere with some of them. I remember once a course participant came up to me and said that she was unable to believe that God would have given us this maladaptive or useless pain, she insisted that all pain was a true reflection of something wrong. Many patients, with pain that is so real in the body are unable to believe that the tissues where it hurts can be anything like normal. For them, hurt must equate to harm, even when a god doesn't come into the picture! On the other hand, sometimes when you simply avoid any explanation of hurt not equating with harm and you just get on with activating the patient using graded exposure and behavioural experiments (chapter GE 2.4) success can still occur. Colleagues of mine working in pain management units strongly testify to this. It's more what we do than what we say or 'tell' that's so important sometimes.

2. Pain is multidimensional, so management has to be! This model shows you where to 'treat' and manage.

3. Passive treatments 'play with processing', which may have a place and be fine as part of a rehabilitation/treatment process, but don't ever make them the central big deal if at all possible. Making them 'not a big deal' however is very difficult. The best way I believe is to think rehabilitation, think shopping basket, think getting the patient going at a pace that's appropriate to the problem and its natural recovery and deal with all the barriers to recovery as best you can. It's OK to do those passive favourite techniques/approaches, but in the right friggin' context!

4. Models like the one discussed here and the fear-avoidance one can sometimes be usefully modified and explained to patients so they can see the bigger context of the problem they have. Patients need to see that there are a lot of different things that can be worked on at the same time and this is where I'm going next!

Chapter GE 2.7
In Parallel Thinking and Management

If someone comes to see me with a 'musculoskeletal problem' I can break it down into many compartments.

Think of sciatica that's been going on for a month. There's lots to do: I can assess, treat and manage some or all of the following:

- the **pain**

- the **injury or pathology** i.e. put the disc back and free the nerve (joking! – but that's medical model thinking, oh, if you get the chance, read Cyriax's books but take care please!)

- the **physical impairments** I might find, for example, I might find and try to improve: limited SLR, stiff back, limited ranges of movement, weak muscles, muscle imbalance, movement abnormalities, posture, scoliosis, balance and co-ordination, sensory loss/alterations; yin, yang, pelvic malalignment etc.

- the **disability, incapacity, the loss of function** this means get walking and moving again, start a lifting programme, look at what's needed for work and start a graded programme and the same for activities round the home and socially and recreationally

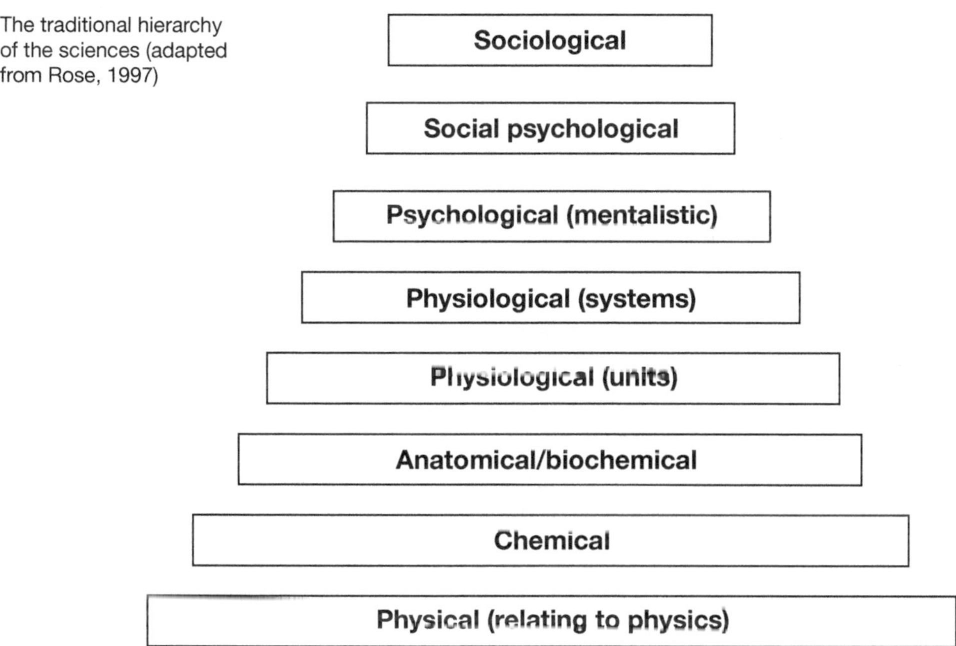

Figure GE 2.14 The heirarchy of explanatory levels

- the **level of concern and anxiety about the cause, solution and future of the problem and of their lives.**

Let's look at it another way... what I call 'the hierarchy of explanatory levels' relevant to pain and related disability. It encompasses all the various possible therapeutic disciplines. I got this idea from Steven Rose's book 'Lifelines'. In the book he showed the 'traditional hierarchy of sciences' (figure GE 2.14). I've also written about this at length in an essay:

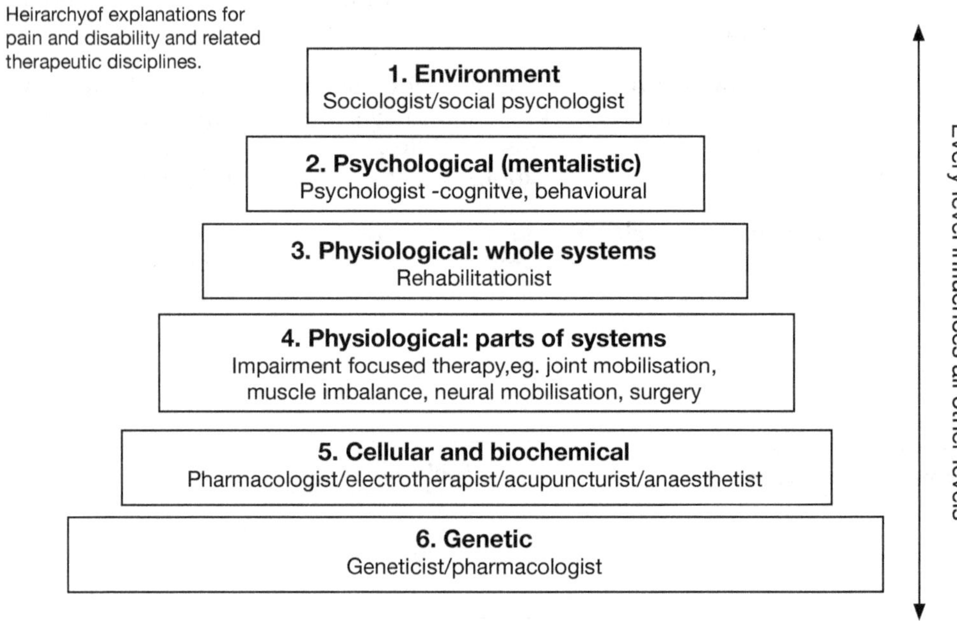

Figure GE 2.15 Heirarchy of explanations for pain and disability and related therapeutic disciplines

Gifford L. S. (2013) 'The Patient in Front of us: From Genes to Environment' In Gifford LS(Ed) Topical Issues in Pain 2. CNS Press, Falmouth.

Figure GE 2.15 is applying the traditional hierarchy of sciences to all the various dimensions and possibilities for pain diagnosis, reasoning, treatment and management. It embraces every level, from the broader more nebulous environmental influences at the top, right down to the very precise reductionist levels of the gene and all the possible factors and influences there. Therapists of course exist at each level and often remain there, never to peer out of their comfy little burrows to see what's around them and what's above and below.

Let me go through them:

1. At the top level is *'environment'*, here for example chronic pain and

disability may be linked to the patients distress at work, to financial issues, to the way their family reacts to them or perhaps to some losses in their social life. 'Manipulate' these and the patient may get better. Sociologists and social psychologists have a claim to pain treatments and management.

2. At the *'psychological'* level, the patient may have powerful beliefs that any physical movement is threatening to their weakened painful state and that rest is the best option for healing; or they may have such emotional turmoil that their interest in any form of healthy activity or life style is non-existent. Educate more healthy beliefs, teach them to appraise better, via graded exposure and behaviour modification, demonstrate that their structural fears are unfounded, help them overcome emotional turmoil and improve their coping strategies and they may get better. Psychologists have an important role in pain.

3. The *'physiological: whole system'* level can relate to systems that may be considered to be faulty in some way. Hence, temporarily or permanently altered function of the nervous system, the endocrine system, the musculoskeletal system, the locomotor system, the visceral system and so forth. From a physical therapists viewpoint this level may more easily relate to faulty or altered gross movement patterns and loss of function – it is here that research and therapy focuses on ALTERED FUNCTION AND DISABILITY (in the older clinical reasoning literature we used the term *'general physical dysfunction'* in a synonymous way (for example, see Gifford 1997; Gifford & Butler 1997, Butler 1998). The patient with back pain may be unable to bend and this affects the ability to dress, to sit comfortably, to drive their car, to sit at the desk for work. Treatment may focus on graded functional programmes and exercises and goal setting to gradually improve flexion and to pace up sitting and bending tolerance. For the sprained ankle, treatment may focus on normal gait or in starting a gradual and progressive weight bearing programme. Rehabilitationists are central to this level of management.

4. The *'physiological: parts of systems'* level can relate to more specific findings. For example, the joint, the ligament, the tendon, the muscle or muscle group, or a specific nerve. Issues might include loss of range, increased mechanical sensitivity, muscle imbalance, even loss of structural integrity. This level relates to an IMPAIRMENT focus by the researcher or clinician (in the clinical reasoning literature the term *'specific physical dysfunction'* was used in a synonymous way). Altered function at this level might be addressed by manual therapists, surgeons, or better – specific exercises, for example.

5. The *'cellular and biochemical'* level looks at pain from the perspective of changes in the tissue environment and changes in cells and pathways in the nervous system. For example, inflammatory chemicals in freshly injured muscle or ligament, alterations in neuropeptides or receptor populations

in nociceptors and nociceptor pathways subserving the injury, or altered immune functions, altered neuroendocrine reactivity and so on. This paradigm for pain offers help via chemical manipulation of organ and tissue physiology, of chemical and neurological pathways as well as of the cellular environment – hence the pharmacological claims to the management and treatment of pain. Involvement at this level for physiotherapy might be via electrotherapy, acupuncture or perhaps manual therapy. Think direct tissue effect, but also via changes in processing and the ever-present top-down effects too.

6. Currently, the lowest and most 'reductionist' level of possible practical value, is the *genetic* level of research, thinking and intervention. For further discussion here see my essay: 'The patient in front of us: From genes to environment', in Topical Issues in Pain volume 2.

The goal of 'In parallel' reasoning is to drive everyone out of their safe little therapeutic and intellectual burrows in order to get them safely above ground looking at each other and talking things in common! Now I reckon a pain-genetics researcher wouldn't have a whole lot in common with four or five levels away. Could you see a geneticist talking comfortably with a psychologist or a sociologist or an anthropologist even...? 'Er, what on earth has humanity and culture got to do with gene expression and phenotypic switching... yeah, how you going to treat that then... eh? You gonna' give culture steroids in the water supply or what?'

Look my big point **each and every level influences all the others** like it or not? The brilliant bit is that physiotherapy is in a unique position to embrace all the disciplines in our treatments, managements and interactions with patients. Unique is the word and the way, praise be to whomsoever you want to and let's get stuck in!

I'm strongly arguing that if you can change something at any one of these six levels you are very likely to change the other levels too. A patient with on-going back pain is struggling with finance, the possibility of losing their job and their family relationships are suffering. After several weeks of a negotiating with his employer a 'return to work' occupational physiotherapist has managed to get the patient more appropriate hours and a less stressful position. The employer now understands much better that the patient is working hard at getting their fitness back, needs to pace activity and rest and is very keen not to lose their job, which they were very good at. As a result, the workplace has welcomed him back, the atmosphere is good and he's coping very well. His self esteem has improved, he looks forward to work again and he's performing far better with his exercises, fitness tasks and general function at home. 'Home' sees light at the end of the tunnel and is a far better place to be. The patient soon starts to improve his fitness and ranges of movement, strength and quality of movement come on in leaps and bounds. Stress levels reduce and humour and relaxation return to life. As the patient gets stronger and fitter his internal physiological status reflects this, his pain processing is far more adaptive and pain becomes less or much less of a problem. He reduces his analgesics and other medications. If it were possible to find out I am sure this fellow's pain and body processing systems will have changed. If these have changed that means his genetic expression will have changed and in turn the microstructure of his neurones and hence their excitability.

That is an illustration of how changing something at the top can filter down to the bottom. But, when you see the changes that occurred, what is really required is appropriate input at every level, and – most importantly, at the higher three possibly four levels. So, why these top levels and not the bottom two or three? Because it so happens that current research supports these levels far more than the lower ones for complex pain state rehabilitation and recovery.

In my career I have always had a vision that one day specialists in pain will be trained at all the levels, sadly, I'm beginning to wonder if it would or could ever happen. The power of biomedicine and the economy it drives are as hard to shift as our dependence on petrochemicals perhaps?

Have a look at figure GE 2.16, a decrepit old model for those of us working with pain and pain related disability. It goes... pain or pathology causes disability, fix the pathology or get rid of the pain somehow and the disability will vanish – the medical model!

Figure GE 2.17 is a World Health Organisation model which adds 'Impairments' to the equations. The arrows are still one way. Figure GE 2.18 the 'Nagi model adds 'Functional Limitation. The British physiotherapist Maureen Simmonds, came up with a bi-directional model figure GE 2.19. At last, an acknowledgement of the influence of one level on another! Lastly my view on it figure GE 2.20 which adds pain and tissue mechanisms to the pathology and most important of all the term 'psychosocial factors' overseeing and having an impact on the whole lot. It simply recognises the importance of the person and their brain's hold over how impaired, functionally limited or disabled a given individual in pain may be. It's simply top-down before bottom-up!

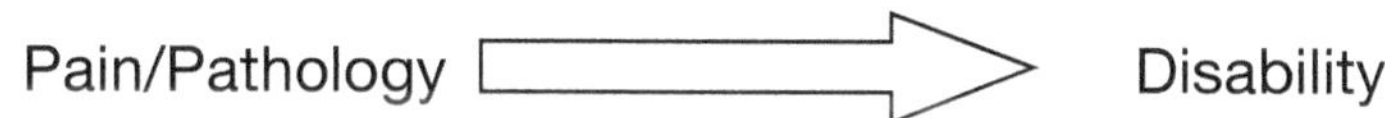

Figure GE 2.16 The medical model

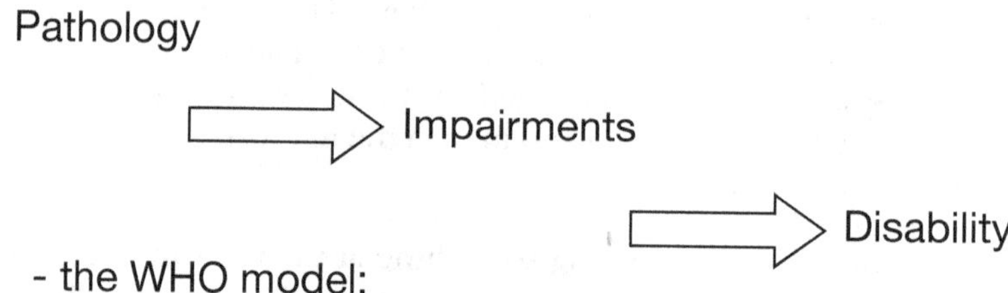

Figure GE 2.17 The WHO model

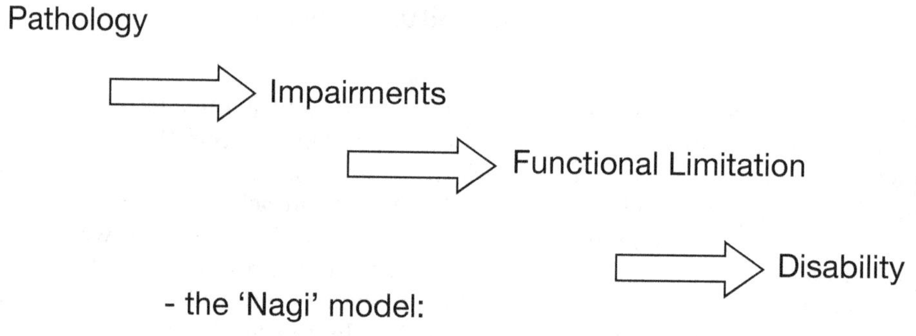

Figure GE 2.18 The 'Nagi' model

A therapist is hardly going to shift a patient from functional limitation and disability to a situation of fit to participate if their beliefs, attributions and emotions are stymieing the process... 'Look if I start lifting, moving about more and getting involved with any kind of work, I'll be back at the Drs again, the disc will go and I'll be back on the waiting list for an operation...'

I now hope that I've persuaded you that if pain is multi-level or multi-dimensional then management has to be too. Further, think back to the placebo chapters— where a drug given without the patient's knowledge has very little impact—even

Pathology

Impairments

Functional Limitation

Disability

- Maureen Simmonds' bidirectional model:

Figure GE 2.19 Maureen Simmonds – bidirectional model

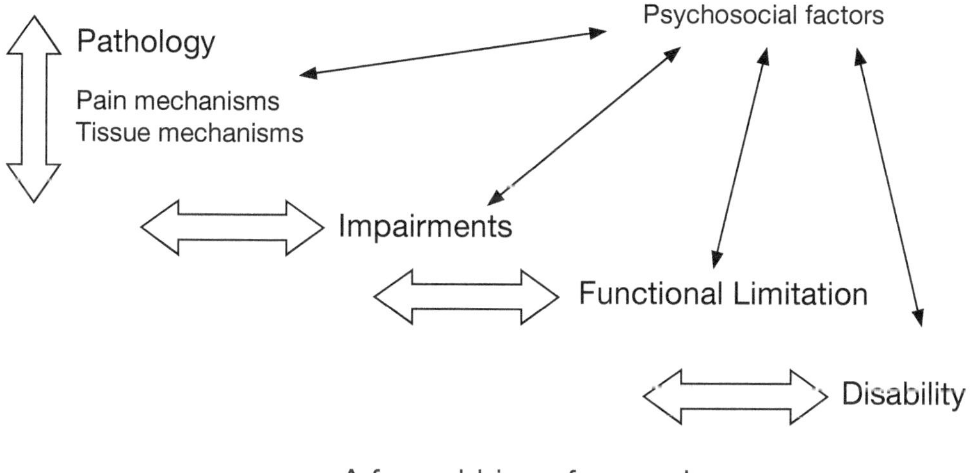

Figure GE 2.20 The bidirectional model – plus some add-ons

very strong drugs like morphine. So, those who are stuck down at levels five and six and also those many therapists at level four – think about it! If you are not including the higher levels in your interactions you're biologically on a par with the hidden drug infusion. If you want to make your thing work better, like it or not, you have to include the brain and the individual whose brain it is.

The terms impairment, disability and handicap are discussed at length in: *Main C. J. and C. C. Spanswick (2000). Pain Management. An interdisciplinary approach. Edinburgh, Churchill Livingstone.*

In the Shopping Basket Approach in section 4 I will discuss how I deal with these terms.

929

Chapter GE 2.8
The Biopsychosocial Model

When you've got disillusioned with tissue based 'fix-it' courses why not buy or borrow the books below and study them. Also, find and go on some well taught practical biopsychosocial/yellow-flag courses as well as courses on Cognitive Behavioural Therapy (CBT) for physiotherapists. Just because you talk to your patients a bit and do a bit of explaining doesn't mean you're now using CBT. The best thing is to sit in on a CBT pain management programme

Read the following:

All the Topical Issues in Pain volumes – but in particular if you're making a start, volume 2 and the 'how to do understand it and do it' chapters by Paul Watson and Nicholas Kendall. Plus there's a brilliant, if not essential, chapter in Topical Issues in Pain 3: chapter 8, 'The distressed and angry low back pain patient' by Paul Watson and Chris Main.

The Back Pain Revolution. By Gordon Waddell.

Understanding Pain for better Clinical Practice: A psychological perspective: by Steven Linton.

Pain Management: An Interdisciplinary Approach. By Chris Main and Chris Spanswick.

This is a vast topic and one which more and more undergraduate physiotherapists are hopefully being trained in or at least being made more aware of. However, it looks to me as if there are only pockets of interest and still great resistance for 'physical' therapy to embrace what many see as the soft and squidgy world of sociology and psychology. What I hear a lot of is this, 'I deal with acute musculoskeletal pain, that stuff is pretty irrelevant to my practice,' or something similar. One of the worst is: 'Most of the pains I see are 'mechanical' and therefore only require mechanical treatment!'

Those who think like this need to go back to the beginning of the last section and read Steve Linton's 'Seven Features of Success' and read about the key things that prevent chronic pain and chronic pain related disability.

CUTTING OFF THE THINKING-FEELIING-REASONING PERSON FROM PAIN IS IMPOSSIBLE, EVEN WHEN IT'S ACUTE!

Look at the MOM, look at the Fear Avoidance Model, look at Chris Main, Chris Spanswick and Paul Watson's Model of Disability and THINK AGAIN. I've gone as far as saying, in a nice tongue in cheek way mind, that if you're resistant to the inclusion of the individual in all aspects of pain and rehabilitation the best advice is to go look for another job. As I've already suggested try dentistry, the patient can't talk when you've got their mouth jammed open!

Enough ranting!

The psychosocial 'onion', as it's sometimes termed is shown in figure GE 2.21, with a clinical illustration in GE 2.22.

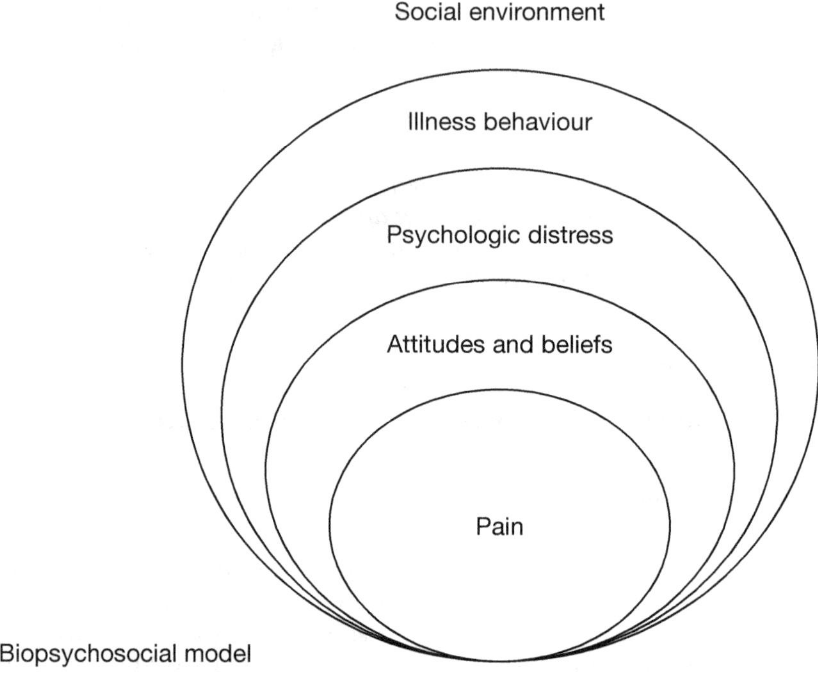

Figure GE 2.21 The psychosocial 'onion'

So, there are three things here from me, and there's more how to do it – in the 'Shopping Basket' sections and clinical examples later on.

1. Psychosocial factors are the best predictors of a poor outcome – this is in great contrast to physical factors, which are actually poor at predicting. So it's not the extent of the damage, the extent of the degenerative changes or the degree of pathology; it's much more down to how an individual reacts to the situation they find themselves in. Thus, someone in the early stages of their problem, who has high levels of pain, is highly distressed and/or angry about the pain and the situation they're in, who believes that they should rest, be physically careful and not go to work or do normal functional things until the pain has gone; who is fearful of causing more damage by getting going, is resting and doing nothing to help themselves and who is encouraged to be like this by their family, their Dr/therapist and their work – is very unlikely to get better quickly and is highly likely to become chronic pain disabled.

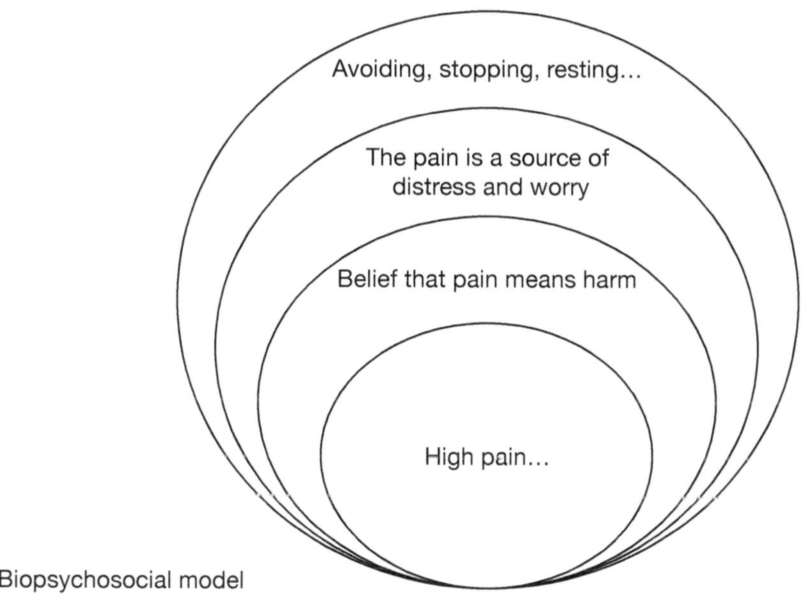

Figure GE 2.22 The psychosocial onion with a clinical illustration

2. These factors must be addressed as soon as possible in the evolution of the problem. The trouble is these days is that early management is so 'treatment' orientated rather than 'rehabilitation' orientated; and it's not until the patient isn't getting anywhere that 'other' factors start to be thought of, let alone addressed. Steven Linton's work already alluded to is huge testament to this.

3. An 'In parallel' type management approach is required. The 'manual therapy/ insert guru's name approach', to me, epitomizes the uni-dimensional 'In-series' approach here. My experience was with Geoff Maitland's approach; with the one technique at a time, the reluctance to give exercises, the passive nature of the intervention, the heavily weighted balance of the treatment session to the treatment technique and its constant evaluation by asking about pain while observing movement; rather than to sound advice and reassurance, to graded functional return and simple goal setting. The way I fit 'passive' therapies in will be discussed and illustrated later in the clinical examples and the 'Shopping Basket Approach' that I advocate.

Section GE 2
Read what I've read

Asmundson G.J.G., Vlaeyen J.W.S. and Crombez G. (Eds).(2004) Understanding and treating fear of pain. Oxford University Press.
... and a very practical chapter tucked right at the end of the book...

Campbell G.E., Goodchild N., Charlton B.G.(2005). Depressive symptoms in injury and illness. PPA News issue 19: 22-23.

Charlton B.(2005). The malaise theory of depression: Major depressive disorder is sickness behaviour and antidepressants are analgesic. PPA News issue 19: 17-22.

Cyriax J. (1978) Textbook of Orthopaedic Medicine Volume 1. Bailliere Tindall. London.

Cyriax J., Russell G. 1977) Textbook of Orthopaedic Medicine Volume 2. Bailliere Tindall. London.

Diamond J. (1991) The Third Chimpanzee. Harper Collins, New York.

Gifford L.S. (1997) Pain. In: Pitt-Brooke (ed) Rehabilitation of Movement: Theoretical bases of clinical practice Saunders, London 196-232

Gifford L.S. & Butler D.S. (1997) The integration of pain sciences into clinical practice. Hand Therapy 10(2): 86-95

Butler D.S. (1998) – articles that relate to clinical reasoning and specific and general physical dysfunction...

Gifford L. S.(2013). Preface. In: Gifford L. S. (Ed) Topical Issues in Pain vol 1. CNS Press, Falmouth. vii-xi.

Gifford L. S. (2013) The patient in front of us: from genes to environment. In Gifford LS(Ed) Topical Issues in Pain 2. CNS Press, Falmouth.

Kluger Matthew – study on fever in lizards.

Main C.J. and Spanswick C.C. (2000). Pain Management. An interdisciplinary approach. Edinburgh, Churchill Livingstone.

Martin P. (1997) The Sickening Mind. Brain, behaviour, immunity and disease. Harper Collins, London.

Nesse R.M. And Williams G.C. (1994). Evolution and Healing. The new science of Darwinian medicine. London, Phoenix.

Oka T., Oka K. (2007) Age and gender differences of psychogenic fever: a review of the Japanese literature. BioPsychoSocial Medicine 1:11

Roberts L. (2013)Flagging the danger signs of low back pain. Topical Issues in Pain 2, Gifford L.S (ed) CNS Press, Falmouth.

Rose S. (1997) Lifelines. Vintage, London.

Sapolsky   R. M (1997) Junk Food Monkeys and Other Essays on the Biology of the Human Predicament
(Now called 'The trouble with Testosterone and other essays on the biology of the human predicament.) I think the title was thought too offensive for the US market? Into stress and understanding life? These essays are a must read!

Topical Issues in Pain 1-5 (2013) CNS Press, Falmouth.

Ursin H. and Eriksen H. R. (2001) Sensitization, subjective health complaints and sustained arousal. Ann N Y Acad Sci 933: 119-129

Vlaeyen J.W.S. et al. (2004) Fear reduction in chronic pain: Graded exposure in vivo with behavioral experiments. Ch 14 In: Asmundson et al (Eds) Understanding and treating fear of pain. Oxford University press: 313-343

Von Korff M. and Moore J.C. (2001) Stepped care for back pain: activating approaches for primary care. Ann Intern Med. 2001 May 1:134(9 Pt 2):911-7.

Waddell G. (1999) The Back Pain Revolution. Churchill Livingstone, London

Watkins L. R. (2000). The pain of being sick: Implications of immune-to-brain communication for understanding pain. Annual review of Psychology 51: 29-57

Watson P.W. (2013)Topical Issues in Pain 2. Gifford L.S.(ed) Authorhouse, Bloomington.

LOUIS GIFFORD ACHES AND PAINS

PAIN BITS AND PIECES!

Chapter GE 3.1
Pain: two moans! Pain is smart! What we can learn from injured toddlers!

Pain: two moans!

First moan – through all the years of reading about pain I've always been a bit annoyed by authors saying something like this:

'Pain is a warning, it is a message of danger that the individual or the part affected should stop what they are doing, or at least take great care of it while it is vulnerable – pain means stop, rest, be careful, be guided by the pain and it's best to avoid.'

What annoys me is the 'pain means stop' bit. This type of statement makes me think that the individual who wrote it, or says it, hasn't paused to think about pain and what it does to them because the pain message is very often, get off your butt and MOVE! Remember 'botty rot' my Dad's word for the discomfort you get when you sit for a long time. Remember too those amazing human 'statues' and how our natural reaction to them is 'that's a form of torture'; not moving hurts and when you're injured, not moving can hurt even more! Healing tissues need movement and your pain system actually asks you to move. More shortly!

Second moan – is that I get annoyed with the guru teachers of the world, who tell us clinicians how to do it, when in actual fact they stopped treating patients many years ago. They 'peddle their wares' and tell us little naive clinical 'saplings' what we should be doing with our patients. To balance this; there are many who haven't seen patients, who do research, who think about the implications of their research and who openly admit to no longer doing clinical work, but tell us a great deal and make sound suggestions that may help in the clinic. I know several who are of craftsman quality in this respect.

Recently I started a blog and I've had a great many emails and letters from therapists frustrated that the profession hasn't moved on and that what I was writing about and questioning over ten years or more ago is still in the same state today. I'm so often asked; how on earth is it possible to 'change' their colleagues' attitudes to pain problems? How do they move them away from continually looking for answers in perceived impairments of the musculoskeletal tissues? How do they persuade them to see a bigger picture? Well, my experience in the early days, back in the mid 1990's, was that I was frustrated in the same way. I believe that what made the big difference – what persuaded therapists to see a different perspective and then make changes to their own practice, were demonstrations with 'real' patients out the front of the class! I particularly asked for chronic problems. The sessions were never set up in an atmosphere that I would 'cure' patients, but they were designed for…

a) **the therapists watching…** to see how information was extracted from the patient; the kind of communication skills required; the unravelling of a pain narrative; the multidimensionality of the problem; the barriers to recovery; the unhelpful attributes and fears the patient may have about their problem (often related to previous therapists input or iatrogenics); the issues of family, work and treatment for the patient; the type of physical examination appropriate to the patient's presentation; the discussion and observation of illness behaviour issues; the initial 'setting-up' of the patient's understanding to enable the possibility of change in attribution to more adaptive perspectives; the discussion of a route they could take to get to a better place, also and importantly, some appropriate physical practice and lots more depending on the patient.

b) **the patient…** to allow the patient to clearly understand that the session in front of the class was never going to make them feel difficult or awkward; that it was not going to 'cure' them; that it was most likely going to give them more information about their problem; to suggest and discuss with them some different perspectives and potentially different therapeutic routes to follow; it was going to give them a chance to express and discuss the frustrations and problems they were having.

I have to say that the first time I did it I was anxious that it would all end in tears and be highly embarrassing – for me and for the patient! Yet, the patients were amazing and they always illustrated the issues and points that I'd been making in the lectures. Patients revealed the most incredible things, the therapists watching were stunned by what they heard and a great many reported afterwards that it was witnessing it all 'live' that helped them see the need for change in their own practice. So the only real way to get your colleagues to change is for them to witness a different approach. Second best, in my opinion, are explicit and detailed case histories or parts of case histories as I've presented here in this book – but not the simple 'they-had-this-and-I-did-that' ones.

If you go on courses where the lecturer tells you how they fix everything and the case histories they patter off are all wonderful – yet when you go back to your patients and try for yourself, it doesn't quite seem to happen the way they said…! Well, perhaps you need to get those whizz-kid guru type fix-everyone teachers to agree to coming and doing some patient demonstrations?

In my career I did all the reading, the theory, the practicing of techniques and I was totally devoted to doing my very best with all the tools and information I was given and I could find. But the best learning was seeing it in action, seeing skilled therapists doing their thing. I've been lucky, maybe I was in the right place at the right time, but I got to watch in particular: Shirley Orme on Walton Hospital's orthopaedic wards teaching and making quads exercises relevant, getting patients going and confident – nice patient communication; Paul Chadwick, also then working at Walton Hospital in Liverpool, a great manual therapist, watching his hands communicate and the patient feeling safe and confident with what he did; in London at St Stephens' Hospital, Peter Wells, Joan Blair and Agneta Lando – again, skilled hands and skilled communication, plenty of patient mileage and plenty of amazing discussions. Then later in Adelaide, Geoff Maitland, inkling out the most exact and precise detail of a patient's history or of their physical examination, 'making it make sense' as he put it and then back in the UK observing the skills and craft of 'Cognitive Behavioural' therapists working with the worst chronic pain patients and seeing them change their terrible habits of movement, their pain behaviour and their maladaptive thinking in remarkably short periods of time, without even touching them. Suzanne

Brook particularly stands out.

So, get your guru to demo and if they refuse, get sceptical and go find another guru! It is my belief that the best guru isn't a guru, he, or she are probably quietly working away in the a department or treatment room right next door to you, so my advice is – don't pay a fortune to some so-called expert from overseas – go and watch, listen and discuss with those physiotherapists around you. Most confident therapists love to teach, demonstrate and discuss! Good clinicians have no fears and are keen for you to observe and learn. Beware the show-offs though. Also, if you want to change your colleagues, don't get all 'know-all' and cocky, the best thing is to try getting to the stage where you feel you're confident enough to take a fresh patient, completely unknown to you and take their history in front of a few colleagues; then discuss what you've heard, keeping the patient in confidence of everything discussed and for them to voice their opinion, about your opinions!

Pain is smart!

Back to pain! I want you to keep a few of your own pain experiences in mind for a minute and see what you think.

Let's ask some simple questions. What's pain for? Why do we have pain? What happens to us when we are in pain? What's our response? There are a great many answers, but for my purpose here's a list:

Pain...

- protects while we recover...

- makes us stop doing, or be a bit cautious... and...

- makes us start doing... makes us try out movements...

- **Pain is by nature inconsistent**... one minute it's stop and rest, the next it's get moving... it makes us restless

- it makes us moody and feel sorry for ourselves

- it makes us seek help – it makes us slow down

- we may feel a bit fearful, anxious, tense, even angry, certainly grumpy

- pain changes our behaviour

- we show we are injured, it's all about a bit of 'help me,' maybe it's 'keep away from me', 'feel sorry for me', or 'support me'

- pain behaviour... summons help – it gets favours and rewards, or maybe you get ignored and become lonely

- it fulfils the requirement of 'protection' – or low environmental 'stress'

- it focuses our attention on it – so we find out its location and assess how bad it is

- it makes us ponder whether we should seek help or whether it might be OK

- it teaches us to be careful to not do the thing that caused it again, or at least to be more careful – it puts a little note in memory

- pain tells us to not get over-ambitious as we recover, 'make sure you practice those hunting and fighting skills in safety before you venture out again and start off slowly to get your confidence back'; listen to it and if it's working correctly it gives you nature's 'Graded Exposure'!

- so, you see I'd argue that Graded Exposure is an evolved strategy, what better reason can there ever be for doing it?

I love this stuff, its good old fashioned observation and a bit of cheeky, but quite meaningful thinking.

Let's now think about two different sorts of pain, achy pain and sharp pain. Both are a common experience, but to me are rarely, if ever, discussed in terms of their meaning. Think about a typical OA knee or hip and the achy pain and pain behaviour that it drives.

Achy pain:

- achy pain says 'Look, I've had enough of walking right now I'd like to 'take-5' and sit down over there, you carry on, I'll catch up or see you in a while'

- after sitting for a while achy pain says 'I want to move, get up and stretch out a bit and get going again, being still is driving me mad'

- achy pain can make you restless (clever… up to a point!)

- achy pain makes you moody, grumpy, pretty tired, often drained and pretty fed up.

Now think about sharp pain, like the nasty sharp acute neck pain many of us get from time to time. There may be a very low background achy awareness, but the main thing is a nasty sharp pain when you look to the right, or right and left.

So, sharp pain:

- tells you to stop, don't go there, don't do that again – or does it?

- maybe it's 'If you do that movement, just go a bit carefully will you'

- or is it, 'I quite like that, do it slowly, nudge into me a bit, squirm a bit, but it's kind of nice – test me, try me occasionally!'

Sharp 'Ow' with movement – it's so nasty it clearly tells you that the tissue is a bit vulnerable and to not go fast at it. But during healing that sharp pain also likes to be tested; remember that slight pleasure you get out of easing into the sharp pain. Clever stuff, sharp pain looks after the tissue but also gets you to do gentle stretches to it from time to time. The achy pain slows you down but also makes sure you keep moving and don't rest up completely.

Forget thinking of the OA for now and think of any wound or strain pain problem, but think too that pain is different messages at different times.

Acute instant pain *at the time of injury* (or potential injury) has the purpose of trying to limit damage. You're going over on your ankle. The whole thing is in slow-mo – you let the leg go relaxed and try to go with the direction it's going in – you fall to the ground; a few bumps and bruises but because you fell with it the inversion strain wasn't so bad. Lucky you were young and fit and didn't mind taking the 'falling-over' option. What if you're older and a bit fragile? That's not an option –it's try not to fall if you can help it – the old ankle twists badly as a result, but that's better than a broken leg or hip!

A last thought for this section.

Over the years, you may have noted that some patients are very pleased when you find their pain, that's one thing, but also, some love it when you get your fingers stuck into the area of tenderness. They want you to 'get at' the pain and hurt them! Other patients it can be the exact opposite, while they're pleased you've found the pain they become very agitated and don't like it at all if you start digging your thumbs into it. Pain seems to have the ability to know what it wants. Well, perhaps, but we mustn't forget that this feature may well be driven by the patients attitude, beliefs and fears about their problem.

What we can learn from injured toddlers!

The fundamentals of good 'treatment' may come from observations of hurt toddlers and their mothers.

So, let's take a little side step and observe something: how injured children and their mothers behave – thinking in evolutionary terms!

A child does something, falls over and screams. The scream of a child is to most human ears a terrible sound and very hard to ignore – brilliant! It attracts attention to the little 'me', who's in trouble. The yelling draws adults in to try and help – in particular the parents, most often the mother, unless the father's the one who's always around. The kid screams for their mum, someone they know and trust. If you've ever tried to go to the help of a fallen toddler you will have noted how distressed they get if you're not their mum or dad. A stranger just won't do and often even dad won't do.

So here's the first treatment rule: ***accept help from someone you trust/seek help from someone you trust/has a good reputation etc***.

(Treatment 'rules' are shown in bold)

Right, mum arrives, what does she do instinctively? She picks her little tacker[1] up saying, 'What's the matter darling, where is it, what have you done?'

Well I've also seen mothers screaming, 'Oh my god, oh my god, what on earth… Oh get a Doctor, where's the paramedic? Oh my god'… for some minor fall, haven't you? No? I was just making a point about acute 'modern maladaptive behaviour'.

The 'adaptive' mother reaction is all about what us primates do naturally, in order to begin to manage and treat injury and pain. We/mum **finds the location** of the pain, we **investigate** it. Just like you do with your patients, you put the pain location on the body chart. It's good to think that what you're doing is a highly evolved behaviour isn't it?

Back to the blubbing kid – he indicates the little scratch on his knee and mum has a good look, she pulls up his shorts a bit to see if there's anything else and has a general once over. She **finds out what's wrong** – she does a **physical assessment** and makes a **diagnosis.** In 'MOM' language, it's an 'is it good' or 'is it bad' 'scrutinising' moment if you like and the assessment was the 'sampling' bit! As mum assesses the situation she's actually quietly **reassuring herself** that all is going to be OK, that it's nothing much. As I see it, this is exactly what we all should be doing with our patients – looking to see if anything bad has happened in the first instance and in the second, **building evidence to reassure ourselves that what we're finding is going to get better**.

If there's nothing serious the next thing, just as the mother would do, is to begin the process of **reassuring the toddler/patient**, as opposed to the 'obligatory', medical model driven diagnosis of something wrong. If it's not a serious disease or broken, then it's over to nature and biology and your job is to create the best conditions for best recovery. That, in a word or two, is the nub and reality of what any of us can hope to do. When therapists are really cool, they're good at facilitating turning the patient's pain 'fear' and 'anxiety' dimmer switch down. Good mums do it well.

Thus, once the mother has reassured herself it's all OK, she instinctively sets about reassuring her child. (With the patient, in this modern day and age, sometimes that can be the hard bit, more later!) Mum starts the reassuring process, 'There, there, it's alright, it's only a little scratch, you'll be fine, it's going to mend, you'll be fine.' I bet you can think of those kids who scream, throw a tantrum and stubbornly go 'No it won't be fine. I'm hurt badly. I want a pasty and an ice cream.' It's just like with patients!

Now the good mother should just ignore all that and start the next phase, stroking, kissing and putting on a plaster perhaps, the **treatment 'fuss' phase** has begun. Note that the mother instinctively does the 'dimmer switch' down stuff – she's using the good old **'pain-gate'** for a bit of pain and pain behaviour modulation as well as

---

1 - 'Tacker' is Australian for young child!

'**distraction**'… via stroking, talking, touching, holding, soothing, patting the back, cuddling close – as well as a bit of **direct local stuff**, that little plaster on, maybe some of mum's soothing 'cream[1]'… and a bit of fuss – then more patting and then a bit of tickling and bit of giggling and bit more of this and that.

(I hope you can all see the 'placebo' in brilliant action here?)

Mums and a great many social mammals (like primates, elephants, wolves, dolphins and whales), instinctively **hold close, cuddle and stroke** and often the stroke is on the back, mid thoracic area. Most of us love it. Maybe it's a 'hard-wired' 'nice' spot and therefore well connected to pleasure and pain-off processing mechanisms?

So, with your patients, hold close, cuddle and stroke, talk soothingly to, rub their backs; that's it, you've got the idea – **touch!**

The neat last phase of the 'adaptive' mother's approach to her wounded child is a subtle shift from distraction to **withdrawal of the treatment and finally back to normal activity**. For some it can take a little while, for others it's very quick. Thinking patient, this is where time is very important.

As the toddler starts to stop yelling and whimpering and becomes calmer following the treatment the mother starts bouncing little Henry on her knee; gradually to start with to gauge the reaction and when that's OK, slowly getting more vigorous, then adding in a funny face, blowing a few raspberries, turning him upside down and generally playing with him. The addition of fun and humour is a big one – for the kid and when appropriate, for us with patients too.

Have you noticed that some of the best clinicians are the ones who have a great sense of humour?

What we are doing is shifting the mood from down and out, low in spirits, concerned, anxious, frustrated, whiney, angry, to a calmer, better mental state. De-stressing, allowing the healing biology to work at its most efficient – and getting back to normal activity as soon as possible. Anyone who cared to come and observe in our, or any good clinic, is very likely to witness plenty of fun and laughs from time to time and lots of action. Odd that, when the place is dealing with pain! There are certainly more laughs than tears.

Note the term 'withdrawal' – the mother instinctively and gradually gets away from the child, so that she can get on again and the kid stops bothering her – job done! Children, like adults, vary in how long they want to hang around, little Henry might soon want to be off and out again, fearful he might have missed some fun action with his mates – others might keep dragging away at mum's skirts or legs, for ages, just like patients!

Note how much time it can take for the good parent to work through all this and get the child out and off again? But think of those parents who are impatient, that

---

1 - My mum used to use either Vaseline or Nivea as 'treatment'

instantly 'reward' the kid with a big lump of chocolate in front of the TV. That's a treatment method that promotes further crying and bawling surely? Is that you in your clinic with the patients? Can't be bothered to go through the **listen, look, assess, diagnose, reassure, treat, distract and humour and the final withdraw and get going again phases**? Stick the patient straight on the machine and keep pinging in those needles –hardly without a word?

Hmm? Hard work being a 'mother (treater)' isn't it? Every kid, every patient is different and for some the process speeds along nicely, others it's slow and if you don't get it right they'll hang on to those skirt tails!

I cannot pass on from here without a needed but cynical comment about economics – which is that therapists are very likely avoiding getting quickly on to the 'withdrawal' phase. I get mad that *clinical providers treat for far too long and that the skill of 'treatment withdrawal' isn't taught in musculoskeletal and pain modules – it is a considerable bugbear for me.* OK, grump over… let's wind this up now.

My point here is that an acute injury plus early achy and sharp pain instigates a fairly stereotypical, assess and diagnose, then reassure self, reassure child/patient, distract/ treat, withdraw and return to activity process.

What about the adult, or the situation for a child where they're out and about and a parent isn't around. Now it's often more of a 'do-it-yourself' process. The child falls over, they wimper a bit, a stranger offers help, they balk at this and hey presto, up and away again back with their mates. Or, they sit there wimpering a bit, they then do a bit of a self examination, reassure themselves, give it a rub, get up and get going with their mates again.

Moral of the story… every human needs mates to play with if they want to get better quickly!

This last section is dedicated to my Philippa – who when asked how she might go about treating a patient will say… 'I just kiss them round the neck (clockwise in the northern hemisphere and anti-clockwise in the southern) and give them a cuddle!'

It's a new form of treatment – called 'The Primitive Approach!'

Chapter GE 3.2
Pain and illness behaviour!

Waddell's book: 'The Back Pain Revolution' is essential reading. No ifs or buts, buy it, read it, study it.

I'm going to start this with an example of 'the-patient-I-used-to-dread'.

These patients are actually the ones that stimulated me to find out more about pain. They are the ones that are described inadequately, or not at all, in the medical literature; they are generally feared and misunderstood and considered time wasters and users and abusers of precious resources. They are what I've come to call 'the hardest patients on the planet'. Physiotherapists dread them because they make them run late; they don't make sense at all on standard pain charts; they have multiple problems and... and... 'We only deal with one problem at a time.' Or, as it was at Geoff Maitland's practice and many others in Adelaide back in the 1980's – the patients used to get charged 'per area' treated. So if the patients came in with neck pain, back pain, pain down one arm and leg, their bill would get quadrupled and still they'd only have a twenty minute time slot!

Here we go: this was back in the 1980's at Geoff Maitland's practice. The patient is Mr Grubb – a 35 year old ex-policeman now on disability payments.

You pop your head into the waiting area and say, 'Come in Mr Grubb, I'm Louis, follow me.' Mr Grubb doesn't move; his eyes sort of rotate towards you and then his neck follows with a jerky tremor-like movement; he's got two elbow crutches and a lumbar support on the outside of his shirt. It's all soiled and scruffy and it's riding up round his ribs. His eyes frown and he begins to shuffle forwards in the chair. There are grunts and groans. Eventually he gets up, leaning forward dramatically on the crutches, one crutch then moves forward, the opposite leg follows, then the crutch – the arms shake as they clench the grips. The other patients stop what they are doing, most are aghast and feel that they should be somehow helping him. You come over closer to help, even though you don't really want to. You're thinking 'Oh no, why me, today or all days, I've got twenty minutes and it's going to take five minutes at least to get this guy into the cubicle, then what the fuck do I do.' You swear inwardly again and curse the awful time pressure. He starts to speak after about four paces.

'I've got all my tabs with me and I've got the surgeons and the rheumatologists' notes in my back-pack.' Then he looks up and I think he's going to look into my eyes, but he looks blankly passed me and stops. 'Could you just pull the support down a bit Louis, it's riding up and starting my thoracic outlet pain up.' He pauses after I've done this; then starts to move again, a bit like a bulldozer stuck in low gear – his left leg starts to wobble and he drops down at the hip shifting to his left as if a slow motion fall is about to occur, or he's compensating for the movement of the ship we're not on. I subtly get in the way and he presses lightly against me and regains a bit of equilibrium He's very tense and totally absorbed by the formidable task of each step.

Eventually he gets sat down, but has to get up again for a pillow to be placed under him.

Twenty minutes later I've got the pain chart, twenty minutes after that I've got the history, twenty minutes later I've heard every living detail of each of his pains. There's no area of the body that hasn't got a pain. None of it fits any standard pain map or referral pattern; pins and needles over the whole of his back and buttocks; numbness in the lower right arm, the back of head and both legs and on and on.

I've now got three patients in the waiting room. I tell him to book in again tomorrow when I've got more time at the end of the day, but before he goes I'll have a quick feel of his back. Taking his shirt off seems to take an hour. I leave him sitting and put my hands on his back, he jerks and shrieks out, I move down a little, more noise and more tension. 'You're clearly in a lot of discomfort Mr Grubb. I need to have a lot more time with you, so let's see you at the end of the day tomorrow when I'll have as much time as I need with you.'

Thankfully, he's OK with this and fifteen minutes later I'm starting the next patient, totally messed in my head and wondering how I'm going to deal with all the 'waiting room waiting anger' that's heading my way.

I'll come back to Mr Grubb later.

Gordon Waddell and his 'illness behaviour' construct is as good a place to start this off as any. Waddell defined 'illness behaviour' as:

> *'Observable and potentially measurable actions and conduct that express and communicate the individual's own perception of disturbed health.'* (See chapter 10 of the Back Pain Revolution) Or, *'Illness behaviour is what people say and do that expresses and communicates that they are ill. It depends on how they think about their illness.'*

Gordon Waddell, a Scottish orthopaedic surgeon, has been a source of much controversy and debate. He is well known for the somewhat pernicious, Waddell 'non-organic' or 'behavioural' signs and symptoms. As they have been used by many so called medical 'authorities' to determine whether patients with back pain are on the one hand, 'real' or 'organic' or on the other, wagging it, over-egging it, malingering and making it up for some kind of gain. In other words they're 'non-organic' meaning not real, or more true to the term 'non-organic', not part of the living world. Maybe they're 'mineral'!

To get Waddell's series of behavioural signs and symptoms into context it's important to understand the history of them. Laudably, Waddell as a spinal surgeon was keen to only operate on those patients who would do well. He wanted to come up with some way of being able to distinguish between those who'd succeed and those who were likely to have a poor result. Remember this was way before any 'yellow-flag' predictors were ever researched or published. He came up with his 'non-organic' series of signs and symptoms, put them to the test in the late 1970's/early 1980's and found that they were actually very good predictors. He presumably refused to operate on the Mr Grubb's of the world and a good thing too because they invariably do badly. The problem though, was that it was like a rejection process – 'Organic?' 'Yup, you're real, come this way.' 'Non-organic?' Sorry you're a mineral, can't help you, bye.'

It was interesting that Waddell, possibly influenced by better informed psychologists, later changed the term he used from 'non-organic' to 'behavioural' signs and symptoms.

Waddell's behavioural signs and symptoms strictly only apply to low back pain and sciatica, but if you've been a good observer of patients over the years the presentations described for low back pain can be generalised, but not the tests obviously. As far as I'm concerned it would be a pretty dumb physiotherapist who can't sniff out this sort of maladaptive pain behaviour in all pain regions of the body. As you may gather I prefer the term 'maladaptive' pain or illness behaviour – but even that term is arguable, which I'll discuss.

Read the following signs and symptoms through. I want you to think of your own patients, as well as what I might have found with Mr Grubb if I'd asked about the symptoms and done the tests for the signs. If you want to think in a 'reductionist' hard biomedical reasoning type of way – don't. But if you can't help it, best think of the massive generalised maladaptive processing that must be going on here. A big point is that if you just think processing, you're actually likely to think change the processing and all this will get better. Don't go there, you're wrong. That's like thinking that because it's a neural processing problem amytriptyline or gabapentin will fix this guy's movement and pain problems.

Here we go...

The Waddell 'non-organic or 'behavioural <u>symptoms</u>' are (pretty much self-explanatory):

- pain at the tip of the tail bone (that may seem surprising!)
- whole leg pain – 'stocking' distribution
- whole leg numbness – 'stocking' distribution
- whole leg giving way (note Mr Grubb above)
- complete absence of any spells with very little pain in the past year
- intolerance of, or reactions to, many treatments
- history of emergency admissions to hospital with simple backache

The 'behavioural <u>signs</u>' are:

- **widespread tenderness on palpation** – not in any typical pattern – what Waddell termed, 'non-anatomic'

  Testing is done by light pinching of the skin in the painful area as well as deeper pressures. At an extreme, this is the patient who has massive back pain but hurts when you touch anywhere from the occiput to the big toe plus or minus variations in between.

- **axial loading test positive for back pain**

This is simply pushing down with a few pounds force through the top of the head or the shoulders and the back pain or the sciatica/leg pain being provoked. As Waddell says, this just doesn't provoke normal back pain, even in the presence of serious lumbar spinal pathology (I can vouch for this statement being true!)

- **simulated rotation**

Have the standing patient put their hands down by their sides. From behind, the examiner holds the hands against the patients' hips and passively rotates them turning the hip/pelvis. This effectively cuts out any spinal rotation. A report of pain indicates a 'behavioural' sign.

- **distracted SLR and 'distraction tests'**

You should be thinking that these tests look as if they are designed to trick the patient out, and you're right. The important thing is the interpretation of them and the consequences for the management approach that is most appropriate. More discussion is promised shortly.

Use the SLR as an example: when you test these sorts of patients with the standard passive SLR lying down there's often a massive pain response after a matter of only 10-20 degrees. What you do is repeat the test in a different way some time later. For example, they may be standing up again, whereupon you ask them if they'd mind getting back on the plinth again but this time to be sat up with legs along the plinth so you can 'have a feel of their back'. So, the patient is now in a more or less fully tight SLR/ hamstring/sciatic nerve stretch position. If there's little or no response the test is judged positive. Another way of doing it is to get the patient to sit up with legs dangling after the limited and poor SLR test lying. In this position you do reflexes and test foot and knee muscle strength for your neuro, plus you might say... 'I'm just going to check your knees Mr Grubb' and then you quietly fiddle with the knees and at some point bring them up into extension. As most of you will know, full knee extension in slump sitting brings on low back and leg pain in most patients with a 'genuine' SLR of 20-30 degrees when they're lying down. The other thing an alert therapist should note with this 'distraction' thinking is that patients, when examined formally, will demonstrate poor lumbar spine ranges and report a lot of pain – they do a lot of grunting and grimacing and tense up. But, on the other hand when undressing and taking shoes, socks and pants off many actually manage well. The key words are discrepancy and inconsistency. More discussion shortly!

So this test is deemed positive when the normal lying SLR is massively limited and painful, yet the patient is able to sit in long sitting or allow their knees to be extended as described.

- **regional weakness**

I'll use Mr Grubb here, but I'll bring him forward in time from me being in Geoff Maitland's practise to when I'm wiser, have a far greater declarative knowledge base and hence, I am a much better reasoner than I was back then. This is what happened when I tested Mr Grubb's lower limb muscle groups. First of all, albeit slow and tense, he managed to get himself up off the chair and into the waiting room. Thinking muscle; that means he has enough strength and good enough neurology to produce the movement; that he's likely to be weak and deconditioned isn't being argued.

Now when I examined his muscle power I had him sat up on the couch with legs dangling. I tested his reflexes first up and they were brisk and normal. Note that reflexes are the one clear sign that cannot be messed with by the brain! The only way a patient can stop a reflex is by tensing up. So you have to get them to relax or let-go – then you can truly test them. Anyway, that's by the bye, so now I start by testing the quads and I ask him to take his leg forward slightly from the dangle position – what happens? The movement is jerky and uncontrolled. Straight away I know a static resisted test is pointless. The result of me asking him to build up resistance against my pressure is going to be jerky giving way. I know because like a great many observant clinicians the response is commonplace. Power comes on then goes and comes on again. And yes, it doesn't seem to make neurological sense but it is a consistent finding.

Now if you're not sure, you must spend time treating neurologically damaged and neurologically abnormal patients – something I did early on in my career and something I'm very grateful for. Centrally neurologically damaged patients for example have spasticity, tonal changes and flaccidity, whereas peripherally damaged i.e. neuropathies with muscle weakness, just cannot hold against your pressure, the weakness is a smooth giving way. With patients like Mr Grubb it's usually all the muscle groups in the region of the pain that are like this. For me now it's merely a non-worrying observation that gets popped into the shopping basket. Meaning-wise, it tells me that I am not fearful of disease or damage in the patient in front of me. I'm dealing with a massive multidimensional problem that it is pointless searching for some kind of classic tissue-based diagnosis.

- **regional sensory change**

I am instantly reminded of the finals examination patient I had on the Adelaide Advanced Diploma in Manipulative Therapy course – passing the exam with flying colours was my aim. I wanted to be a member of the celebrated 'MTAA' – the Manual Therapy Association of Australia. I had one chance, fail the exam and you can never retake, that's the pressure there was!

So my exam patient has a folder full of notes to show me. He's not unlike Mr Grubb and I get the – 'Remember, fifteen minutes for the subjective Louis then get on with the assessment', whisper in my ear from my examiner (sorry Pat, I think this may have been with you!). It was absolute nuts, this bloke needed two hours at least to listen to before doing anything 'physical'. Talk about squeezing a patient's 'pain-everywhere' problem into a frigging facet joint! I was seriously hacked off, not just with the patient they'd given me, but with the whole set-up and all within about a minute of the bloke sitting down (I wasn't equipped to deal with this either). After twenty minutes of being nowhere near doing a decent 'subjective' I got the whisper, 'Do your neurological Louis...' Again, this guy was just like Mr Grubb, all grunts, groans and jerky stuff, lots of pain reaction and illness behaviour.

Then I did the light touch and pin prick; this wasn't anything like the 'stocking' distribution/ numb everywhere altered or lost sensation that Waddell describes; but patchy bits here, there and every-bloody-where and because the fellow was so pedantic I couldn't be quick. If I'd drawn the numb areas onto his legs he'd have looked like a leopard probably. The point here is to know normal disease related patterns of neurological sensory deficit, both via CNS disease or injury and via peripheral nerve and nerve root. Sensory deficits for peripheral nerves and nerve root problems tend to fit pretty well into standard clear cut patterns. Remember the one and a half fingers for ulnar nerve, but also the C8 nerve root distribution which is rather vaguer but still along the medial border of the hand/ forearm and into the little finger. Loss of sensation for CNS problems can be in a glove or stocking distribution however, so some care is needed.

As far as my exam patient was concerned to me, the whole exercise was pointless. I did it though and I passed. When I think back about this type of patient, I realise that physiotherapy and especially manual therapy, had absolutely no idea about this type of patient – what their symptoms and signs meant and how they should be managed. Forcing them into a 'facet joint' diagnosis just about sums it all up.

Often when I recall that exam patient I wish I'd marched out of the cubicle grabbing the examiner on the way and told her what I thought about the whole set-up and inappropriateness of manual therapy for this type of patient. But I wasn't quite old enough and definitely not wise enough!

Now some 'be-careful' points that are of importance:

1. One or two of these behavioural signs and symptoms are commonly found in more straight forward presentations. I'm thinking of the sciatic patient who's been seen by the vicious orthopaedic surgeon who rammed the patients leg into full SLR without any warning and made them worse for two weeks afterwards. Those folk are naturally jumpy and tense when you pick up their leg for an SLR. Every finding must therefore be taken in a bigger context. A big deal for a positive behavioural label is when these observations and tests are plentiful and combine with lots of other signs of 'overt' pain behaviour. Waddell states that three or more signs and symptoms '… are reliable and consistent over time and correlate with other features of illness behaviour.' Think of things like; 'bracing', 'guarding', 'rubbing and holding', 'grimacing', 'sighing and grunting.' For me, they're all things to simply 'put in the shopping basket' so they can be thought about and possibly addressed when or if appropriate in management.

2. The **distraction** aspect is of interest if you think in terms of how movements are processed. A patient who bends normally to get their shoes and socks off is processing movement in terms of a well ingrained habitual movement, it's a goal orientated movement. A patient who's been primed by a therapist to think about their pain and then asked to bend forward and seek the pain as they do so is processing the back movement in a completely different way. So, function may gate-out pain; focused attention on pain with movement gates it right back in; that's good biology and to some extent it's normal. It's evidence of the normal and amazingly fickle nature of pain. It needs to come and go for survival. The key thing for us is to reason whether what we are seeing is adaptive or maladaptive/unhelpful. In the context of other information, for example the early few moments of observation and interaction with Mr Grubb, it's pretty obvious. Note that chronic pain patients like Mr Grubb who have a strong 'illness behaviour' presentation about them, have been to a great many Drs and specialists and that they have put them through broadly similar physical examination routines. It is hardly surprising then, that in the context of standard back movements, pain and pain-behaviour are expressed at high levels.

3. Waddell warns that whatever the presentation, never assume it's 'non-organic' and therefore that there is no need to do important tests and ask important 'RED FLAG' questions. Always be on the lookout for potential bells ringing.

I'm going to have (another!) quick nag about young inexperienced physios who quickly move into 'musculoskeletal' work without having much experience of all aspects of disease, disorder and incapacity. If you haven't clinically experienced the full spectrum of manifestations of conditions like stroke and brain injury; multiple sclerosis; Parkinsons; peripheral neuropathy; tumours; polymyalgia; ankylosing spondylitis; rheumatoid arthritis, for example – it's my strong opinion that you haven't enough experience to work as an isolated musculoskeletal practitioner. It's all very well learning the red flags, but you must have seen them to really know. In my practice I diagnose at least two or three serious disorders a year. It's because I've got time to listen and above all I've seen a lot before. I know when things don't seem to fit a normal pattern. I know the early signs of things like MS, RA and AS and I've seen a great number of rare peripheral neuropathies. It also means that you need to have seen one hell of a lot of 'normal' aches and pains too. I've spent my whole professional life proud to be a simple Chartered Physiotherapist. I really couldn't bring myself to say I was some kind of 'specialist' as many seem to now. To me, that's too arrogant a stance to take (unless you've gone through an examined and validated training programme? There are few around). You never stop learning and even after a massive patient mileage there's always a pattern that seems very unfamiliar. Grump over; maybe I'm just a bit old-fashioned?

4. Lastly here, our friend Mr Grubb and many others who show markedly positive Waddell signs and symptoms should not have some kind of physical problem denied. The vast majority of patients who end up like this had a physical problem and may still have a physical problem, the issue is that their current presentation in terms of the observations of 'behaviour' discussed here can be seen as way out of proportion to the underlying tissue abnormality or disease.

I have decided to quote Waddell verbatim from his book, page 189 of the 2nd edition:

*'There are three situations where you **cannot use the behavioural signs**. You should ignore even multiple signs in these patients:*

1. Patients with possible serious spinal pathology or widespread neurology. You must carry out diagnostic triage and exclude these first. Behavioural symptoms and signs are only 'inappropriate' to mechanical low back pain and sciatica.

2. Patients over about 60 years of age. These responses are common in elderly patients, who behave differently when they are ill. I do not know how to interpret these findings in elderly patients and it is better to ignore them.

3. Patients from ethnic minorities. There are wide cultural variations in pain behaviour. We have only standardised the behavioural symptoms and signs in white patients.

As you've probably realised I have to admit to having the terms, 'adaptive' and 'maladaptive' in my head a lot of the time. It's a useful way to think things through. However, the reality of treatment and management should be that we address the presentation in front of us, with all its little foibles and nuances, in the best and most holistic way we can. The whole point of being able to recognise 'maladaptive' illness behaviour, or Waddell's 'behavioural' signs, is that they help point us towards a pain management, rehabilitationist approach to the presentation and strongly away from one that looks for and wants to treat finicky little physical impairments, or somehow squeeze the presentation into some tissue category like a 'facet joint'. If you do this the yellow flag research is telling us that you're adding to the problem, you're going to be an 'iatrogenic' factor in helping make the patient worse. So the next Mr Grubb who comes in, DON'T go looking for your favourite muscle imbalance problem, tight fascial band, or soothing cranial suture glide and slide. These patients need a different approach and that's why the shopping basket is so useful and why I want to try and encourage you to use it!

Adaptive illness behaviour, what's that? You go over mildly on your ankle and you yell and scream for ten minutes... adaptive or maladaptive? Answer, ask about culture! UK white Caucasian, stiff upper lip, shouldn't be doing that old boy... answer – maladaptive.

Soccer, Premier division, Man United player – the mystery fall, the loss of balance from a wisp of air movement in the penalty box, the rolling over and over and over, the grimacing face, the crafty wink at your playing mate. Adaptive or maladaptive? Ah, easy, adaptive, they get a penalty and win the game. You don't see that in rugby though? Yes, but that's upper class white Caucasian for the most part, stiff upper lip, not traditional, unethical – weak in the face of the enemy, can't be seen to be doing that – that's cheating. Hang on a minute, what about that 'Bloodgate[1]' scandal that deeply embarrassed the Rugby Union in 2009. That was clear cheating...

So pain behaviour following a whiplash, for your pain disability assessment – what about that? Yes, think about the evolutionary rule, 'get as much as you can for as little effort as possible' and you can see why this behavioural expression of 'I'm in pain' crops up so much. It's clearly maladaptive, so is the footballer above, it can and should be considered to be cheating but it can get the subject what they want. Thanks to Gordon Waddell the issue has been spotlighted, investigated, recognised and explained.

Take limping and hopping about in pain – going, ow, ow, ow! Out in the wild and you become easy prey! Luckily illness behaviour comes and goes. It always has done, just like the pain does. It comes when it has an opportunity for gain and goes when it's a hindrance or a liability. Such is the nature of the plastic brain and the sensory-motor system that pain related illness behaviours are best viewed, from the therapist's perspective, as mere 'habits' of movement that are triggered by a variety of situations. If they're going to improve, the behaviours and their antecedents need addressing and treating, much as any other finding would.

In some clinical encounters it's my belief that the patient can be made gently and appropriately aware of some of the test 'discrepancies'. Here's a quick example:

'Mr Grubb, I'm quite confident that given the right approach we'll be able to improve your ranges of movement – some are awful, for example, your back's ability to bend when you're standing, but what's encouraging is that it bends very well when you're sitting. Another one is that your leg stretched out well when I did it with you when

---

1 - Bloodgate – check it out on Wikepedia – it's a bit too complex to explain here...

you were sitting but when you were lying it was awful. I could hardly lift the leg. All this is very common and OK but it tells me that the movements are there and that's excellent news...'

I hope that helps you see what I mean!

The skill is to gradually work on practicing them out – often by doing the 'awful' movements in different starting positions but cleverly working towards the 'awful' starting position. Sometimes significant movement limitations have often been there for a very long time and a great deal of practice is required. My experience though is that given the right atmosphere quite rapid progress can sometimes be made. The therapist must be careful to not make the patient feel awkward or challenged by having the issues recognised, labelled and worked on. The best label to give often revolves around 'tense movement'. I will give some patient examples of dealing with the Mr Grubb types of presentation later.

Finally:

- if you recognise and understand maladaptive pain and its mechanisms, shouldn't you also be able to recognise and accept maladaptive illness behaviour?

- illness behaviour needs to be addressed and treated

- the patient in front of you is what you have to treat – their illness behaviour is a finding that may require management, directly as mentioned above, but also indirectly, for example by using appropriate behaviour reinforcement and extinguishing skills and techniques.

GE SECTION 3 · PAIN BITS AND PIECES!

Chapter GE 3.3
Picking up some pain management and psychology skills

Now if a psychologist read this they'd probably shudder, although I'd like to think maybe they'd be pleased that a physio is trying to make use of some of their methods and skills, particularly as there's such good evidence for it.

My thing, as I said in the preface to these books, is that I want to make things practical and useful to therapists and patients. What I write can only be how I've thought about things or how I've done things given what I know – but with the realisation that there are experts who are far better than me out there. I'm at the coal face with the patient. Don't give me the theory of how to extract coal, just show me what I'm to do.

If I had my time again, I'd like to have studied clinical pain psychology and then practiced it for long enough to be really good. Then I'd integrate it and modify what I already do with patients. It's my belief that all physiotherapists should receive CBT training to a good practical standard at undergraduate level.

I've been in contact with many CBT trained physios for a number of years and I've watched and read a lot, picking up useful things in my 'self-taught' kind of way. I've dropped the confusing and difficult stuff, also the things that sound good but that I just haven't been able to see how to use, or haven't been at all comfortable doing in the setting I was in.

My main CBT experience, thanks to physiotherapist Vicki Harding, was that I was lucky enough to have participated for a week at the INPUT chronic pain management programme at St Thomas' Hospital in London. I sat in with the patients and did all the classes, the activity and exercise pacing as well as observing all the psychology, physiotherapy and occupational therapy. It was brilliant, an eye-opener and a big 'ah-ha' moment in my career. And I'm hugely grateful for the experience.

This book is about what I do with my patients. It has clearly been influenced by pain psychology and CBT programmes. I'm not going to give a crash course in it, but a little summary of some of the things I witnessed and might just help anyone who is naïve as to what goes into CBT programmes. Mostly I want to highlight what I found very useful and add a few comments where helpful.

Individual assessments

I sat in on a patient with RSI related chronic pain being interviewed by a physiotherapist and functional difficulties were being investigated.

> She could write for ten minutes, anything more than ten minutes and pain would increase, there were no problems with less than ten. To the question: 'How do you know when to stop?' she answered that it was pain contingent.
>
> Typing was zero, or two to three seconds and increased pain markedly. Note the discrepancy between this and writing. Circuits that fire together

wire together of course, typing was powerfully linked to pain, whereas writing was quite a lot weaker as it wasn't a major part of her work.

Walking for five minutes was observed. And the time to walk a corridor lap, as well as overall distance (number of laps), was measured. The therapist had a sheet with a grid to fill in the results on. Laps up and down a corridor (twenty metres) were timed and the patient was told that she could stop if she wanted to. The therapist also recorded the number of steps taken per lap and the use of the wall while turning, as well as the number of times she used the chair (i.e. a recording of pain behaviour). I'm sure breath holding, grimacing and grunting could also be recorded, but it wasn't necessary for this lady. The test was repeated at the end of the programme and significantly increased; in stride length, confidence, use of chair and wall, time per lap/speed and overall distance. The initial results were also reviewed so the patient got plenty of positive feedback and reinforcement regarding her progress.

The patient was asked to do a writing test. This involved copying words from a sheet over a one minute period. Notes were made of observations: for example that she was very tense and the writing was laboured.

She was asked to do as many sit to stand exercises as she could for one minute. I can't recall the exact instructions but it was made clear that she could go at whatever pace she wanted and could stop anytime. The number was recorded as well as the pain behaviour/quality of movement.

She was asked to type for one minute – with similar instructions. The key message from the physio was that they weren't doing the tasks to exacerbate her pain but to get baseline measurements of what they could do at the start of the programme. My notes indicate that she managed to do fourteen words in one minute and that she wasn't a touch typist.

Next, the number of steps she could climb in one minute was recorded. The pain management unit had a set of stairs with rails that were five steps high. She went up and down them for the minute. Again, pain behaviours like pulling on and grasping the rail, stopping, grunting and groaning were noted.

Lastly she was asked to do arm circling for one minute and the number were recorded.

Comment: it's one thing for the patients to tell you what they can and can't do but it's another to actually measure functional activity. In fact with chronic pain patients it is vital, because it gives the patient and the unit feedback about progress or lack of progress. The lesson for the standard musculoskeletal physiotherapist here is this – no 'How's your pain?' talk, forget that completely. These patients have been assessed by just about every medic and scan or x-ray they'll ever need. The focus is on, not only on coping and managing their pain better, but also on getting function and fitness back so they can get some semblance of health, self-esteem and self confidence back again.

The typical physiotherapist dealing with pain states in private practice, or in out-patients departments in the NHS:

1. Will ask about the difficulties the patient is having with function, but won't get the patients' estimate of how much they can do (well maybe a bit…). They won't get them to actually do some of the things they're having trouble with, to observe and test them and are very unlikely to actually get some measure of their capability in the way illustrated here.

2. Will often give out exercises to do – often standard printouts on a sheet of paper, without actually doing them with the patient. This is usually due to the emphasis on looking for the problem, assessing the standard ranges of movement and the various physical tests deemed to be required and then getting on with some form of treatment to make a change to them. Exercises are invariably felt necessary but only squeezed into the last minutes of the consultation. The result is that they are very poorly done and hence, given little emphasis. The patient is left with the impression that the 'treatment' is the main thing because that was where the emphasis was during the session

   If exercises are given, they are unlikely to be actually done in the session and even more unlikely to be reassessed when the patient returns for the next treatment. Patients merely get asked how the exercises are going – the clothes are then off, the range and pain assessedand on with the fiddle-faddle-flim-flam!

That won't do, even for acute and sub acute patients, who haven't got the broad reach of yellow-flag issues that the more on-going and stubborn problems have.

Pain management integration into one to one physio sessions suggests a bigger emphasis on:

* knowing functional capabilities, then observing and measuring them

* the design of appropriately relevant, graded and paced exercises to help address functional deficits where required

* following activity and exercise input up by reviewing and performing them; this provides an opportunity for using reinforcement techniques to help encourage helpful movement quality and extinguish less helpful

* re-measuring and comparing to baseline are part of feedback and will reveal difficulties and hurdles to get over.

The above approach is very appropriate to Mr Grubb from the illness behaviour chapter.

Learning from the first group and meeting staff on the CBT programme

This is what happened when I observed. There is much here to pick up for the one-to-one therapist. The advantage of working with groups is clear. Note that the level of information given out is not that accurate, but the message it gives is what's important. Note the simplicity of the material. I'd like the reader to think about how to make their own explanations as brief and clear wherever possible. Not to necessarily dumb it all down but to make it meaningful and easy to grasp. If the patient requires further detail it can be given but patients rarely do. A massive recurring theme is that the tissues are strong enough to do a lot more physically and that pain that goes on a long time doesn't parallel the degree of damage or disease.

So…

Staff and patients introduced themselves and the patients were asked to give a very brief history of their problem to the others.

'Dr in charge' introduction

The group was first addressed by the 'Dr in charge' (happened to be called Charles). He highlighted the following; don't compare yourself to the others; we know you are in pain; the programme is stressful – we know it is for you and we understand. There will be classroom stuff – listening and learning as well as practice. The key is for each of you to find different ways of managing pain – you are here to get what you want out of the programme. Don't feel shy to get up and move about anytime.

The notion that 'pain does not mean damage' and that 'hurt does not mean harm' were underlined.

'Too much pain does not mean too much harm'.

There was an introduction to 'fear-avoidance' thoughts using examples of acute and chronic pain and explaining what medicine meant by these terms. Remember to most people, acute pain means nasty sharp pain, to medicine, acute pain means pain that's recent and hasn't been around very long. Examples used of acute pain were appendicitis and the basic mechanisms involved were discussed; as well as a simple cut of the skin and common sprains and strains and here the relationship of pain to injury/damage in all these was reasonably close. This was contrasted with chronic pain where the relationship was not so clear.

Typical healing times were given, for example skin healing after an operation being around two weeks (not true, but more importantly is functionally true as we've seen in earlier chapter) and bone around six weeks to three months. Charles then told the group that there was nothing wrong with their healing and that bones were one of the slowest things to heal, being six months maximum. He then highlighted that the average pain history of the group was four years – the message was: tissues healed but pain stayed on and that the reasons for this were complicated.

This is all good stuff coming from the Dr – in the eyes of patients he's '<u>Mr to-be believed</u>' – the 'top of the tree' man. What I mean is that most ordinary folk tend to believe a Dr rather than us lower-ranking professionals! In other words the physiotherapist, psychologist, OT, nurse – you know what I mean!

He then discussed scans and highlighted that there was a tendency for medicine to keep looking for damage to explain chronic pain, but often the scans and other tests were negative, or showed very little. He contrasted this with chronic pain like rheumatoid arthritis, where there was plenty of evidence to be found with scans and tests but that this was a disease.

He then asked the group for examples of acute pain with no damage and immediately got – headache. Brilliant, scan a patient with a headache and what do you find? Yup, no damage, nothing on the scan! Then came – cramp; no damage and awful pain. Someone said 'Then someone twists your arm' and everyone laughed... Neuralgia! Again brilliant.

He next explained how important understanding all this was and that **how our thoughts underpin how we act.** He gave the example of being told your spine was 'crumbling'. And that a perfectly reasonable thought with this might be that the more you used it, the more it would crumble and the more it would degenerate. You would tend to 'take care of the pain' and be 'very gentle with it'.

Then he moved on to talk about a 'spiral' into secondary problems, using the example of a soccer player who injures their knee and rests for six weeks. After six weeks, what happens? The muscles waste away and the joints stiffen, hence he now has secondary problems.

Another example he used was to compare two forms of management. 'Take two people who strain their back. One goes to the GP and is given pain killers and told to rest. They're then re-examined three years later and it's found they have an MRI scan showing 'disc degeneration. They're in a great deal of pain and their activity levels are very low. The second person, same age, same injury goes to a physio who re-activates them, gives them stretches and exercises and gets them back to full function over a period of a few weeks. Three years later this second person is scanned just like the first. Their scan shows the same or no degeneration, they've little or no pain and they're fully active and functioning.'

'Look, people's backs manage for years with no medical care!'

He went on...

'On the other hand there are those who do push and push and that, yes, sometimes those people do get pain.'

He then says the word 'habit' and continues, 'Give a patient a stick for a year, then take it away and they really struggle, they've forgotten how to walk normally!'

He talks about habits of movement, of tension, of being careful and that habits like these aren't at all helpful, just like the stick, especially if it goes on too long. Unlearning it and learning to move in a more normal and relaxed way can be very helpful.

He then uses a nice term 'loss of trust' and that many patients hear a whole pile of different reasons for their pain and don't know who to believe – they lose their trust. Further, if someone in pain feels that there is still damage, again, they 'lose their trust' in their own body and as a result can't function normally for fear of hurting or setting things back.

Charles emphasised that the view of all the staff on the programme was that with on-going pain a big issue was more the secondary problems and not any injury or permanent damage.

The participants then asked questions which were always answered in reassuring ways avoiding the notion of continuing and worsening damage.

There was lots of discussion about x-rays and wear and tear. Charles pointed out how a great many people have awful x-rays and little or no pain, others have awful pain and pretty normal x-rays. He used the example of '30% of normals, have abnormal spinal scans'. But also, 'joints are very resilient' and that the term 'wear and tear' was not a useful term; that joint function, with clear degenerative changes, can be hugely improved and that nothing could be done to cure wear and tear anyway; that current research was showing that regular exercise and normal movement slowed the wear and tear changes and kept the joint tissues in a fitter state than if they had rested.

After this he explained the over-activity/under-activity cycle; that activity was so often pain dependent and the importance of setting achievable baselines and quotas for exercises and activity building.

The psychology and physiotherapy introduction to the group

Next up was Neil, the psychologist. He was much more interactive than Charles. Charles was great, but he didn't use interactive skills – he was much more didactic, telling and teaching rather than drawing things out of the group and getting them working out the answers to the problems presented. It's a small criticism but if you look at the material covered, to an extent it has to be taught and it worked well in setting the scene. Importantly, looking round the room while he was talking, I noted that he held everyone's attention. When you think about it, that material should be of great interest to a chronic pain sufferer. Pleasingly, Charles' material was reviewed again in more detail during the physio sessions and here there was more of a chance to spend time and discuss issues raised further.

Back to Neil.

Neil writes the word PAIN in the middle of the whiteboard and states, 'Pain has effects on the quality of life' and then asks the question, 'What effects? Give me some that maybe have affected you?'

The group's good; they're coming up with excellent stuff and as they call out Neil adds their point to the whiteboard. Circles it and links it with a line to 'PAIN'.

'Self confidence goes...!'

'I've stopped planning ahead... I live day to day, it's tedious.'

'Social life plummets!'

'Sex!'

'Work.'

'Sport.'

'Changed my personality... I used to be a party animal...'

'You get all isolated and you feel depressed.'

'I get mad and frustrated quite a lot.'

'Pain is engulfing, you lose love...'

'Sometimes you feel suicidal.'

'Guilty, for being so useless and unhelpful.'

'I do very little, but there's no leisure, there's no spontaneity anymore.'

'No feelings of peace or contentment.'

'I don't feel I want to see or talk to anyone quite a lot of the time.'

The board is covered... Neil looks up 'I guess you all share in quite a lot of this?' He pauses as they raise their eyebrows and nod in agreement. I remember feeling that there was an atmosphere of unity or of closeness coming over the group. For the first time their inner anguish was being recognised and that they weren't alone – 'Amazing, others had the same experiences' and the therapists understood all this and had seen it all before. The therapists too were united in their beliefs and understanding of the patient – they were all '**singing from the same song sheet**'.

Neil then said, 'As you already know, on the programme we can't get rid of the pain[1] but we can help all of the things on the whiteboard here. Essentially, we can improve the quality of life, we can look at all these things and many more that crop up and then focus on them and learn how to deal with them and cope much better.'

He then asked the difference between a 'psychologist' and a 'psychiatrist'.

No one really knows.

'A 'psychiatrist' has a medical training and uses drugs to help things like anxiety, depression and problems with mood. A 'psychologist' looks at learning and thinking skills and new behavioural habits. We use learning skills rather than medication – we help you to learn skills that will help you work things out better, how to be more balanced in your thoughts and decision making for example. We want to help 'empower' you to help yourself more too.'

Neil stepped back and now the physio, Vicki, came to the front and gave an expanded explanation of the 'over' and 'under-activity' cycles and also explained pacing. She reviewed the stretching and exercises sessions that they would all be involved in and how pacing would be used to start them off and get them more active and fitter, each at their own speed. Some simple demonstrations were done and reactions to exercises were discussed and normalised.

The group then split up with each patient sitting with a clinician in order to discuss 'one-to-one' their thoughts and impressions about what they had heard. I sat in with Neil and a female patient, Mandy.

Off she went, 'What I'm hearing here is totally different to what I've been told – for two and half years I've been doing the exact opposite of what's been told just now, who's telling the truth?'

Neil responds rather like a politician would, not committing to a likely unproductive discussion of who's right/wrong but being a bit evasive and smart, by saying that the biggest selling point of what they were all saying was to give it all a go and to let her own experience be the judge.

Mandy then said that she was told that if only she'd had treatment earlier it would have helped and that she had to go back to work. She had moved. But then she'd put on five and a half stone in weight and again, 'Who am I supposed to believe?

---

1 - This is not entirely true because a great many of those who successfully complete pain management programmes and go on to becoming far more active, even re-gaining employment – report less pain. The key thing is that pain management programmes want to steer the patient's focus away from pain relief to dealing with and improving on all the other things involved. If patients remain focused on pain relief and a fix for their problem, they miss a huge opportunity to help themselves here.

Why wasn't I told about pacing and moving?' And so on.

Neil quietly, as psychologists tend to do, emphasised just giving it all a go and seeing what happened. They weren't recommending throwing anything away but that the process was one of changing things slowly and that a key message to start with was – *a little every day, starting really at low seemingly easy levels and learning to relax while doing the movements.*

(Ah-ha! – you can see where I got 'start easy build slowly' from!)

Learning from the psychology sessions: situation, thoughts, feelings

The first session the patients had with Neil was called 'Changing Thoughts'. It was actually more about the links between thoughts and feelings/emotions. To start with it was similar to what he'd done on the board in the first session before the physio.

He got the following from the group when asked about the impact of pain: irritability, depression, stress, anger, mood, frustration, isolation, dependency, anxiety, not understood and guilt.

The he asked another question.

'Where do feelings come from?' and he again went to the board and put up three columns.

'Let's think of a common situation – you're at home in bed and suddenly you hear a crash downstairs!'

In the first column at the top left he writes SITUATION and under it he puts 'crash in the night'. At the top of the second column he writes the heading, THOUGHTS and asks the group for what they might be thinking.

Off they go...

'There's a burglar.'

'Cat.'

'Left the window open and the wind's knocked the pot-plant over.'

'Someone's downstairs and they've fallen over.'

'Clock fell off the wall.'

'That ghost is back!'

'Earthquake!'

'The end of the world!'

'Gas explosion!'

'That's the bread board slipping into the sink again.'

The ideas dry-up and Neil puts the word, FEELINGS in the third column and for each of the above possibilities they give the associated feelings they might get: fear and anxiety, annoyed, worried, concerned, terrified and relief are what they come up with for the various situations.

He then does another **Situation**…

'A friend walks right past you in the street who would usually stop and say hello.'

Thoughts and **Feelings**?

He gets this…

'They didn't see me – disappointed.'

'That wasn't nice at all – annoyed, saddened and angered.'

'They're maybe worried about something – concerned, intrigued.'

'They've gone off me – rejected, worried and sad.'

'She's won the lottery – envy, anger, disappointed, bitch!'

'She owes me money – angry, annoyed.'

'Lost in thought – never mind.'

'In a hurry – snubbed, unimportant.'

The discussion goes on and gets summarised. Feelings are not so much about the direct result of a situation but more about a result of our **thoughts** about the situation. In the above situation of a friend passing without saying hello, one person might be angry, another hurt, yet another understanding or concerned.

He does another…

Situation: physio session doing an exercise and getting an increase in pain.

Thoughts and then **Feelings**:

'I'm weak – useless.'

'I'm damaging myself more – concern, fear.'

'This will stop me doing anything for a few days – depression, fed up, can't see the point, angry with the physio for letting it happen.'

'It's not too bad and I'm making progress – hopeful, positive.'

Neil points out the impact of thoughts on feelings and also what might be needed to help. For example, if a patient is thinking, 'I know these exercises are damaging me more' they're more than likely going to be fearful and possibly upset or angry as well. What can be done? The answer could be either, they stop and avoid what they're doing, or the physio may be able to give them reassurance, or maybe make a simple adjustment to the exercises in some way, or alter the quota of exercise. Or, you may just find that it doesn't quite turn out to be as bad as you thought it might. (Remember 'disconfirmation' from earlier on?)

Neil introduced yet another one.

This time, his goal was to illustrate how the same situation can give a whole range of different thoughts and feelings. And that quite often the feelings we get, even though we can't seem to help it, are unfounded and not necessarily helpful.

The **Situation** was sudden turbulence on an aeroplane. Immediate **Thoughts** might be 'We're going to crash' with the awful **Feelings** of dread and even terror!

But… put two people in the same situation and some feel elation while others may feel incredibly frightened.

On the plane – this is how a psychologist would want you to deal with it.

Ask two questions:

First, 'What evidence is there on the plane that everything is OK?'

Second, 'What evidence is there that it's going to crash?'

Pause, think and look. Pull all the evidence together and 'Ah, the cabin crew are serving tea, there's been no message on the tannoy, everyone else looks quite calm and hey, the wing hasn't fallen off the plane, and hey, I can't get out of here anyway – when your number's up, your number's up.'

So, it's reasonable that the initial reaction is instant fear (straight to the low road!), but after a minute or two and thinking about it the problem becomes more manageable and you feel a bit easier even though the situation is still the same.

Key? Thoughts and evaluation of the thoughts restores balance.

One of the patients pops up with, 'The trouble with trying to change the way you feel all the time, trying to stay positive all the time, is it's so draining and it almost becomes a negative thing.'

Neil agrees, but the trick here is **not to keep trying to force your emotions but to become aware of your thoughts**. He acknowledges how hard that is but emphasises that it gets easier with practice.

Then he says, 'Last one for this session.'

Situation = increased pain. **Thoughts** = 'I'm doing damage.' **Feelings** = anxiety, frustration.

Here's the question 'Is there any evidence that you are not damaging it?'

He gets the group to give answers...

'You're still moving!'

'The physio has reassured you.'

'There's no swelling.'

'A thousand other people have done this programme and not damaged themselves.'

'Many pains occur without damage.'

'What's the feeling like now?' Again they come up with answers...

'Re-assured.'

'Less anxious but a bit concerned.'

'Pleased'...

At the end of the session the patients are given a sheet with the **Situation-Thoughts-Feelings** columns already on, plus a column in which to rate their pain on a 1-10 scale.

The instruction is:

Please fill in one example each day at times when you notice your pain increasing, or notice yourself getting upset or worried. The thought can be any repeated idea, or something you say yourself, or said to someone else, or an image that keeps coming into your head. Also write down the feeling or feelings at the time – like feeling worried, or fed up. Rate your pain from 0-10 as usual, where 0 is no pain and 10 is pain as bad as it could be.

The patients have now been introduced to the idea of thinking and reflecting – becoming aware of their thoughts and that alternative ways of thinking can be helpful and that finding alternative ways of thinking can often be very rewarding and empowering.

Importantly, they are not being 'told' what to think, they're gaining the tools that enable them to work out what's best to think.   Also, that by challenging their habitual thinking and introducing new ideas, they can help themselves to change feelings and emotions.

They have to practice and learn this skill!

In later sessions Neil spends time with them going through their sheets and finding out how they dealt with the situations they were in. He's also able to find out those who get the idea and those who struggle and who he needs to spend more time with.

Learning from the psychology sessions: 'Making Changes'

The next session was called 'Making Changes' and introduced the 'problem-solving' model with the purpose of 'finding solutions'. Neil used the example of keeping going with exercises.

The method is simple:

1. **Specify** the problem.

2. **Generate** solutions.

3. **Evaluate** the best solution.

It was the good old three column thing again and he used the situation of having friends round for a meal and there's a power failure. Neil now went 'suspend judgement' before coming up with a solution. He wanted them to stop and think and come up with up to ten possible alternative solutions, each one to be evaluated before picking the best course of action.

The point was that we all have rather habitual ways of thinking, we're often only on one track and don't see other possibilities. We jump in head first.

So: **suspend judgment, generate alternative solutions and evaluate each one – before picking the best one or one or two** was the nub of what he wanted the group to grasp and start to practise.

He then came up with another example, after four or five weeks at home you're getting bored with the exercises.

Generate some alternatives and evaluate – this is what they all came up with:

- do them somewhere else – novel, feels different, but might get ridiculed!

- put on the TV or radio, music – takes your mind off them

- involve friends – good fun and they're encouraging too

- change the order – makes you think and feels different

- break them up don't do them all at once... makes it easier...

- incorporate into daily routine – again makes it easier and thoughtless, you focus on the task not the exercise

- give yourself a reward – makes you feel good for the achievement

- hire a personal trainer – supporting and social too

- do them with your partner – it does them good too, which feels good for you, they can see what you're doing and how you're getting on

- go see the therapist and get some new less boring ones – good idea!

Neil now discussed 'Rewards' or what psychologists call 'Reinforcers'.

A comment from me: good physiotherapists do this all the time. For example, we naturally tend to praise and encourage patients when they make an effort at a movement or exercise, or if they learn a more normal way of moving that we are trying to teach them. Reinforcement encourages a repetition of the behaviour or task being attempted and we are all influenced by it. Reinforcers may be subtle, via encouraging smiles and nods, eye contact, our body language or more openly via words of encouragement, like 'good' and 'well done'. I've sometimes found myself saying things like, 'You know what, I'm actually thrilled you can do that now, you've made my day!' Sometimes there's even a 'high five'. What's important is that the reinforcement is appropriate and taken in the right way by the patient. Psychologists are usually a lot more reserved with their reinforcement!

Neil explains to the group that reinforcers are rewards, like buying yourself a magazine, or organising a social night out with your best friend; but that they can also be less tangible, for example reflecting on your achievements; reaching a simple goal with the exercises and then mentally patting yourself on the back. The key is that the reward should make you feel good.

The group now looks at another problem.

Specify, this time the problem was 'feeling discouraged with goals – goals seem so far off.'

Generate, looking for solutions to this...

'Break into sub-goals.'

'Rewards!'

'Chat with the professionals.'

'Change the goal to something more achievable.'

'Look back and review progress.'

'Shoot yourself.'

'Discuss your goals.'

'Get drunk!'

After getting the list, the key **Evaluation** of all these was that breaking things down into easier chunks was probably one of the best solutions, clearly a 'Graded Approach'.

In the next session with Neil he reviewed the Situation-Thoughts-Feelings introduced in the first session, with an emphasis on making more helpful thoughts and challenging unhelpful thoughts. An almost key 'mantra' to use in the face of any challenge was the statement, **'I have resources'**.

The example was…

'A spider running towards me.' **Thoughts** = 'It's going to bite me!' **Feelings** = anxiety!

This 'challenge' could be met with…

'It's probably more frightened of you.'

'Spiders don't bite in this country.'

'Step on it!'

'Put a jam jar over it.'

Neil acknowledged that all this doesn't get rid of anxiety 100% but it does make it more manageable.

He now introduced a simple case history. A welder who one day at work had an accident and ended up completely blind. Neil then put two columns on the board.

On the left, **Thoughts** – immediately after the accident.

On the right, **Thoughts and Outcomes** – two years later.

To start, a list was generated under the 'immediate' heading. Most of it was all about his 'losses.'

After this the group turned their attention to the 'two years later' column on the right. Here they listed the outcomes and a great many were very positive.

Here are some of the examples they came up with...

'Loss of job' – 'Re-train.'

'What would happen to his family?' – 'Help with benefits, plus new job coming.'

'His own independence was gone' – 'Now had guide-dog, so reasonable independence regained.'

'Can't see the kids grow up' – 'True but other senses give a great deal.'

'Won't see friends' – 'Yes, but interact and also make new friends.'

So, the initial thoughts in the left column were understandable but in the right column, two years on, he'd generated a different perspective. For chronic pain this type of approach is used to help generate more realistic thoughts and solutions about a given situation. Sometimes it helps to think of time going by in a situation and gradually working out solutions to help you to adjust and manage.

Situation: failing an exam!

Thoughts: I'm a failure!

Feelings: depressed, useless, shocked and angry!

But is it true that I'm a failure because I didn't pass? How else could we think that would be more helpful?

'I've passed other exams.'

'I can re-sit it.'

'There may have been other reasons for failure.'

'Other people who I respect have failed too.'

'I deserved to fail with the amount of work I did, if I work harder I will pass next time.'

Neil emphasises two questions to ask when thoughts pop up and negative feelings result:

'Are the thoughts I'm having realistic?'

'Is the way I'm thinking helpful?'

He acknowledged that how we think about and challenge our own thinking can be very individual and that this whole exercise was not about minimising or trivialising the situation but that the key was trying to get a realistic perspective on the situation.

An aside from me: what was interesting was that quite often I'd sit in with individual patients, where they'd be discussing a problem with one of the other therapists, it could be the physio, or the OT and across the board the patients were not 'told' or simply 'given' a possible solution to their problem. For example, one of the patients asked the physio about difficulties she was having doing a sit-up exercise.

'I can raise my head, then I go to lift my shoulders and the pain just canes my back, I'd like to give this exercise a miss unless you can tell me what I should be doing?'

'How does doing it make you feel?'

'Annoyed and a bit disappointed I suppose.'

'Have you thought about any possible solutions?'

'Well no, except stopping it for a while.'

'Well, that's a possibility, can you come up with others?'

There's quite a long pause while the patient ponders, then she smiles and says,

'Neil's been having a go at you hasn't he!'

After a smile, the physio encourages her to come up with something.

'I could come up and raise just one of my shoulders I guess.'

'Yes' (she has an expression of encouraging more...)

'Can I lever myself up a bit perhaps...'

'Good, keep going...'

'When I did it on the bed it was much easier than the hard floor — how about having some pillows behind my head and shoulders?'

'You've done well, what do you think I could say now?'

Patient smiling and looking pleased that she's come up with answers. 'Go try it and see how I feel.'

'Spot on: Specify Generate-Evaluate!'

The patient has a very pleased smile and as she gets up she's repeating, 'Specify, Generate, Evaluate...'

Note this was an excellent chance for the patient to learn how to generate alternatives rather than give up. Also, by the therapist not telling the patient what they might do (or 'should' do – as some physios might feel), they were getting the opportunity to think and find a solution for themselves. Note how the therapist reinforced her solutions, but that the biggest reinforcement was the pleasure gained from coming up with good self-generated solutions.

A big problem with learning new skills in one classroom is that they're not generalised to being used elsewhere. But in the pain management situation, as I said before, everyone is singing from the same hymn sheet – the whole team knows what the others are doing and can, as here, reinforce earlier learning and help the generalisation process. Patients need enough practice so that when they're at home they instantly know that they have to try and work it out for themselves. Clearly if the patient's are completely stuck, the therapists may make suggestions but only to seed the process as far as possible.

The next thing to note is that standard physiotherapy is often all about the 'correctness' of an exercise like a sit-up. The fact that this patient couldn't do it would more than likely lead to a 'give that up, do this' approach with standard physiotherapy interaction. It gives the patient no chance of the finding a solution for themselves. A major problem is that many physiotherapists and exercise therapists are schooled in specific and so-called 'correct' ways of doing exercises. The idea of the patient adjusting an exercise to make it easier to do or more achievable is something of an anathema. 'No, stop, you can't do it like that, you must do it like this' or words to that effect are just not tenable here, or for me in any part of pain rehabilitation. Sorry, the best way to exercise is the way the patient finds they can do it and enjoy doing it. The only time I ever instil a degree of 'correct technique' is with lifting and during heavy loading for example. I can see the point in correct technique with top athletes and those who push their bodies to the limits but even here a degree of latitude is surely important.

In the next of Neil's sessions he did many more examples of Specify-Generate-Evaluate, most of which were relevant to the patients and their problems.

He specified the following problems to which the class generated solutions…

Forgetting to do exercises; put a list on the fridge; involve others; think of it as a new habit; ping it on the computer; put something out of place that you'll see; use an alarm; make a list of tomorrows' tasks and leave by the bed or on the fridge door…

Being interrupted during exercises; tell them to bog off; have a do not disturb sign; don't answer the door; tell them to call back in ten; have them come in but continue; stop and finish off later; tell others when you're doing them…

Back then it was 1997 – so no mobiles! But the telephone was discussed, with the obvious solutions generated…

Lack of motivation; give yourself a day off; get a friend or family member to support you; find and use a reinforcer; look at progress; change environment; re-read the manual from the programme; give yourself a fine…!

Note this last one, give yourself a fine, brings up the notion of punishment and its effect on behaviour. What fascinated me when I was observing the clinician-patient interactions was how the therapists dealt with any behaviour that could be considered 'maladaptive' – like the grunting, sighing and moaning about the pain in the exercise class, or all the self grasping and gripping during movement. All the therapists used the principles of behavioural psychology (or more correctly 'operant principles'), which were to remain neutral or ignore maladaptive responses by using body language, for example, by simply ignoring and not making any comment or by avoiding eye contact. But, when there was an effort to change, there was always reinforcement – eye contact, nodding, 'well done' and other words of encouragement. The 'operant' way of looking at maladaptive responses is to use 'removal of reinforcement' to bring about 'extinction' – rather than saying anything or using punishment.

In my experience with patients, these techniques soon become ingrained as I practiced them but also I found myself feeling rather naughty in that I would sometimes be quite explicit. 'Mr Grubb, remember one of our agreed goals today was to walk in as relaxed a way as possible – if you do one thing now, I want you to focus on smooth easy breathing.' I soon realised that when I did this sort of thing, I was 'telling' the patient and this was typical of a 'medical' approach – rather than a behavioural/operant technique and for a long while I felt as if the psychology gods were going to come crashing down on me for this. Not any more though, the key is to use a technique or approach that helps for that patient as far as possible and gets a shift in the right direction. In the right atmosphere 'Your bloody grunting and gripping yourself again Grubby, come on, you'll never get the chicks by going on like that!' Can raise a laugh and also be very productive! Psychologists I don't think would ever dream of being so cheeky and explicit! The big thing here though is that Mr Grubb was a very difficult and 'serious' chronic pain patient. His habits of behaviour were well engrained, they were his outward expressions of his desperation for the world to see and sympathise with so, me being explicit like this was actually not appropriate and likely to have a negative impact. On the other hand, a great many acute and sub acute patients who show this type of behaviour only need it pointing out to them once or twice. When this happens they quickly realise that they were getting into bad tension habits and mostly make big efforts to normalise. You have to ask the question of the patient's behaviour: is it ingrained and maladaptive? Or, is it only modestly maladaptive and on the way to becoming an unhelpful habit? Can I tackle this by being direct? Or, should I be more subtle in my communication to begin 'extinguishing' it? It takes many patients and a lot of thoughtful mileage to do the right thing at the right time.

A classic 'operant' example of manipulating behaviour is the baby crying in the middle of the night. What do you do? Get up, grumpy, but always lovingly go cuddle and rock them until they go back to sleep? Lovely, baby wakes the next night – off they go again and the cuddles and rocking may reinforce the crying behaviour.

Sometimes things can get incredibly out of hand. The example of the mother who could only get her youngster back to sleep in the middle of the night, for the first five years of their life, was to go out in the car and drive her round for an hour! Blimey! Kids rule you, eh? Well, they're smartly wired up to get as much as they can if you'll let them. So the fix is to gradually withdraw the cuddling and rocking or car driving. It's going to be hard because the behaviour will often get worse before it gets better – that's louder and longer crying and that is probably set to break you into miserable little pieces. No wonder we so often take the 'easy' route and give in!

Psychologists emphasise that the best way to change behaviour is by using reinforcement techniques. Reinforcement can facilitate adaptive behaviour; withdrawal of reinforcement – rather than punishment, is used for extinguishing maladaptive behaviour.

I've just thought a bad thought here. Some of you may remember the dog trainer and TV personality Barbara Woodhouse who was famous for saying 'Walkies' to the dogs she was training. This was back in the 1980's or even earlier. (Check her out on Youtube!). There was one programme dealing with 'dog' behavioural problems and all these owners had brought in their problem moggies. Well, one little dog was the supreme mother-f***ing neighborhood yapper. The slightest noise, especially pots and pans and this offensive dog would yap non-stop and then wouldn't stop. Out came the dog and its owner and Barbara started banging some pots and pans and the dog went off on one. Yapping away non-stop – the audience were groaning and the owner looked embarrassed. Eventually the dog calmed a bit and Barbara banged the pans again and off it went. This time she gave the dog this almighty whack across its snout, stared into its eyes with an, 'I'm going to kill you if you do that again' look and it instantly went 'eow' and shut up. Then she banged the pans again and off went the dog with a bit less enthusiasm though and it got yet another sudden and very unexpected whack and a look. Barbara repeated the pans plus the look about three times, the fourth time dog does nothing – it just sits and looks a bit forlorn. Sorted! It's good to compare this to the techniques and attitude of the 'Dog Whisperer' – who usually finds fault with the owner and changes their behaviour to sort the dog out!

What therapists also need to realise is that 'pain talk' is also a form of pain behaviour. A major problem in my experience is that <u>therapists need behavioural training too</u> – to stop their own constant enquiries about pain with the patient! I've been here before I know. But, we used to be required to get the patients to track their pain after the treatment, that night, the next day and so on until the next appointment. What's the word? IATROGENICS! What kind of behavioural outcome will that get? And what better way to learn your pain than being asked to concentrate on it 100% of the time.

To finish off: a few useful psychological terms, a bit of discussion and some little practical tips that I gleaned.

Fears and Phobias...

Discussed in the earlier chapter, but two things:

1. A great many of us tend to overestimate the danger – think of some of the things that make you frightened, they're usually ridiculous.

2. Most of us underestimate our ability to cope.

Catastophising...

This is when we make a disaster out of something that is only a 'problem'.

Doug leaves your treatment rooms and goes home. All the pains he's had for months come back, and he says to himself, 'It's no good, I'll never get this right, the treatment can't help me, it must be worse than they thought. I'm going to go mad, where are my tablets? I'll phone the Dr again.'

Thoughts can occur in 'chains' or 'cascades' for example, you're late for an appointment...

'They won't want to see me.'

'They'll get cross with me.'

'They'll think I'm pathetic.'

'They're going to start hating me.'

'I'm useless, what's the point.'

'I might as well give up and die.'

With pain, the end result is often things like 'I can't cope, I'll never get better.' Inevitably the pain gets worse.

Psychologists deal with it by using the Situation-Thoughts-Feelings to start with and then plenty of practice with the Specify-Generate-Evaluate.

In the not-so chronic situation – the post treatment flare and the waxing and waning of symptoms needs explaining and normalising, see the 'Toblerone recovery' from section 13. I used to hate the patient coming back with, 'I don't know what you did to me, but it's been the worst ever'. The reality is often that they were good for a day then it got worse.   I like the patient to come back with, 'That Toblerone thing you explained was the best and most reassuring thing you said last time. My pain went ballistic for about a day but instead of going shooting back to the Drs or ringing you I remembered what you said, did some of the relaxing exercises, kept taking the tabs that work and it settled by the evening and the next day was pretty good.'

These patients clearly aren't catastrophisers, if they were even the reassurance of the Toblerone explanation wouldn't have helped. Information is one thing, but patients also need to learn that when they're in a situation they need to be able to **Generate** some alternatives to the way they are thinking and then try them out or **Evaluate** them. It's not always easy.

Expectations...

Take the three 'fighting' words: **should, must, ought**.

I **should** be able to cope...

I **must** fight the pain...

I **ought** to be able to manage...

An individual can be wracked with pressure and demands that are unrealistic and simply cannot be achieved.

Take for example, 'I **must** fight'. A phrase, that will lead to overdoing and consequent disappointment even anger. Keeping expectations at a realistic level is vital and an important phrase is '**working with the pain**'.

It's interesting and surprising to note that levels of depression with chronic pain are much higher compared to those with spinal cord injury! If those with chronic pain continue to try and 'beat' their problem they are invariably setting themselves up to fail. The tyranny of the **shoulds** and **musts**! The dangers of black and white and all or nothing styles of thinking need to be emphasised. The proven way to go is simply via continuous building, small achievements, learning and building skills and the importance of recognising progress. Unfortunately, depressive thinking tends to be the exact opposite!

Locus of Control and Coping Styles...

Most therapists and Drs assume that all their patients want is for us to give them something or do something and 'fix' them and if they don't, the patient will not be satisfied and leave disgruntled. This is not necessarily so. One of the most basic questions to ask a patient is what their expectations of physiotherapy are and what they want to get from treatment. What you get sometimes is very revealing!

This is typical. 'I know what I don't want and that's having my bones crunched. What I really want to know is what I've done and whether you can help me?'

We need to check the patients understanding of their problem and its recovery and also get a feel for their 'locus of control'.

There are two broad types (extremes!) at either end of a spectrum:

1. Those that believe that 'outside forces' or 'forces beyond their control' are

responsible for the problem and are responsible for curing their problem. These people are said to be 'passive' copers. They want you to fix them and their beliefs may be firmly fixed in the power of medicine/physio/manipulation/machines/acupuncture/traction/god/prayer/the healer etc. People who have this type of coping style are said to have an **'external locus of control'**. Their prognosis for recovery (especially if they have an on-going problem) may not be good unless their beliefs and hence their 'locus of control' can be helpfully changed to a more internal one. Good therapy tries to get these patients to 'engage' in helping themselves and being active in promoting their own recovery and well-being. A great many chronic pain sufferers often have difficulty here and may be quite resistant to helping themselves and making helpful changes in their lives. Others grasp the opportunity and can do surprisingly well. **Passive copers tend to seek help, they go to therapists. You could argue that therapists rarely see those who have a more 'internal locus of control'.**

2. So, at the other end of the spectrum are those who want to be involved in their own recovery process and who want to take control and have responsibility. These patients are far more **'active' copers and generally recover much better.** They are said to have an **'internal locus of control'**. A big point here is that therapists and clinicians must be careful not to change this internal type into the external more passive type!

'Louis, I want to know what's causing this pain, what's going to happen and what I should do about it—should I keep going and stay active, or is it best to rest for example. I'm also wondering if you've got any clever way of getting it better or should I go and see the Dr or a specialist?'

Note:

Having a sense and feeling of control is a fundamental human drive. To have control is to reduce uncertainty.

Fear often accompanies uncertainty and leads to patients avoiding situations and activities that might be painful or cause pain. As I've already discussed in the 'fear-avoidance' chapter, avoidance leads to loss of health, tissue disuse and deconditioning. If it goes on for long, it results in loss of role in work and home, which then feeds feelings of hopelessness and helplessness, loss of self-esteem (a person's feeling of worth) and self efficacy (belief in one's ability to achieve a goal – think one's 'confidence') and can eventually lead to depressive moods and negative thinking styles. You become low, 'What's the point?' 'Can't be bothered,' – pessimistic and not uncommonly lean towards a catastrophising way of seeing various situations. This downward spiralling of negativity ends with a feeling of the situation being one of utter disaster and pointlessness. Patients who are low in spirits tend to avoid, become passive and lazy and have a very pessimistic outlook.

Clearly, these patients are very hard to help and as a result many therapists take the easy route, 'If they can't be bothered, well I can't,' I'll just stick them on a machine and rub their back – bye, that'll be forty bucks, next patient please. Another rather more serious way of looking at 'If they can't be bothered, well I can't' statement is to acknowledge that to try and instigate change will be a mountain and probably fruitless.

Improving self-efficacy requires a whole host of carefully crafted and drafted cognitive and behavioural techniques in parallel with graded recovery/ mastery and performance accomplishment.

Clearly, lowering fear of pain (show and educate may be appropriate in the non-chronic) is helpful and far better than activity avoidance. A massive issue is to realise that just giving a patient 'pain education' just isn't enough, though done in the right way for the individual patient, it can be. Patients need the proof of what you are saying, remember, they need to experience 'disconfirmation' many times before they start to change their thoughts and feelings about certain activities.

One of the huge tasks of therapy is to prevent patients from <u>developing</u> unfounded fears of movement and activity and also <u>increase their physical confidence</u> in parallel. This is where good examination and good communication come in. However, with chronic pain patients no matter how much examination, explanation, reassurance and attempts to address physical fears of movement and function you do, it makes little or no difference. Good therapists need to be able to determine when such approaches are unlikely to be effective, or when the situation is too much for their level of skill. Many patients need a team based CBT approach, the value of which I've already made a reasonable case for.

Over the years, as I mentioned just now, the most common question I get from therapists is how to deal with, 'They expect you do to something' problem. My reply is, 'Do they? How do you know that?'

Here are two different ways of asking the same question – an important question in the context of the discussion here.

1. 'What do you feel a physiotherapist can offer you or can do for you?'
2. 'Before we start, I'm interested to know what you are expecting from physiotherapy, or what you might get from me?'

Those may appear a little blunt and you may be fearful of getting an answer like, 'Well, why ask me? You're the physio. I was hoping <u>you</u> were going to tell me what <u>you</u> can do!'

Here's one response to this…

'That's fine, the reason I'm asking is that if we work together, if we both can sing from the same song sheet at all times, you'll do much better. There's nothing worse for a patient to come in expecting one thing and the therapist then does something you're not at all keen on or doesn't make any sense to you. Some patients have a list of questions in their head they want answers to, that sort of thing.'

'Ah, I see where you're coming from...'

'A great many patient questions can be distilled into what most people want from their Doctor when the go and see them.'

- Doc, what's wrong with me?
- Doc, will it get better on its own, if so, how long's it going to take?
- Doc, is there anything I can do to help myself?
- Doc, is there anything you can do to help me get over it... maybe you have something that can fix it?

The conversation might not go this way, but if it does it's very helpful. The main thing is to arrive at a position in which between you – you can set an agenda. Here's a simple example of a patient who's got acute back pain:

- reduce pain
- reduce tension when you move
- start getting going gradually
- appropriate mobilisation techniques
- address the findings in our 'shopping basket' – remember the stiff hip, poor leg stretch on the left and your inability to do some simple back and abdominal muscle exercises. I need to help you strengthen your back
- get your ranges of movement back via exercises and maybe a bit of me helping
- etc....

While on the subject of my four 'Doc' questions listed above its good to note that a 1996 survey of first time back pain sufferers found that the patients wanted to understand four things:

1. The likely course of their back trouble and the associated activity limitations.
2. How to manage their back pain.
3. How to return to usual activities quickly.
4. How to minimise the frequency and severity of recurrences.

These concerns ranked higher than seeking a cause for their back pain or a diagnosis.

(Von Korff M, Saunders K, 1996 The course of back pain in primary care. Spine 21(24): 2833-283)

The notion that all your patients want to be fixed or have you do something to them may well be a myth. It annoyed me 20 years ago and it still annoys me today!

On the other hand if the patient does come in and say, 'I've heard you've a fantastic reputation, I've been in pain for years, tried all the therapies there are, you're my last resort, please, please fix me.' You know immediately the patient is likely to be hard to help and difficult to shift their thinking away from fix/cure to one of management and rehabilitation. I'll illustrate one of these in a case history later. I can tell you now though, that with the help of the 'Shopping Basket', these types soon come round to seeing that their problem is complicated and that there is a lot to do. A great many say that they haven't been examined in such detail and had the findings explained so clearly. They often go... 'No wonder all those other treatments didn't help much...'

Another very useful question is to ask the patient about their own understanding of their problem:

'You've told me you've seen a lot of consultants and specialists, also a great many therapists, I'm interested to know about your understanding of the problem?'

In chronic pain patients, what you get is often a biomedical, structural weakness, arthritic, multiple discs out type of understanding, 'The Dr looked at the x-ray and said... the bottom three discs are worn and there's nothing he can do – he shrugged his shoulders and said it was up to me,' or, 'The physio said that when there's wear and tear like the Dr said, the more I do the more it will wear and then hurt. And the only way to go on is to get good at bracing my stomach every time I move.' Arghhhhhh – where's the nearest bridge to jump off!   What on earth are physiotherapy students being taught about the management of on-going musculoskeletal pain problems and arthritis? There's one picture everyone should have on the wall in their clinic

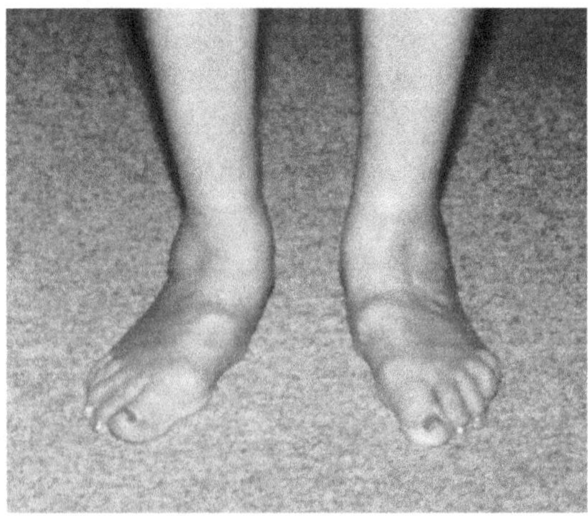

Fig GE3.1 'The lady who walks the cliffs'

and that's, 'The lady who walks the cliffs.' For me she's been the Goddess of helping me to show patients that arthritis does not equate with mobility scooters, electric wheelchairs and stair lifts!

Clearly, 'structural explanations' can be very unhelpful. On many occasions I have written to a chronic pain patient's consultant and quite firmly asked them to tell the patient that his arthritic back/spine, knee/hip is quite strong enough to exercise, get moving and function to quite a high level WITHOUT ANY HARM. I tell the consultant what I am trying to do and where I'm trying to go with the patient. I also tell the consultant what I think they are capable of – for one or two I've said, 'I can see no structural reason why this patient, with adequate input and later training shouldn't be able to run a half marathon. I'm thinking about two year's time!'

Luckily, my firmness and forwardness was always supported (in their heads they're probably going, 'Thank God someone's trying to do something for him, I've nothing left that I can do... If that bloody patient runs a marathon I'll be amazed.'). Some of them did, some of them didn't and in the early days I cocked up quite badly with one or two. The big deal is a full understanding of the most important yellow flags, which are discussed in the following section.

Finally, to get back to where I was a little while ago. The important point is that how can you expect a patient to get moving and do all your exercises, if you've no idea about their understanding of the problem! If they think that every time they move they're wearing out more and more, the movement or exercises you've given them are going to be done with reluctance, processed in the 'fear/tension' 'low road' part of the brain and more than likely be very unproductive!

The moral here – ask the patient, you'll find out a great deal and you'll help them a great deal more than you otherwise would have!

Chapter GE4.1
The 'Shopping Basket Approach' History and introduction

Introduction

The shopping basket approach has evolved from my own analysis of how I think and reason with a patient. In actual fact it was also a reaction to something which drives me mad: the very term 'Approach'– the Maitland, the McKenzie, the Kaltenborn, the muscle imbalance approach and so on. It's a term that drives clinical reasoning into a unidimensional place, whereby the treatment that's given narrowly dictates the clinical reasoning, the assessment and the overall line of questioning. For example, why would someone with an 'ultrasound' approach want to know about psychosocial factors, or how the problem has influenced the sufferers function and activity levels, or even want to try to understand the presentation in terms of biomedical features – if, all they're going to do in the end, is stick an ultrasound machine on the spot where it hurts? Same for Maitland, McKenzie and muscle imbalance; all they require is the basic information that follows a narrow doctrine needed to do the technique.

'Hi, Louis here, it's Monday and you're lucky because Monday is ultrasound day; where's your pain love? Slip your things off; lie down here; show me the spot; bit of jelly; that'll be a bit cold; whoops, yes, right, off we go. Five minutes later – see you on Friday. Friday is laser day!'

'Hi, Louis here, it's Monday' and so on. (Tuesday is acupuncture day if you were wondering!) I have also lectured in Switzerland in 'rehabilitation' centres where patients were booked in for three weeks and received a variety of 'treatments' daily, dictated only by a bell ringing every half an hour – all change!

The 'Shopping Basket' is so named to try to mock this 'approach' thing a bit. Apologies and that's not a very CBT way to start, by alienating the audience! I'm hoping the ultrasound and laser example set a lightish tone to the scene and we can now get up and running.

Last observation then: *one thing I realised a long time ago, is that how anyone reasons is hugely dictated by what they plan to do – the more biased and limited in your skills/knowledge, the more blinkered and limited your reasoning is going to be!*

I hear that nowadays all these 'approaches' are integrating the biopsychosocial dimensions. Well, super, but to me they all are still stuck with the dominance of the physical treatment they are steering the whole thing towards. My suggestion is that you become a 'shopping basket' approach therapist (if you like what I write and reason?). And in only one compartment of it will you find that it is possible to include a little joint 'wiggling' and 'fiddling' if you want to; and overall it is very unusual for any given 'compartment' to be a priority. There's one word that should dominate all physical therapist minds and that is ***Rehabilitation***. It is such a special word and one that is unique to our profession. Please, let's never let it go. It's got more evidence in its favour than any treatment approach or modality ever has or ever will have.

I want to start by acknowledging a great friend, a great thinker and a huge contributor to the world of clinical reasoning. We all owe Mark Jones a huge thank you and a place high up there in the history of rational evidence based physiotherapy. Whether you know it or not Mark Jones' work will have influenced your clinical reasoning at some point. The easiest place to start is with his superb book Clinical Reasoning for Manual Therapists. Chapter 1 summarises it all. Also see chapter 25 on Educational theory by Joy Higgs, and chapter 26 by Darren Rivett and Mark on, 'Improving clinical reasoning in manual therapy'.

The book is full of case histories by the manual therapy 'gurus' of the world – with Mark asking the guru involved various 'reasoning' questions and getting their responses as the case unfolds. Mark is beautiful in his diplomacy with them. I'd have lost my rag, because a great many are not much better at reasoning than my ultrasound-on-Monday therapist! Read them; but it's thanks to Mark's questioning that there is a great deal to learn and ponder. I like it that he ends the book with the 'Improving clinical reasoning in manual therapy' chapter!

Mark started all this way back, just after the 1985 Manipulation course in Adelaide (he was on the course with myself and Dave Butler). He was doing some research based at the University. I remember he came up to Geoff Maitland's practice and videoed him assessing a patient. Afterwards the two of them went back through it and Mark asked him why he was asking the questions and what he was thinking and reasoning in his head with the information that he gleaned. Soon, Mark came up with his now famous 'Hypothesis Categories'.

They were:

1. What is the 'source' of the symptoms and/or dysfunction?
2. Are there any 'contributing' factors?
3. What are the precautions and contraindications to physical examination and treatment?
4. What is the prognosis?
5. What treatment should be selected and what progression is likely?

For manual therapy, or any therapy geared towards a tissue based approach and a passive treatment approach to a pain problem, this was how it was. The answers to those questions were always described in terms of physical injury, tissue abnormality and movement, and biomechanically altered function. Those were the questions we all needed to have in the back of our heads and needed to be able to provide answers to after listening and examining the patient.

Later as Dave Butler and I started to introduce 'pain' and pain mechanisms and a more 'top-down', self-management, multidimensional view of things changes and additions to the hypothesis categories were required. These were committed to the literature in a combined author article:

Gifford L. S. and Butler D.S. (1997) The integration of pain sciences into clinical practice. Hand Therapy 10(2): 86-95.

The clinical reasoning hypothesis categories now became:

* Pathobiological Mechanisms

* Dysfunction

* Sources

* Contributing Factors

* Prognosis

* Precautions

* Management

Pathobiological Mechanisms had the following sub-divisions:

* Tissue mechanism (i.e. what's going on in the tissues? For example, are they: healing, healed, scar tissue, inflamed, etc.?)

* Pain mechanisms (i.e. what pain mechanisms are operating or dominant: nociception? peripheral neurogenic? central? affective emotional? sympathetic? motor (output) even immune?)

The **Dysfunction** category was expanded and defined in terms of the clinical 'expressions' of the pathobiological mechanisms. Hence:

* *general physical dysfunctions:* what would now be termed 'disabilities' or *'activity capability/restrictions' or 'participation capability/restriction'*

   For example, the inability to walk for more than five minutes, inability to type or write or do house work, lift objects and perform work tasks.

* *specific physical dysfunctions*: or what I now call 'physical impairments'

   They're the things that physical therapists find during their physical examinations; like losses of range of movement; pain on certain movements and tests; weaknesses; neurological deficits and also all the little physical minutiae that many physical therapists seem to get obsessed about and go on courses and pay lots of good money to learn about – like muscle imbalance, neurodynamics, an accessory movement not being quite right, a fascial-band restriction, a core stability abnormality and so forth.

* *psychological/mental dysfunctions*: this was an awful term but was an early recognition and germination of the importance of psycho-social factors being important.

So pain mechanisms, or pathobiological mechanisms and a broadening of the 'dysfunction' category were integrated into clinical reasoning and it was an honour for my work to be acknowledged and to co-author with Mark Jones and Ian Edwards the article:

'Conceptual models for implementing biopsychosocial theory in clinical practice,' published in the Journal, Manual Therapy in 2002.

Further thanks to Mark Jones for being so inclusive of my thoughts in his and Darren Rivetts' book: *'Clinical Reasoning for Manual Therapists'*.

Mark, as far as I know now, sees the hypothesis categories like this:

- *activity capability/restriction* (abilities and difficulties an individual may have in executing activities) and *participation capability/restriction* (abilities and problems an individual may have in involvement in life situations)

- *patients perspectives on their experience*

- *pathobiological mechanisms* (tissue healing and pain mechanisms)

- *physical impairments and associated structure/tissue sources*

- *contributing factors* to the development and maintenance of the problem

- *precautions and contraindications* to physical examination and treatment

- *management and treatment*

- *prognosis.*

My view is that this is still quite heavily biased to a 'manual therapy' perspective. My way of doing things never quite sat comfortably with it, although these categories offer a perfectly reasonable way to go about clinical thinking and reasoning.

So one day, sometime in about year 2000 I sat down with a tad of irritable grumpiness about all the various 'approaches' and thought about how I think in the clinic. I came up with a series of simple compartments which I then put in an old fashioned wicker shopping or gardening type basket. It had great clinical utility.

If you take a look at figure GE4.1 you can see the basket and the various compartments. Nice and simple, like me! I like things nice and easy to use – but all encompassing too. The compartments are:

1. Biomedical – which is all about 'think like a Dr' plus quite a bit more.

2. Psychosocial – think psychosocial predictors of outcome or 'yellow flags',

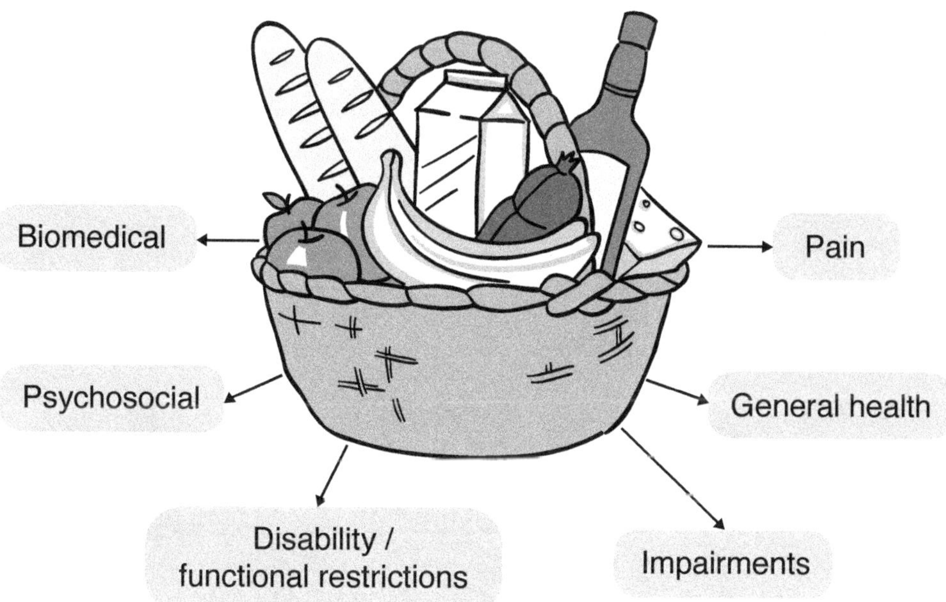

Figure GE4.1 The Shopping Basket approach

that's the now famous ABCDEFW categorisation that every physiotherapist should be taught at undergraduate level.

3. Disability/functional restrictions – everything that the patient reports that their having physical difficulties with in their life, it relates to home, work, social and fitness/hobby activities

4. Physical Impairments – that's the bit that most musculoskeletal physiotherapists are stuck in and feel very comfortable with.

5. General health and fitness – why this? Because it's so important and the evidence so clearly beneficial. I am not an expert here but helping someone get fitter using a graded, paced and goal setting approach is fairly straight forward for anyone well trained with rehabilitation skills.

6. Pain! The category that most clinicians start with. 'Where's your pain?' I've stuck it last for the very reason that a Maitland training gets you're 'needle stuck' on asking about pain. ('Needle stuck' refers to your old vinyl records having a bit of dried up old jam in the grooves which causes a line

of the track to just repeat on and on until you shove the needle on a bit. ... shows how old fashioned I am). I'll never forget having a manipulation exam patient who didn't come in complaining of any pain! I was stymied, gibbering, but luckily managed to eventually squeeze some pain out of him to fill in the time and impress the examiners!

The following chapters deal with each compartment.

Chapter 4.2
The Biomedical compartment part 1

The wave of excitement at the introduction and recognition of 'psychosocial factors', in the late 1990's and early 2000's, almost pushed 'biomedical' thinking into a 'dirty little word' kind of place. It was sneered at as encouraging 'Cartesian' thinking – that the 'mind was separate from the body' and the awful logic that if there was nothing to be found wrong in the body – the complaint was all in the mind. The new fad was to merely use biomedical reasoning to screen for serious tissue states and diseases and, if these 'red-flags' were all clear, then the approach should be driven by psychosocially and rehabilitationist dominated ways of managing the patient's problem. Well fine, but the more I kept thinking about it the more I realised how a biomedical style of reasoning was important to me. For example, knowing what I was dealing with gave me knowledge of natural history and 'normal' progress, or what to expect with progress. Everyday aches and pains that patients came with do fit into broad categories of recognisable conditions.

From the psychosocial perspective acute pain was generally thought of as lasting between three and six months and chronic pain as anything thereafter. Well, that didn't make sense? I was thinking of loads of common musculoskeletal injuries and conditions that go on for ages and eventually get better, yet aren't labelled as 'chronic' and therefore to be shunted off for 'special psychosocial input'! For example a typical frozen shoulder may take anything from eight to twelve months up to three or more years. Dutch physiotherapist Hugo Stam, friend and colleague from Adelaide and Switzerland teaching days, wrote a great review of 'Frozen Shoulder' in the journal Physiotherapy (Stam 1994) (more like this please!).

According to the literature Hugo researched, a typical frozen shoulder's natural history is divided into three overlapping phases: first, the painful phase lasting anything from two and a half to nine months; then a stiff period lasting between four and twelve months; and finally a recovery period that could be as short as five months or go on for up to two years and two months. The total duration reported extended from twelve months to three and a half years, with an average duration time of two and a half years.

To me that sort of information is incredibly useful for your patient. Once a patient knows information like this the vast majority adjust to the situation, get on with life the best they can and eventually the shoulder problem settles, the range comes back and they recover well. Simple guidance from time to time, with good information and reassurance, plus appropriate stretching and strengthening exercises are all that are required. Also, if the therapist has time and the patient the money, it's really nice to have someone give the frozen shoulder a ***nice*** good deep massage and lots of ***nice*** stretching manual therapy occasionally! If I had one, I'd get someone to do that to mine. Pandering? You wait until you get a frozen shoulder!

Further, there are often questions that need good answers like, 'Louis, will this ever come back?' And 'Louis, will I get this in the other shoulder too?' I haven't researched the literature recently for answers here, but in my clinical experience I've never seen a frozen shoulder come back again. However, it's fairly common for the other shoulder to go through it all. I tell patients if they ask that, 'Yes, it does go to the other shoulder in some patients but it isn't very common at all. I've seen about ten in thirty years of practice, that's out of several hundred who haven't.'

Here are some more of my observations (which need verifying): tennis elbow, natural history from many weeks up to eighteen months; carpal tunnel syndrome, eight to twelve months roughly; nerve root problems, three months to a year or even more; ligament and tendon injuries can take months and up to a year. The reader is directed to the physical healing chapters earlier. The point is that we need to be good at recognising a presentation and KNOWING ITS NATURAL HISTORY. This helps us with the word, prognosis, for the patient – the normal outcome. It answers the 'How long is it going to take Louis' question!

But all this must never be viewed in isolation, any given problem's 'natural history' must take into account any psychosocial features present that may influence recovery and outcome. It is interesting to note however that many single area musculoskeletal disorders, that have long natural histories, rarely end up becoming classic chronic pain problems. I'm unable to think of anyone whose chronic pain problem started with frozen shoulder, carpal tunnel or tennis elbow for example.

So I think a much better definition of chronic pain is: 'Pain that extends beyond the expected period of healing'. We need to accept that everyone's healing rate is variable, but a rough estimate of time can always be given, as above.

As you can see, I believe that knowing natural history is really important – it certainly would be if I was a patient and I wouldn't be impressed with a clinician who was vague about telling me what was wrong or at least what was going on. So being able to classify a presentation in some sort of biomedical way is essential as far as I am concerned. What follows are further supporting perspectives which I hope will help you see my reasoning here. Thinking and musing from my metaphorical armchair about 'ideal medicine' leads me to thinking, or more likely dreaming, that it would be pretty cool if the whole of biomedicine could adopt an all embracing approach like this to their craft! Come on educators, get your backsides into gear and get up to date with what we know about pain and musculoskeletal disorders!

So in the biomedical compartment go these sorts of questions for me:

(see also figures GE4.2 and GE4.3)

1. **What's the presentation?**
2. **What's the classic 'Dr' or 'consultant' diagnosis? Be able to give an answer to the question: 'What's wrong?'**
3. **Is the problem mainly one of processing rather than a significant tissue problem?**
4. **Is the pain out of proportion to the tissue health/status/strength/ healing stage/injury?**
5. **Is this a typical 'syndrome', condition or injury with a known natural history?**
6. **WHAT'S HAPPENING IN THE TISSUES? – AND ARE THEY SAFE TO START LOADING?**
7. **What's the normal recovery/natural history of this presentation, what are the rough time ranges?**

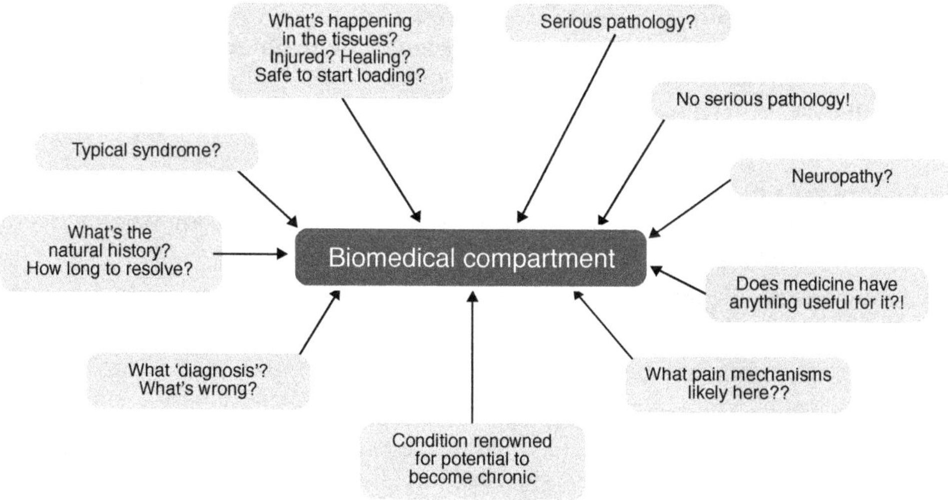

Figures GE4.2 The Biomedical compartment

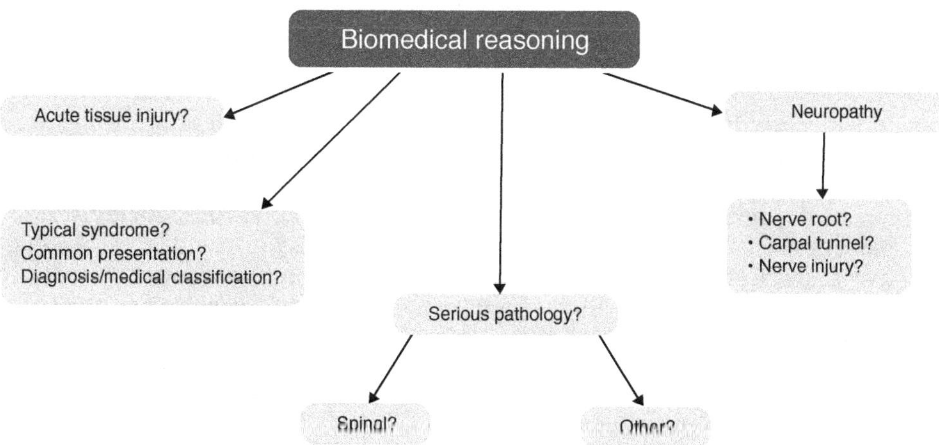

Figures GE4.3 Biomedical reasoning

8. Are degenerative changes present?

9. Is there anything serious wrong, should I send them back to the Dr/ request further investigations?

10. Is there a neuropathy?

11. Does medicine have anything to offer – like operations, injections and medications?

12. Does the condition I'm seeing have a well-known potential to develop into a chronic, ongoing 'pain-disabled' type problem? For example, back pain and sciatica; early presentations of pain following 'office' related overuse or whiplash and RTA type problems.

Right, let's get a bit more organised. I've got two simple figures that summarise the sub-compartmentalisation of how I think we should all be thinking when we're in the biomedical compartment of the 'Shopping Basket'.

I will now review Figure GE4.2. Whenever I see a new patient I want the following questions answered.

Is what's in front of me:

1. An **acute injury**? This is simple and it's all about understanding the state of the tissues, their strength and whether the tissues are safe to start loading and moving. Joint or bony tissue 'stability' is an important question to think about, and of course if there are issues in this respect a decision about medical referral may be important. If the tissues are 'stable' and medical referral is not required then it's rare that some form of movement and graded loading cannot be instigated.

2. A **typical syndrome or common presentation?** The term 'syndrome' is a bit nebulous and may have gone out of fashion rather. 'Common presentation' is far better.

   Some 'guru' based approaches use 'syndrome' style classifications to direct treatment. For example, the 'Postural,' 'Dysfunction' and various 'Derangement' syndromes used by the McKenzie method direct their specific approaches to each. I am not a fan, but as far as these therapists are concerned they see predictable patterns that they say respond in predictable ways. 'Piriformis' syndrome is another 'presentation' that annoys me, because I see so many patients with buttock pain who've spent a fortune on therapy having been told that this is what is wrong. I have seen only one what I would call a true 'Piriformis' syndrome in my whole career and I've seen a great many buttock pains! I have the same disdain for the over diagnosed 'Ilio-tibial tract' syndrome. Those who purport to stretch it and realign it should play with some fresh human cadavers and see how incredibly strong this structure really is. I'll grant that it's not an uncommon area to feel pain but I'm deeply suspect of it being a common source of the problem. The same goes for the sacroiliac joint and all the wacky flim-flam that accompanies it.

   I recall many years ago a presentation called the 'T4 syndrome'. I think it was a top of the head headache combined with bilateral hand symptoms, often with pins and needles? We were told that it responded to T4 manipulation. I saw what I thought were two of these in my early manual therapy days and found that clicking T4 didn't make one jot of difference. I never saw it again

So, 'syndromes' are to my mind controversial, but 'common presentations' are not. I'll make a short illustrative list of what I mean. These are all presentations that have a fairly common set of signs and symptoms and can be diagnosed with reasonable confidence. That there are always exceptions are what makes our work so interesting though.

Here we are:

- tennis elbow
- carpal tunnel
- frozen shoulder
- painful arc/supraspinatus/rotator-cuff presentations
- common degenerative patterns in all joints – from thumbs and fingers to spine to feet, all of them
- collateral ligament and meniscus problems of the knee
- all common joint and muscle injuries
- all common tendon and ligament injuries
- inflammatory joint conditions
- peripheral nerve injuries, neuropathies and other presentations (see 'Neuropathy' category)
- presentations that relate to 'overuse'.

The list could easily be added to and I would like to think that most clinicians of modest experience have probably seen a smattering of all of these. If you'd like me to now give the typical details and natural histories of them I could give my 'experience', but what we really need are good longitudinal studies of all of these, regardless of what therapy they have. We need the narratives and we need far more than what's in most orthopaedic and musculoskeletal books that go through various presentations. I'm yet to see a book of presentation that isn't mere regurgitations of what's been written long ago by some 'armchair expert'. I'm starting to wonder if things will ever improve in this important area.

Serious Pathology?   This is dealt with in detail in chapter 4.3

Neuropathy?   See the 'Nerve Root' sections of the book.

The next figure, GE4.4 shows two lines of reasoning, one into **'Tissue mechanisms'** and one to **'Pain mechanisms'**. The key issue from here is that the clinician should be asking themselves whether the pain they are assessing is Adaptive or Maladaptive. And whether the tissues they are assessing are 'safe to start loading'? Reviewing many of the issues in these two sub-compartments will also help decisions about appropriate 'treatments' and 'modalities'. For example, inflamed tissues may

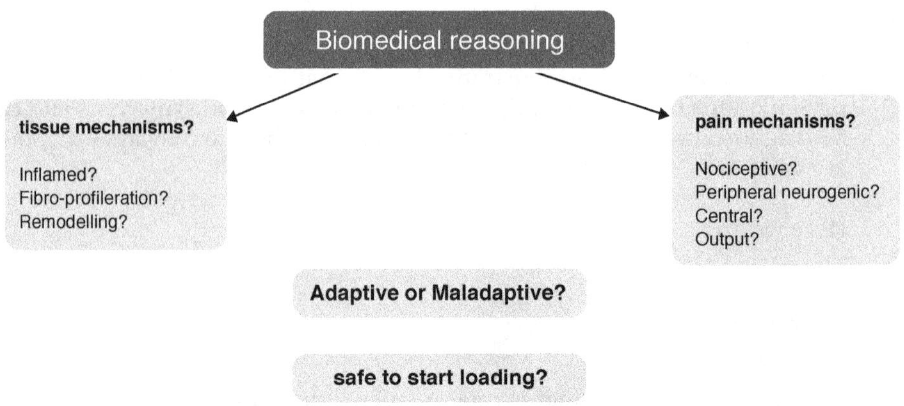

Figure GE4.4 Biomedical reasoning 2

require not only pain control but perhaps a degree of anti-inflammatory medication too, especially if the inflammation is deemed to err towards the 'maladaptive' end of the spectrum.

The occasional patient who appears with an acute and massive joint swelling, for no apparent reason, has just popped into my head. I'm thinking of those puffed up knees or ankles, occasionally wrists too. While it is imperative to think as a rheumatologist would, RA, OA, Gout, even AS, another reasoning perspective is to go: massive inappropriate swelling/inflammation = maladaptive, sound management requires urgent anti-inflammatory management. For a physical therapist we might use all the traditional inputs that we have: ice or heat (yes heat! why not?) if it feels good and helps, do it, massage, appropriate intermittent compression, easy movements, even a bit of ultrasound or TENS. Anything that can produce or enhance an endorphin response has to be of help and 'machines', in the right context can! Yes, they can. Review top-down pathways in the placebo chapters.

Pain mechanisms will be discussed in chapter 4.4.

A patient:
the importance of a medical 'diagnosis'

On reflection a great deal of my clinical life, apart from being involved in rehabilitating injury, has revolved around reviewing, treating and managing musculoskeletal conditions that have underlying joint, bony and soft-tissue degenerative changes. These are the conditions that traditionally see a rheumatologist for drug and injection management or orthopaedics for joint replacement, injection, repair and other surgical procedures. The results have hugely varying rates of success and many have poor support in clinical trials. Occasionally neurosurgeons get involved.

Degenerative joint related presentations have a pattern that is important to recognise. A great many clinicians fail to recognise the 'degenerative' presentation and as a result a great many patients waste a great deal of money on prolonged treatments that are never going to get anywhere near a 'cure'.

Let's have an example to demonstrate what I mean.

Mrs X is 59 years old and tells me she has seen three different practitioners, two were physiotherapists, one a chiropractor. She told me she had spent in the region of nearly eight hundred pound on all of them having a great deal of treatment. And whilst getting some relief, overall the situation was really no better than when it started eight months ago. The pain was in her left buttock and some radiating down the lateral and slightly anterior thigh. It hurt when she walked and she struggled out of the chair after sitting a long time. I could give far more detail, but the point is that:

- physio number one focused on 'piriformis muscle' and fascial release of her 'ITB'

- the second physio had apparently berated the first one and told Mrs X it was all coming from her back and had focused on mobilising various vertebrae and giving her back exercises

- the chiropractor who she saw last and had persisted the longest, started out with a diagnosis of sacroiliac being out and leg length being too short, but after that wasn't helping he moved to her jaw and face – 'for some reason'.

Now with a bit more probing and listening I found that she'd had similar very low grade awareness of the buttock, occasionally leg for about six to seven years and that she had become less and less keen to do any distance walking. She also said she'd noticed having increasingly difficulty with lifting the leg up to tie her shoe laces and that she'd taken to bending to the floor to overcome the problem. When I observed her walking it was quite smooth but with smallish strides due to what looked like a small loss of extension. There was a very slight twist to her trunk too. And so it went on: there was loss of range doing adductor stretch; similarly with left leg back and forward lunge to observe hip extension, lifting her leg to reach the foot was 'heavy and stiff – a struggle, compared to the right. Passive testing revealed marked loss of internal rotation at 90 degrees flexion, flexion adduction was limited and easily reproducing the pain. Think like a Doctor? Why not? She has a classic early degenerative hip problem, surely? What's the need for knowing that is the next question? It's all about the patient and the clinician understanding the nature of the problem, accepting the situation and then getting some kind of joint/tissue/ fitness for life programme going; rather than continually revolving around a bunch of therapists, who long to find their little something, in piriformis, or the back, or the mouth and do something to fix or relieve the symptoms.

This lady's shopping basket would have plenty to do in all the compartments: from pain control and management to general health; improvements in function and activity levels; improvements of joint and related tissue function, in range and strength.

There were several 'yellow flag' related issues – no doubt, and, back in the biomedical compartment some positive information about the nature and best management of hip arthrosis! Isn't that what you'd want to know? It's a classic situation where good positive understanding, combined with a well guided self-management action plan, lead to acceptance, adjustment and the strong feeling of having control back.

I now want to underline the importance of the statement, 'Is it safe to start loading?' I've dealt with this a little earlier in the book, but let's recap. First, think injured hunter-gatherer who, by the way, hasn't access to some medic or therapist saying 'don't do that'. If they have to move, regardless of the pain, they just will in order to survive. Clearly some degree of rest can be dictated by the extent of the pain and the injury, but getting going fairly quickly is vital. Joint, ligament and tendon injuries take ages to heal; the repair/scar process leaves the tissue in never as good a state as it was and if one was to rest for the whole healing journey, the outcome is likely to be quite a bit worse than getting going as quickly as possible. Remember, even an 'unstable' knee to testing can have quite adequate function. Also, the body seems pretty much 'designed' to heal while we stay on the move.

One message is that the healing time/natural history tells us how long symptoms *could* carry on for, but shouldn't dictate the return of function. Use of a graded approach and therefore to get moving as soon as is practical, has to be the best attitude in a great many such presentations. I know orthopaedics wouldn't agree; those guys love rest, especially after some operations. Fair enough, but I see shoulder operations for tendon repairs or on-going painful arcs/impingement type operations. Where the surgeon demands six or more weeks complete rest followed by passive gentle movements and some two months or more before any resisted work is allowed. These patients invariably (if I can generalise) take months/ up to a year to get back to a good strength and range. They invariably get capsular tightening and the equivalent of a frozen shoulder on top of what they had before! I think that's poor, but they'd argue it's the price that has to be paid. I'd argue further that if only the patient had BEEN PATIENT and waited long enough, the shoulder would have settled and recovered naturally (I do acknowledge there is always the exception!). During this time they could have carried on moving, kept some good functional strength going and adjusted activities. The after-reaction of joint 'intervention', while massively accepted by the patient, is often worse than what they had before the op! The argument that it's now fixed is often cited. But I sometimes wonder, having observed and helped a great many patients who don't want to go anywhere near surgery and who have patiently waited – sometimes for up to eighteen months or more and who eventually recover extremely well.

My line with patients who ask me about these shoulder operations is to be open. I always say that given enough time most problems like theirs do get better but they have to be patient. And I also point out that the surgery doesn't instantly fix the shoulder, it leaves it weak and stiff and it takes almost as long as nature can. BUT, I always say that the results are excellent. I occasionally put them in touch with a patient who had a similar problem, who had surgery and did well and also with one who didn't have surgery and did well – so they can assess for themselves! I make sure that they ask the one who had surgery how long the post-surgical recovery took and what it was like.

Think of skin when you think of the 'is it safe to start loading' question. The answer, even though it still may open the wound and bleed a bit, is very soon, well almost immediately!

Chapter 4.3
Biomedical compartment part 2: Serious pathology

Serious Pathology

Important books to read, study and review:

Red Flags: A Guide to Identifying Serious Pathology of the Spine, 1e (Physiotherapy Pocketbooks) by Sue Greenhalgh MA GD Phys FCSP and James Selfe PhD MA GD Phys FCSP (22 Feb 2006)

Red Flags II: A Guide to Solving Serious Pathology of the Spine, 1e (Physiotherapy Pocketbooks) Sue Greenhalgh MA GD Phys FCSP and James Selfe PhD MA GD Phys FCSP (2009)

The Back Pain Revolution. Gordon Waddell.

This is vital. I'm going to be rude here: clinicians, including many Drs, are very poor at this. On the Graded Exposure courses I taught I used to get a clean flip chart page ready and write, 'Low back pain red flags' at the top and say to the audience, 'Come on, give them to me – shoot, don't stop, I'll write them down as you shout them out. But it was always a dreadfully slow and laboured response.

Pause... er...

- 'Night pain'...
- 'Loss of weight'... pause...
- 'Cancer history'... long pause...
- 'Unwell'... longer pause...
- 'Steroids'...
- 'Non-mechanical pain'...

That was about it usually. Hmmm! How can you be expected to be able to reassure patients that there's nothing seriously wrong and that it's safe to start loading and get moving if you don't know the major key signs of sinister pathology?

Here's the clinical rule: you can't drive on the road without passing your driving test... So, YOU'RE NOT ALLOWED TO TREAT PATIENTS UNLESS YOU PASS YOUR RED FLAG TEST WITH A SCORE OF 100%. I'm not kidding!

Also, you not only need to have learnt this red flag stuff you really need to have seen it for real in the clinic or hospital.

I always loved these definitions of the 'four levels of competence'. I think it was Michael Shacklock who told me about them...

1. 'Unconsciously incompetent' – you're crap and dangerous and don't know it. Let's hope someone tells you.

2. 'Consciously incompetent' – you're crap and dangerous and know it. That's

a bit better, you can do something about it.

3. 'Consciously competent' – well OK, but you're 'cocky'. Like all the therapists who are promoting themselves as 'specialists' after a mere 3-5 years of limited experience. Warning, you may well be unconsciously incompetent.

4. 'Unconsciously competent' – wise? Well, perhaps.

An early example from a lifetime of case histories...

While working at Geoff Maitland's clinic back in 1986, a young lad of about 13 years old was referred to the practice by an orthopaedic surgeon, for 'spinal manipulation'. The youngster was complaining of arm pain and some pain in his thoracic region, across his back at about level T7-10. There was no history of trauma and he was otherwise fit. The spinal orthopaedist had reassured him and his parents that a bit of good manual therapy would do the trick. The referral note actually stated: 'Please Manipulate' on it. Thankfully I asked him about numbness and paraesthesia and he mentioned pins and needles in his hands and some in his feet. He said that his hands and feet had slightly odd in feelings too. His Dad, who was in the cubicle as well raised his eyebrows, he'd not mentioned this before. It turned out that the lad loved rugby and he hadn't wanted to be stopped from playing, so he'd kept quiet about these things. He was otherwise fit. There was no loss of weight, tiredness, general feelings of being un-well etc; and he was going to school as normal.

I went on and got all the usual details of his symptoms and symptom behaviour, all the aggravating and easing factors etc. etc. Anyway, I asked him to pop his things off and as I watched his hands struggled to coordinate undoing his shirt buttons and taking his shoes and socks off. I then focused on an extensive neurological examination; all reflexes were markedly brisk; finger tip to nose and heel along shin with eyes closed were quite poor; he had difficulty maintaining light moving hand to hand contact; his balance wasn't good, when tested in detail and he'd lost sensation in his hands and feet. He had marked clonus.

I sent him back to the surgeon with a letter requesting he have a closer look and even check the cord in the lad's cervical spine. Two weeks later his father came to see me. They'd found a tumour in his son's neck!

That was the first of many instances over the years where my competence with sniffing out serious disease was put to the test. A major factor in my ability to hear the alarm 'bells' ringing was my time working as a newly qualified physiotherapist on neurological and neurosurgical wards. Treating and seeing neurologically damaged patients and many other serious pathologies and diseases. If I had carried on with this young lad and under pressure of time, I could quite easily have manipulated his neck or thoracic spine and missed these vital clues.

What were they?

1. Under 20 years of age and no history of trauma.

2. His pain was pretty much non-mechanical and symptoms were constant, like many 'nerve' (central and peripherally generated) pains.

3. There was widespread neurology.

4. Thoracic pain for no apparent reason.

Let's review the full classic list but I would strongly urge all therapists to study the books cited above. And get good general clinical experience; take time to listen to patients; and do thorough physical examinations; so you know the clinical presentations at the 'worst' end of the spectrum. In musculoskeletal practice we tend to see the early signs of those more severe pathologies.

Here's the list. Please learn it off by heart and have it in mind with every patient, every time:

(my comments are in italics)

<u>**RED FLAGS**</u> – **learn and learn and learn again...**

- presentation age <20 years (think serious pathology or structural problem like spondylolisthesis); or onset >55 years (serious pathology e.g. spinal metastases or osteoporosis)

- violent trauma e.g. fall from height, road traffic accident
  (consider age of patient – a small fall can easily fracture in the elderly, note minor trauma if on steroids, or postmenopausal with osteoporosis, think possible collapse of vertebral body. I have seen vertebral crush fractures from small heights in younger people too)

- constant progressive non-mechanical pain (unrelated to time or activity, spontaneous onset, gradual onset, gradually worse, no relief with rest or exercise, no position of ease, worse at night etc.)
  (But note, many neuralgias and nerve root pains are like this – often being ghastly at night and no position of ease being found in bed or anywhere else!)

- thoracic pain (in Waddell's series of 900 patients – 30% of patients referred to hospital with thoracic pain had either serious spinal pathology or osteoporotic collapse or a vertebrae)

- a previous history of: carcinoma, rheumatoid disorder, TB or any recent infection

- systemic steroids (may cause osteoporosis)

- drug abuse, HIV

- systemically unwell (likely to be serious disease. BUT, the absence of fever does not exclude infection. The lumbar spine is a common metastatic tumour site for breast, thyroid, lymph nodes, abdomen and prostate.)

• weight loss is the most significant symptom here
(I have to say from my own experience, weight loss has only come when the disease is at its worst and very obvious!)

• persisting severe restriction of lumbar flexion
(this is not ability to touch toes, because some people with no lumbar spine movement can do this, see below)

In Waddell's series of 900 patients this was the most important 'physical' sign. Here 50% of their patients with this sign had either serious spinal pathology or an acute disc prolapse. 70% of patients with spinal infection had it. But, flexion was normal in 30% with infection, 81% with inflammatory disease and 91% with spinal metastases. Spinal pathology can be present in the thoracic spine without any restriction of lumbar movement. REMEMBER THAT A NORMAL PHYSICAL EXAM DOES NOT EXCLUDE SERIOUS SPINAL PATHOLOGY. *(I have seen one patient in my career whose flexion was in this category. Unlike the majority of acute low back pains, whatever position this patient was put into flexion was still acutely painful and severely limited. Acute low backs may be very restricted standing, but often find curling up on their side or even curling up from all four's comfortable very relieving)*

• widespread neurology
(It is my opinion that neurological examinations are done very badly, avoided and done with poor technique and little interest. Sorry, you need heaps of practice or you'd fail with me as your examiner. It's one of the most reassuring things we can give to the patient and one of the most reassuring things for our own confidence. It's my opinion that knowing normal losses of reflex with ageing is important: loss of calf and triceps reflexes in the elderly seems fairly normal to me – nice research project for someone?)

• structural deformity
(this relates mainly to trauma in my experience, but occasionally to pathological fracture. Check age and general health)

• investigations when required: ESR >25mm *(think RA and polymyalgia)*; plain x-ray *(for vertebral collapse or bone destruction for example)*

So the whole idea of the notion of 'red flags' is to sort out (or triage) what's called 'simple back pain' from more serious disease, where medical investigation and input may be required. Simple back pain clearly shouldn't be medicalised and categorised as some kind of abnormality or 'disease'. Medical input here is ideally confined to pain control; then quick referral for the appropriate rehabilitation, where care is taken to deal with any important psychosocial factors, plus encouragement and guidance to keep going as much as possible and return to full function.

I agree, but I feel that the inclusion of all the other shopping basket compartments provides a bigger, better and more informed picture.

The 'red flag' literature relating to the low back not only delineates serious pathology as above, but also describes three other presentations: nerve root pain, cauda equine syndrome and spinal inflammatory disorders. The delineation is important because medicine does, or can have something to offer here, but not to the exclusion of good rehabilitative physiotherapy that embraces the shopping basket style of approach!

Here they are, again my comments in italics.

Nerve root pain:
(see the nerve root section of the red flag literature; to me this is very basic and written by those who haven't really listened to the patient. However, it is adequate for 'classic' sciatica!' i.e. for General Practice – the key is that for a Dr it helps them decide whether or not the patient is worth referring to a spinal surgeon. For us, knowing if a nerve root is involved tells us that progress is likely to be slower – see nerve root section of the book)

- unilateral leg pain greater than back pain

- pain generally radiates to foot or toes

- numbness and paraesthesia in the same distribution

- nerve irritation signs – reduced SLR which reproduces leg pain *(see nerve root section for more detail and discussion; for example, often, especially in the older sciatica, this sign isn't limited or only slightly. Distal symptoms provoked with extension can be more common)*

- motor, sensory or reflex change – limited to one nerve root.

Gordon Waddell in his excellent book, 'The Back Pain Revolution' adds the following points for sciatica:

'Give guarded positive messages' (p290 in my edition of the book):

- no cause for alarm, no sign of disease

- conservative treatment should suffice – but may take a month or two *(or 3 or 4 or 12...! see nerve root section of the book)*

- full recovery expected – but recurrence possible.

Cauda Equina syndrome:

- difficulty with micturition

- loss of anal sphincter tone or faecal incontinence

- saddle anaesthesia about the anus, perineum or genitals

- widespread (> one nerve root) or progressive motor weakness in the legs or gait disturbance.

Decreased or absent sensation in the peri-rectal region should be tested with pin-prick and light touch. Dulled or loss of sensation may occur in the buttocks and thigh regions too. Lack of voluntary contraction of the external anal sphincter is a positive sign.

These patients require urgent referral to a spinal surgeon. *(I have seen one case of these in my whole career, a physiotherapist who had been on a Brian Edward's 'Combined Movement Course'. The young girl was examined for purposes of demonstration and repeatedly but into a position of standing extension plus rotation plus side-flexion. At the time she felt pain in her back and both feet went numb. Within an hour or so her left leg went weak and numb and was giving way. She later became incontinent, though not permanently).*

Inflammatory disorders of the spine:
(Ankylosing spondylitis and related disorders)

- gradual onset before age 40 years

- marked morning stiffness

- persisting limitation of spinal movements in all directions

- peripheral joint involvement

- iritis, skin rashes (psoriasis), colitis, urethral discharge

- family history

Lastly here, for the sake of contrast, it's worth including '**simple mechanical backache**' as given by the low back pain guidelines (e.g. RCGP (2000) Clinical Guidelines for the Management of Acute Low Back Pain. Royal College of General Practitioners, London)

Note that the term 'mechanical' is used simply to indicate that the pain behaviour can be related to physical activity.

This is **simple backache**:

- onset generally age 20-55 years

- lumbo-sacral region, buttocks and thighs

- pain mechanical in nature – varies with physical activity – varies with time

- patient well.

I like the positive messages that Gordon Waddell lists:

- there is nothing to worry about

- backache is very common

- no sign of any serious damage or disease

- full recovery in days or weeks – but may vary

- no permanent weakness

- recurrence possible – but does not mean re-injury

- activity is helpful, too much rest is not

- hurting does not mean harm.

I would like to note the following:

> The most important information in all this comes from a careful clinical history. Never be bullied into 'doing the subjective in fifteen minutes and then getting on with the physical testing'. I never do anything until I've taken an adequate history. Interestingly, I know Geoff Maitland would be the same. In other words go on for however long it takes.

> A normal physical examination or x-ray does not exclude serious pathology. Routine spinal x-rays do not detect osteoporosis until there is 30% loss of bone mass; the most virulent disc infection may not show any x-ray change for several weeks. Metastases may take many months to show up on x-ray. A lateral x-ray of the lumbar spine will only detect a focal lesion when at least 50% of the cancellous bone is destroyed.

> The famous spine researcher, Alf Nachemson claims that if there are no red flags on careful clinical assessment then x-rays only detect significant spinal pathology once in 2,500 patients! He said 'There is a great risk that minor changes revealed on scans and x-rays are false-positive findings but that they drive clinical management. They can also make patients very upset – unnecessarily.

> THE KEY IS CAREFUL CLINICAL ASSESSMENT. In other words, don't get on with the 'physical' and 'treatment' until you have really listened and asked about potential red flags. Investigations supplement the decision made clinically.

In general day to day practice, the whole purpose of this material is to enable us to say with confidence to the patient that, 'There is nothing medically serious wrong with your back' and 'That medicine does not have a specific treatment to fix or mend your back, but it does have pain killers that do have their place.'

Some final points of importance:

1. In your head, always ask the question 'Does this patient and their problem require the things that Drs and specialists can offer?' However, a word of caution. There is a great danger that therapists send patients back to the Dr/specialist because they are 'treating' the patient with modalities and they're not getting anywhere with them. Sadly, the patient, who probably needs a more multidimensional perspective and approach over a longer time frame, is put back into the very system that perpetuates unnecessary and unhelpful 'medicalisation'. I believe that a great many therapists have a poor understanding of natural history and the time recovery sometimes takes. They treat their patients four or five times over a two to three week period. And when nothing much changes – they send them back to the Dr with a letter that says, sorry, unable to help. One of the worst offenders here was a hospital in Switzerland where I used to go and teach a couple of times a year. Patients with 'musculoskeletal' pain problems were brought in as 'in-patients' – with three weeks 'treatment' funded by their insurance companies. The hospital and all the clinicians involved had three weeks to work the miracle; then the money stopped and the patients were discharged! The end result was that patients had 'therapy' schedules that went on all day long. On the list were things like: various massages, hydrotherapy, exercise classes, manual therapist, masseuse, rheumatologist, drugs, injections, orthopaedics, injections and scans and x-rays and decisions about surgery. On and on, day in day out, for three weeks. You could almost hear the tills going after every session!

   When I went there to teach, they'd bring in these patients for me to assess and demonstrate with in front of the group. They were invariably chronic pain sufferers, but quite often nerve root problems, which hadn't a hope of getting better in the time let alone with all the treatments. Ghastly? Yes!

2. Sometimes referral to a specialist, for 'reassurance' that nothing is seriously wrong and that physiotherapy is the most appropriate management, can be very useful. You have to have a wise specialist though. If you made the mistake of referring a patient to a specialist in Switzerland, they'd more than likely be operated on the next day! (My observation!). If you want the specialist to say to the patient:

   'There's nothing seriously wrong. What you have isn't appropriate to anything I can do. Surgery is an absolute last resort and has no guarantees – keep going with the physiotherapist, do what they ask and be patient.'

   ... you have to get to know your specialists and be good at writing letters and asking them to do this for you. I've tried to educate some of my local specialists and they're a lot better than they used to be!

3. Remember inappropriate referral to a specialist can be a factor in making things worse.   Avoiding surgeons can save the patient from getting the 'bad degeneration' or similar 'structural' anomaly or diagnosis pointed out!

4. Remember too that just about all chronic pain problems we see have been subjected to many tests and often many procedures with little of significance found. More 'high-tech' screening, more referral and more biomedical intervention is likely to be ineffective and unproductive, keeping the patient in a futile 'find the cure' journey. These patients need rehabilitation, preferably CBT, in a pain management setting.

Chapter 4.4
Biomedical compartment part 3: Pain mechanisms

Pain mechanisms

In the mid to late 1990's when clinical reasoning was expanding to include 'pain mechanisms', it was all the rage to consider and categorise the patient into one of the following 'mechanism' brackets:

- nociception

- peripheral neurogenic

- central

- 'output' – sympathetic, parasympathetic, neuroendocrine, immune, emotional, motor...

On our taught courses we summarised the features of each, especially nociceptive, central and peripheral neurogenic. 'Output' – like altered mood state, emotional reactions, motor responses, pain behaviour, altered movement patterns, illness behaviour, sweating, blanching etc. were seen as consequences of the other pain mechanisms; but it was acknowledged that sympathetic output and changes in muscle tone could reflect back and influence the nociceptive/sensory system and thereby drive and exacerbate pain. We also recognised that low mood, anxiety and pain feed off one another.

It's interesting that the pain 'mechanisms' categorisation of pain, actually adds a 'processing' dimension for consideration that's unheard of in the traditional biomedical model. Think about it and you see that it would be helpful if general medicine also adopted a similar diagnostic reasoning pathway! Here's the Rehab or Pain consultant with our maladaptive pain behaviour patient, Mr Grubb.

'Ah, Mr Grubb, we've run all the 'tissue tests' now and found nothing to really explain the amount of pain you have. What we do know is that you have nothing seriously wrong with your muscles, bones, ligaments and nerves where you feel the pain, and all other systems in your body are healthy. What this means is that your symptoms are most likely to due to some kind of pain 'processing' problem. Think of it like a computer that's acting up a bit. (*This is one of my old ways of explaining pain to patients and I sometimes still use it*). Imagine pressing the X key on the computer keyboard three times – in normal processing you see three X's come up on the screen. Now, say the processor starts playing up a little and again you press the X key three times, but this time the X's come up in a really large font and just keep on scrolling down the page – that's a good way of thinking about the cause of your problem. Think of it simply as an electrical fault perhaps. We know that very similar things can happen for the processing of pain messages – they get 'amplified' and they can keep going and going all the time when it's absolutely of no use. Now, medicine has no simple fix for this, but the clever thing is that given the right inputs there's a lot that can be done to help. Your 'processing' system can improve. You need to see a good physiotherapist with pain management skills. What they get you to do will help your body to get fitter, move more normally and also may help to improve your pain processing systems. There's no guarantee that your pain processing will change, but there is a guarantee that you will be able to do more, feel more in control and feel a great deal fitter. What we've actually found is that patients who are successful with the pain management programme often do report their pain as being a lot less or that it's far more manageable and that they cope with it far better.'

If every referring consultant was like this, wouldn't it be more helpful!

Now back to a few problems with 'mechanisms' diagnoses.

One is that therapists and clinicians seem to love to 'label' and have management driven by that label, for example, the patient's got 'central mechanisms', which to me is just as bad as, 'it's a disc' or 'it's a sacroiliac joint' etc. Yes, this is a 'biomedical' section and that's what tends to happen when you think biomedically – there has to be a one issue label or diagnosis. Like, 'It's stress!' The plea is to think all-mechanisms-all-the-time, but that sometimes some or all of the mechanisms can become maladaptive. Think multi-mechanism/multidimensional and see what you come up with in all the various shopping basket compartments?

Let's take a look at how the features of '**central mechanisms**' were presented in the old days...

Here are the 'typical' features of 'central mechanisms' (I do like this list by the way. It's the interpretation that irks a bit).

1. A lack of consistency in symptoms – one minute they are high, the next low and for no apparent reason; one day good, then bad for days, again for no obvious reason. The weather gets the blame for example. Also the pain moves around, bad in the back one moment, later bad in the legs and then a headache. In the old manual therapy days we used to try to force these pains into some 'mechanically patterned' behaviour. If you ask the patient for long enough they'll always mention some physical activity that they _think_ promotes the pain – the ironing, the washing-up, making the bed, an awkward movement. The enlightened therapist finds, that yes, these things are often _associated_ with stirring the pain up but that it's _inconsistent_ and that's another feature worth noting.

2. Symptoms do not fit within the normal boundaries set out in physiotherapy and medical textbooks! At last an answer to all those 'annoying' patients I suffered in my early naive years during and after first training and later through all the manual therapy! The pain is all over the place and therefore 'impossible!' Make sure you read the discussion of Waddell's non-organic symptoms and signs from earlier and reflect on central mechanisms too – because this aberrant processing physiology does explain it much better than any other model. We have a biomedical and physiological explanation for crazy pain presentations. It's not from the tissues. It's from processing excesses!

3. So symptoms are often *weird* and unsettling, especially to the newly qualified and relatively naive therapists. Can you recall my fisherman patient who described his pain as a wire trace threaded round his scapula and that it felt like it was being constantly pulled one way then the other? That was extra weird. But there are a great many patients who have seemingly quite reasonable problems, but when you really enquire there's something about them that is odd and that doesn't fit with normal patterns and presentations. It's maybe the way the pain behaves for example. To feel comfortable with maladaptive central pain mechanisms and serious pathology presentations requires plenty of patient mileage.

4. Everything hurts! Also, there's often huge reactivity to harmless forces and movements. Every physical test you do, if you focus on the patient's pain response, hurts out of all proportion to the forces used. A massive amount of pain to movement related information can be gathered with some patients, in others their ranges of movement may be quite unrevealing.

5. Examine them today it'll be this, repeat tomorrow, it'll all have changed. Again, it's the inconsistency flag. Note though, if you were to ignore the pain response in those that hurt with every move, the feel of the joint movements, the range and everything else you care to test – are largely quite normal. Yes, normal, but you have to forget about the pain and just feel, move and watch the joint. That the movement can be tense and jerky is another aspect of this presentation.

6. So, a good thing to emphasise is the futility of 'going after' a particular fault in a particular tissue, or what might be called 'impairment-hunting'. What I've liked to call the 'if you look you will find' problem. These patients are full of little (probably on the verge of imaginary) impairment minutiae if you want to find them. Every test hurts; but knowledge of central mechanisms explains this and should drag us away from the tissues and the impairments to see a much bigger more important perspective.

7. Therefore therapists who are ignorant of central mechanisms and chronic pain presentations will 'find' a great deal and find it very difficult to unravel. The message is to steer well clear of testing tissues only; move up a level in the 'management hierarchy' to 'function and movement quality and then up again to psychosocial considerations.

8. Many of these patients suffer from lack of a clear physical diagnosis, or reasonable explanation, they feel rejected by the medical profession and a great many practitioners too. They are misunderstood and often feel neglected and angry as a result. 'No one believes me, they think I'm making it all up' is a common statement.

9. These patients have a great deal of 'baggage', just open up and listen to their past and current histories, the pressures and the emotions.

10. Their responses to standard treatments are predictably unpredictable! One time it's fantastic, you'll cure them; the next time they're in agony and they're filing a complaint.

11. Neurological testing can be difficult, but reflexes are easy and invariably normal for their age.

12. There are heaps of abnormal movement patterns, pain behaviour, fear avoidance etc.

13. The list could go on and on. The point is that the pain and pain behaviour are out of all proportion to any 'damage' or 'disease' process.

What's good is that pain mechanisms gives us a 'biomedical' explanation, albeit one that only considers neural or information processing. When the reality is that it encompasses all of our hierarchy of levels, from the lowly gene and its activity all the way through the psycho-social and on up to the wider environmental influences and factors. Thus, what irks me about the label 'central mechanisms', is it being used in a unidimensional way and without the word 'maladaptive' attached to it! My point is that 'central mechanisms' occur in all pain states—actually within less than seconds from onset—but are, for most of us, quite adaptive.

Another thing that irks me is the description of '**nociceptive**' and sometimes '**peripheral neurogenic**' mechanism when they're related to pain like this: 'Both nociceptive and peripherally evoked neurogenic symptoms have a familiar pattern presentation, with a predictable stimulus-response relationship, enabling consistent aggravating and easing factors to be quickly identified by the therapist.' I agree, but also strongly disagree – sorry. The following example and discussion illustrates why the statement I've just written: '...familiar pattern presentation, with predictable stimulus-response relationship, enabling consistent aggravating and easing factors to be quickly identified' – should be strongly challenged.

You may remember this from section 5? Case studies of amputees have demonstrated pain 'memories' of painful diabetic and decubitus ulcers, gangrene, corns, blisters, in-grown toe nails, cuts and deep tissue injury (Coderre et al 1993). Many pain presentations that are clear cut, mechanically patterned and have stimulus response consistency – can still have a clear maladaptive 'central mechanism'. I can think of many chronic sports injury type pains that are well past the normal healing time, yet still suffering high intensity precise mechanically patterned pain. These problems I am quite happy to deem to be of a maladaptive nature and most likely driven by maladaptive central mechanisms/engrained cell assemblies.

The big message from this 'central mechanism' categorisation is:

• that hurt does not mean harm and, like most things musculoskeletal, unless there's very severe damage or a surgeon demanding rest it's actually safe to start graded loading...and...

- to think about healing times and whether the presenting symptoms have gone on too long for the tissue healing, PLUS, whether the PAIN IS OUT OF PROPORTION TO THE DAMAGE DONE AND THE STAGE OF HEALING.

The **peripheral neurogenic** mechanisms and presentations are discussed in the nerve root section of the book and one tends to think that nerves are relatively rarely injured so that they cause upset in some way. I tend to agree, it's only an unfortunate few who get nerve root type pains and even fewer who get neuralgias stemming from peripheral nerve trunk injury. However, think about cutting the skin or straining anything, sensory nerve fibres and their terminals are highly likely to be torn, over-stretched and otherwise injured in some way.

Should we actually be assuming that some form of nerve injury is likely to play a part in most of the pain presentations we see? Maybe. The point though is does it matter much? As I discuss in the nerve root chapters of the book – pain/nociception deriving from injured nerves can be particularly pernicious and long lasting in some nerve pain prone individuals. It may therefore be one mechanism that explains why some relatively simple injuries end up becoming so intense, long lasting and resistant to treatment and rehabilitation. Consider the frequently very simple antecedents of complex regional pain syndrome? Often their story is of a simple knock on the skin evolving into a major pain syndrome.

Whatever the case is for now, the involvement of peripheral nerve in nociception is an arguable conjecture worthy of attention but not to the extent of getting too worked up about.

Nociception is what I used to call 'nerve end pain' because it derives from the mechanisms, discussed in earlier chapters, which drive the firing of sensory terminals in the injured tissues. Nociception relates to tissue injury, tissue inflammation, sensitisation and firing of nociceptors. Think adaptive, as in cut skin and sprains and strains and maladaptive. For example, too much inflammation going on, as in various rheumatoid conditions, including OA and degenerative changes. Remember, on-going inflammation is destructive. Explain this to patients and they become more willing to take NSAID's in a positive way.

So what are typical features of a nociceptive mechanism?

> Think classic acute pain – of injury or any musculoskeletal pain problem. But, and a big but, you need to know what has gone before. Could what you are seeing now be an old problem, an old central imprint that has merely rekindled? I can think of many 'acute' low back pains that were re-emergent old problems, precipitated by very minor physical acts that to me must have significant central representational components. Cell assemblies kicking off, which give the illusion of re-injury. Could that be possible? Well yes, but how do we know for sure? We really don't, but the forces involved in triggering it may be a clue and of course the question 'Is it safe to start loading?' is key – whatever the confusion about what might be going on. It is very rare that a spinal problem can't continue to be

loaded for fear of significant damage. Apart from the potential for nerve root damage of course.

Think typical healing pains and note the pain quality and behaviour, as the tissues transition from acute damage/weak/inflamed through to early repair to repair and remodelling. In the early stages, think constant ache with protective mechanically patterned sharp pains; also joint and tissue 'stiffness' feelings that make you go slowly with movements after rest; then as time goes on, the lessening of the constant symptoms to the more sharp and protective with near end range or over-loading. Note that the vast majority of normal healing pains improve with movement but that they also build up with excessive movement.

Morning stiffness is often used as a significant marker of inflammatory joint disease, as in the likes of Ankylosing Spondylitis, Rheumatoid arthritis, Polymyalgia, Psoriatic arthritis and even lowly osteoarthritis when joints are in an inflammatory phase. Common-or-garden strains and injuries also seem to show the same pattern, but significantly watered-down. *(Louis left a comment in the margin, 'What are common-or-garden strains that need watering down!' I think he was having a pop at his own language? Sorry, I couldn't delete it!).* Generally the stiffness frees from within a few minutes up to around a maximum of about thirty minutes. If I ever get patients who report significant morning stiffness for around an hour or more I'm suspicious of something more significant.

From the more benign presentations, think of acute sprained ankles, some acute low back pains and common muscle overstrains.

The classic symptoms of swelling, warmth and redness are sometimes obvious. Good responses to NSAID's can be quite helpful, but don't forget these drugs target the 'cycloxygenase' pathways in the arachidonic acid cascade (see section 15), they block prostaglandin formation for example; and prostaglandins are significant neurotransmitters in the brain. In other words, there's no such thing as a well localised drug! Just because an NSAID helped quell a patients pain doesn't 'prove' it was due to inflammation in the tissues, it could have influenced CNS processing. Damn!

My spin on this is that a nociceptive mechanism is always likely to be part of the symptom presentation. In chronic on-going pain states, think of the tissues as being fully healed but, that is likely to mean scar tissue; or, because they haven't used their musculoskeletal tissues normally for a long time, that they're deconditioned, weak and unfit. Review the 'vulnerable organism' (chapter GE 2.3) – when you're weak and low, you hurt more easily... normal afferent traffic from tissues, including a 'normal' nociception buzzing into the CNS will get access to consciousness far more easily and hence have the potential to cause pain. It's maybe that the chronic pain sufferers' central body monitoring system has become super-sensitised to listen to the tiniest of 'gripes' from the tissues. A bad and sad habit is one interpretation!

Finally in this biomedical overview, don't forget to ask yourself the simple question: are there any other interventions available that can help in the management and treatment of the presentation? Most chronic pain conditions require a multidimensional approach, which can include medical management, usually some form of pain control. But be cognisant that good pain management uses the medical part of the input to promote 'de-medicalisation' (see chapter 3.3) and if at all possible and where the patient is willing, they help the patients cut down or even completely come off all medication. Another goal for the patient is to make them more self reliant, to be able to work out what they need to do in flare-up phases, rather than continually go tearing off to the Dr's all the time.

A basic human drive is to feel and be in control; useful information helps patients to gain control, adapt to the situation and in so doing reduce uncertainty. It is through biomedical research that sound knowledge comes.

A major goal then is to **reassure**, you first, then the patient, that there is nothing seriously wrong with them!

Case history: Tanya, where some biomedical knowledge is helpful

Tanya is 47 years old. She fell off a stool at home while putting curtains up and fractured her right lower end of radius. The fracture was impacted. She was put in a plaster for five weeks after reduction of the fracture. She had a 'terrible time' with the plaster and had to take a great many pain killers due to the agonising pain. She had great difficulty sleeping.

It's now four weeks since the plaster was removed. Her hand is swollen, the skin is red and shiny and hot all the time. It is often sweaty. The wrist is deformed and has only one third of normal range in all directions and movements are horribly painful. She holds it up to ease the constant aching pain and says that the whole arm has become hypersensitive. She protects it all the time from being knocked. Light stroking of the skin causes horrid pain and a sudden reflex increase in tension. She is developing pain in the whole upper arm and her shoulder movements are stiffening.

Questions:

(These sorts of questions are typical of what I used to do in 'reasoning exercises' breaks in my courses. If you look at the questions many relate to what the patient would like to know too. I have to say that when I was a frustrated manual therapist, all those years ago, all I wanted was to be able to give much better answers to patient's questions about their condition. I gave absolutely crap answers then, but they're much better and more informed now. Thanks to reading a lot, the emergence of pain mechanisms and a great many good papers and studies that have been done.)

The following questions are included because to some degree they require biomedical knowledge.

List any contributing factors why is it going on so long?

1. High levels of distressing pain from the get-go. (This is a yellow flag, see next sections. But also think, high afferent barrage on an 'accepting' nervous system = maladaptive central neuroplasticity i.e. 'maladaptive central mechanisms' with big 'top-down' influences. For example, distress about the pain and the situation). This patient just wasn't given any adequate explanations; her complaints were basically seen as a nuisance and largely ignored.

2. She could be 'genetically' predisposed to high pain response? (See nerve root section).

3. Further yellow flag type issues are: poor sleep and poor coping, over-protective, fear-avoidant and poor early management – at the physical and the 'personal' level too.

4. We know the typical natural history of wrist fractures and sometimes, in a few unfortunate patients, they just do this sort of thing. This is an important statement for the patient to know. That fractured and immobilised wrists sometimes are very troublesome, while in plaster and afterwards. But, THEY DO GET BETTER!

What tissue mechanisms are operating?

There's likely to be a *maladaptive inflammatory response*. Think possible triple response, neurogenic inflammation, immune response may be excessive or not enough with lack of adaptive 'controlling' mechanisms. These patients typically don't respond to standard anti-inflammatory medications, even though they're pressured to keep taking them.

Oedema, increased tissue pressure, hence poor/altered interstitial circulation, circulation pooling and zones of hypoxia/ischaemia, or 'oxidative stress'. Likely to be high levels of oxygen free radicals (in animal studies the introduction of oxygen free radicals are known to produce oedema, increased skin temperature, impaired function and pain behaviour). Free radicals are pro-inflammatory and their excessive production may lead to destruction of healthy tissues. Of interest here is work by Veldman, who showed quite marked improvement in these sorts of patients using 'oxygen free radical scavenger' drugs. Vitamin C is a known scavenger. Veldman showed a marked prophylactic effect of it on post Colles fracture patients – reducing the incidence of post Colles fracture reflex sympathetic dystrophy (now it would be termed CRPS type 1) from 22% to 8%. (See Topical Issues in Pain 3 page 66-67).

What pain mechanisms are operating and is there a 'pain' diagnosis?

This presentation is classic early 'complex regional pain syndrome' – CRPS 1. In the bad old days the poor old sympathetic nervous system got the blame. Thankfully more broad reaching perspectives have emerged. It's now clear that contributions from all pain mechanisms have to be considered – there must be nociception going on, there must be huge afferent barrages from sensory fibres into the CNS. So, maladaptive central mechanisms are highly likely, at all processing levels, with plenty of downward 'facilitatory' currents too (Shane's family!) given the emotional state of the patient and their levels of concern (think worry/attention/pre-occupation/over-focus and so forth).

It doesn't look as if there's any frank nerve injury. Hence, the 'peripheral neurogenic' mechanism, while quite possible from minor nerve terminal trauma, is less likely to be operating in a more gross and obvious way. On the other hand, nerve branches in the area of oedema/inflammation may well be (must be?) affected by the chemical milieu. From the 'output' mechanism situation it is perfectly reasonable to assume that some sympathetic-nociception link is operating, but also immune control and neuroendocrine too. The bottom line is that 'maladaptive' processing is likely in all the categories all the time! It may be worth reviewing the 'Sympathetic' chapter earlier (section 12).

What are the sources of the problem?

To me this is almost a daft question, because as should be self evident from what I've just been discussing, sources are, local, proximal, central, emotional, attention, output – outer-space! You name it, it's from everywhere! The notion of finding a 'target' to treat in the biomedical sense is a nonsense; even if you could magically heal the wrist and give it back its full strength and range of movement it still may hurt horribly. Help with pain control and inflammation etc. is fine but usually in these patients little helps. In the old days these patients were often given a 'sympathetic block' using guanethidine. Mick Thacker and I reviewed the evidence for blocks in chapter 4 of Topical Issues in Pain 3 – the evidence is poor and these procedures seem to be rarely done these days in the UK. In my experience I have never seen a patient who has had a good outcome, sadly it's usually worse. But check the Blumberg's 'sympathetic-block' case histories in section 12, they may have some mileage! However, one wonders why a great deal more support for these interventions hasn't built over the years or been far more forthcoming, those Blumberg case histories were way back in 1994.

Is there anything seriously wrong?

No, even though it is agony. The pain is out of all proportion to the damage done.

A great many CRPS researchers are starting to use the term 'disorder', 'disease', 'impairment' or 'dysfunction' of the pain or nociceptive system. This may be helpful in that it's an indication of medicine shifting a little, but as far as the patient is concerned it could be quite disconcerting and worrying. You can imagine a Dr or consultant going: 'Sorry Tanya, you've got a disease of your pain processing system, there's nothing that can be done'. *(Louis, at the beginning of this chapter, makes a case for the referring consultant/Dr to talk 'processing' problem to the patient. But with Tanya he then acknowledges the difficulty of explaining pain processing and possibly doing more harm. Unfortunately I can't discuss this with Louis further. I suspect our conversation would have acknowledged that Mr Grubb's and Tanya's problems were at different stages in time and also the huge difficulty of changing all our perceptions about pain!).*

Do you have enough information to make a diagnosis?

Well, as I mentioned above, I would hope most clinicians when reading the case history would have been going this is common in my clinical experience. I've seen this before. It's CRPS like and it goes on for ages but gradually gets better. Also think, 'Quite often, the less physio fiddling and forcing the stuck stiff joints these patients have, the better they do!' They're ideal candidates, one would have thought, for the 'graded motor imagery' type of approach? Although, I have to say that I've had zero success with this and fear it misses the bigger more complex multidimensional picture!

Can you answer the following patient questions?

1. I was shocked when this happened to my arm. Why has it happened? I thought it would all be fixed when I came out of plaster?

2. Is it going to get better?

3. Why is it still swollen?

4. Why does it hurt so much when I put it down by my side?

5. Am I best to use it or rest it?

Mick and I wrote and discussed in Topical Issues in Pain 3, chapter 2 the potential mechanisms underlying complex regional pain syndrome – one of them was 'immobilisation and disuse'. In researching this I came across a paper by Butler, Nyman and Gordh (2000) titled, 'Immobility in volunteers transiently produces signs and symptoms of complex regional pain syndrome'. I also came across a paper by Ushida and Willis (1996) from the eighth World Congress in Pain. These researchers immobilised rat wrists in full flexion for three to four weeks – in some of them they broke the forearms before immobilising. Nice! The results showed, an increase in mechanosensitivity i.e. touch and movement allodynia, just like our patient here. The rats also showed central 'plastic' changes in the dorsal horn relevant to the immobilised areas. Even immobilisation for one week increased sensitivity to heat, cold and mechanical stimulation.

In the Butler et al (2000) human study twenty one normal volunteers had their wrists immobilised in plaster for four weeks. Here are some of the results:

- all subjects showed a temperature difference in the skin compared to the normal side. Ten showed an increase and eleven a decrease and the range of difference was between 0.5 and 2.7 degrees. In three of the subjects this persisted for longer than two weeks

- sixteen subjects had decreased range of movement of the thumb; twelve had altered sensation to sensory testing or whom four had summation to pin-prick – meaning that every time the subject was 'pricked' the sensation felt got more and more intense; another four however showed hyperalgesia – it was more painful than the same stimulus on the normal hand/wrist

- pain was present in seven; burning in two and aching in five

- eighteen reported stiffness and fourteen had symptoms of a 'neglect-like state'

- six subjects had abnormal sweating, seven had skin, hair or nail change and one had abnormal swelling

- there was a big variation in sensitivity to environmental temperature changes, some more and others less e.g. when cold, some had cold pain; two thirds showed a decrease in sensitivity to increased temperature, yet others showed an increased sensitivity – they detected warmth earlier

- some of the above changes lasted many weeks but most were back to normal by four to five weeks.

You may be wondering why I've put this in here and how they relate to those patient questions. Well it helps answer them. And its biomedical information at its best – telling us what happens to normals when they're immobilised.

So in answer to question 1: 'Why has this happened to me?' We can simply say that 'Unfortunately this happens quite commonly following a wrist fracture that's been kept in plaster for several weeks. The figure usually given is around one fifth of patients. There are two things: the break you had of the wrist creates an inflammation and a healing reaction that sometimes goes a bit over the top and secondly, the immobilisation you had to have. We know that if you put normal volunteers in plaster for a month, some of them will end up with symptoms just like yours – swelling, sensitive, hot, super-sensitive, stiff and so on.' So, NORMALISE IT!

Question 2: 'Is it going to get better?' Again, normalise it and give the patient a rough idea. 'Well, all those normal subjects who had their arms immobilised got better. Most took around four to five weeks but some a lot longer and they didn't even have a fracture! Now what's happened to you often gets seen by physiotherapists and in my experience they do get better but it takes time and patience. A rough guide is anything from three to four months to over a year – which is a bit of bad news but still good news too. The important thing is that your fracture has united well. It's not going to break; it's going to get gradually stronger and stronger, especially if you gradually start to use it. I'll help you and I'll show you what you can do and hopefully you'll start finding out what you can do to...' (and so on...)

Question 3: 'Why is it still swollen?' Again normalise it. Use the 'normals' experiment above; swelling is a normal part of healing; swelling also occurs in some people after immobilisation, some more than others etc.

I'm hoping you may remember the earlier discussion I had about the positive aspects of oedema. That it is the body's way of diluting vast concentrations of inflammatory chemicals and in a sense, detoxifying the environment? Cast immobilisation clearly prevents this; and keeps high concentrations of inflammatory chemicals in the damaged and surrounding area due to the pressure. This is not particularly healthy for the tissues and also not healthy for sensory processing, in that it'll keep it firing and thus have the potential to cause central plastic changes.

Question 4: 'Why does it hurt when I put my arm down by my side?' Again normalise it in terms of swelling and increased pressure on highly sensitised tissues. Getting relief putting your arm up and it being worse with the arm down is called the 'orthostatic' sign. You can tell the patient about this. And as time goes on, when you gradually bring the arm down repeatedly, the situation usually improves as it desensitises. A graded approach to desensitising is vital.

Question 5: 'Am I best to use it or rest it?' Think of it like this: 'Is it safe to start loading and moving?' The answer of course is yes and it's not just the tissues where the problem is. It's the general and local circulation; the whole arm and her body needs to get going. In fact, as anyone with any clinical experience will know, the more you fiddle with these wrists and insist on pushing the range of movement the more sore and aggravated they can become. Further pain modality treatments often make them worse too. It's all extreme allodynia, with potential for becoming chronic CRPS syndrome. So, a good answer to her question is that it needs both. But to start with the best thing is for her to get going. Hence a graded walking programme plus any regular home exercises like sit-stands, step-ups etc. – if willing to do.   From here, gradually move towards using and moving the arm, then getting the hand/forearm going – of course the order can vary and it can all be done at once. But the main message is movement and function is good for recovery; but keeping the pain high and nasty isn't, so a balance has to be sought.

I hope the reader noted that Tanya has plenty of yellow flags:

- high levels of pain and sensitivity, spread of pain

- distress

- bad experience with treatment

- behaviour towards resting, avoiding and protecting

- poor sleep

- time it's been going on and worsening situation

Yellow flags will be dealt with in more detail in the next chapter. I think it is worthwhile having another case history!

Case history 2: Roy, where some biomedical knowledge is also helpful!

Roy is 69 and not very fit. His right knee has been troubling him for about a year. It's worse in the last three months. He's been getting more discomfort, more stiffness and finding it harder to get going in the morning and after sitting. He says he can't get comfortable in bed and that it often aches all the time. He gets sharp pains if he does awkward movements or quick movements. Sometimes the knee feels swollen.

Physical examination reveals a moderate varus deformity (slightly 'bandy'), loss of full extension and about six inch 'heel to buttock' loss of flexion. There is a modest effusion. If you look at the knee it is obviously 'degenerate,' it looks like a typical OA joint.

The Dr has had an x-ray taken and told him its 'wear and tear'.

Possible Questions:

1. What's the syndrome/presentation or diagnosis?

2. What tissue mechanisms? Adaptive or Maladaptive?

3. Pain mechanisms? Adaptive of Maladaptive?

4. Patient questions:

- Have I got arthritis?

- Is there anything you can do, or should I see a surgeon?

- What are osteophytes?

The first question: **What's the syndrome/presentation or diagnosis?** If Roy hadn't already been to a Dr or specialist and he'd asked me what was wrong and I would have said something like this:

'Roy, if you took your knee to a knee specialist he would probably give you the diagnosis of 'wear and tear'. What he really means is you've got what's often called 'degenerative joint disease, or osteoarthritis but they don't like to use these terms for fear of frightening patients into thinking they've got some ghastly disease. It's their way of trying to stop the patient leaving the consultation imagining walking sticks and wheelchairs. All the terms mean the same thing.' I continue.

'We think 'wear and tear' is a bad phrase too because it makes you imagine that the more you use it the more it wears away, when in fact good use and keeping fit has been shown time and again in trials to help in keeping the joint healthy. While rest is fine, too much is not; your muscles go weak, the joint stiffens even more, you get generally unfit and the knee structures become deconditioned. So, even a degenerative joint needs and benefits from movement.'

Let me show you some pictures of bad arthritis which are actually are attached to very active patients. The first one I call 'the lady who walks the cliffs' (figure 4.5) and the second I call 'Mr Tombstone' because he makes gravestones,' (figure 4.6).

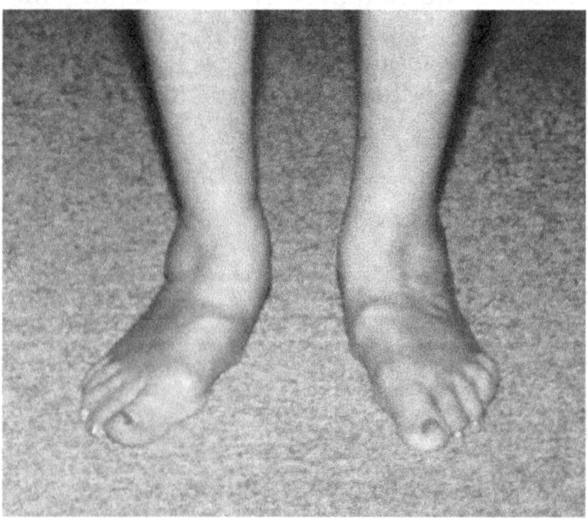

Figure GE 4.5 'The lady who walks the cliffs'

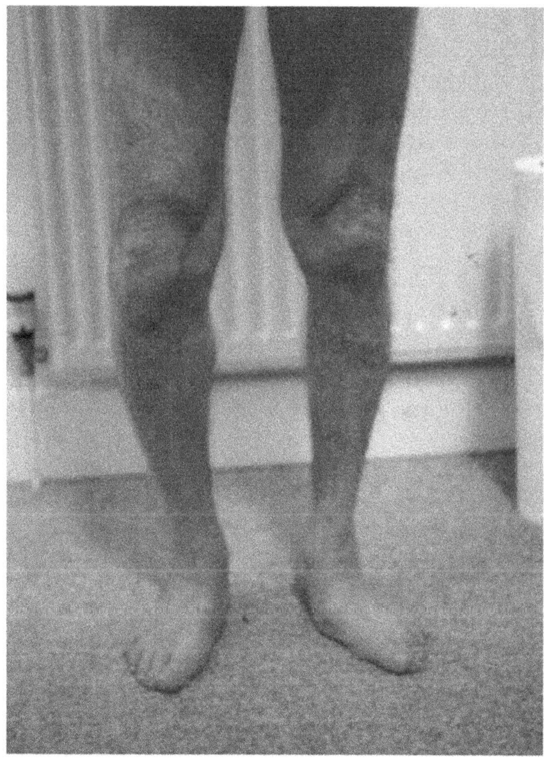

Figure GE 4.6 Mr 'Tombstone'

I then discuss the obvious OA in the feet, the collapsed feet, the bent (varus) shape of Mr T's right knee etc. and relate their fairly simple presentations, but particularly how active they both are. I also tell Roy that the 'cliff walking' lady came in for a hip problem – not a foot. 'Mr Tombstone' for a neck and shoulder problem and that he'd, in passing, asked my opinion about his right knee and feet! These are two examples of 'glorious' wear and tear that haven't stopped functioning. You could take pictures of arthritic hands and do exactly the same; you could have a set of spinal x-rays with marked degenerative changes from patients who are very active – remember Wallace who did his 1000+ exercises reps per day?

In this little discussion with the patient hopefully I've answered his first question, 'Have I got arthritis?' With the introduction of the yellow flags one of the categories that we are alerted to is the 'A' or 'Attitude and Beliefs' of the patient with regards to their problem (see following chapters). What the patient understands about their problem certainly impacts how they organise their life and respond to physical challenges. However, it seems that diagnostic honesty has been avoided for fear of giving the patient the wrong message, or more correctly a message that has the potential to create fear and avoidance and a great deal of anxiety. For example, this response: 'Arthritis means I'm going to get worse and worse and become a burden and a cripple' – which is also an example of catastrophic thinking. This information can be detrimental and disabling to some patients. When a patient comes to me, via Drs and consultants, saying things like 'I've got arthritis, I don't walk more than fifty to a hundred yards,' or 'I limit the number of times I go up and down the stairs to save my knee' – it's clearly unhelpful. I also had this once from a patient who had neck pain: 'My physio told me that my upper two cervical vertebrae are unstable.' This lady hadn't turned her neck more than 10 degrees right or left for over two years. What was meant by 'instability' I have no idea, but it certainly stopped normal 'thoughtless-fearless-movement' in a neck that should have been perfectly capable of it and was eventually!

For me, I prefer diagnostic honesty, so long as it is not given in an isolated way that leaves the patient with concerns and fears, or has the potential too. For this reason I spend ample time making the situation clear and the potential, realistic, future and then get on with practicing what I preach – which is action and therefore getting the best function possible with the least amount of fear.

Let's now review the patient question: 'What are osteophytes?'

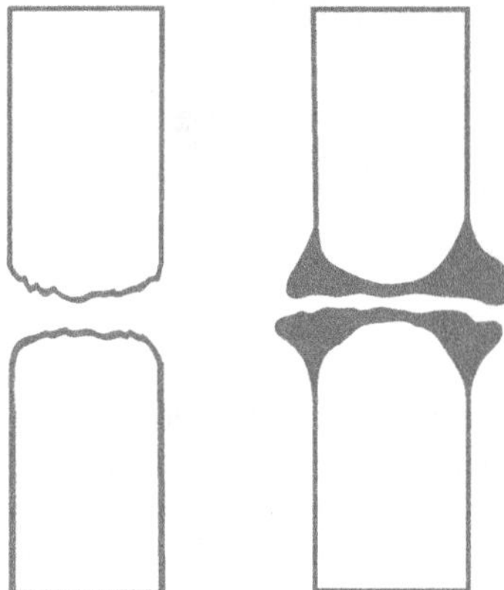

Figure GE 4.7 Schematic figures of a normal knee and an OA Knee

Well, medicine sees osteophytes as a sign of disease but a biologist sees them as a remarkable attempt by the body to adapt to changing circumstances. Think like this and draw diagrams as you explain. See my crude figure of a knee (figure 4.7) and note that in the left joint the femur surface is normal, with normal nice thick cartilage on the joint surface. On the right the tibia's cartilage is thinner and rougher, typical of a joint with degenerative changes going on. Now, because the weight bearing cartilage is thinner it seems that the joint becomes aware of this and in response attempts to spread the load. So, the bone grows out sideways to make the weight-bearing surface a bit bigger – similar to the way osteophytes grow out in the spine to support and stabilise an ageing and bulging disc. In both cases the ultimate outcome is a stiffening of the joint. This is NORMAL. But as we all know, it's good to maintain fitness of the joint by moving it and nicely stretching at comfortable joint limits to prevent further stiffening and keep the joint as healthy and functional as possible. It's also good to maintain strength as 'the lady who walks the cliff' and 'Mr Tombstone' do – by carrying on and being normally active over the years.

So Roy gets to understand what osteophytes are and why his right knee is larger and slightly mis-shapen, very much like Mr Tombstones. It's easy to tell Roy that degenerate knees change their shape, some bowing out (varus) other peoples going knock knees (valgus).

Let's now follow on from this with his question: **'Is there anything you can do or should I see a surgeon?'**

Roy is not very fit but he does 'potter' in the garden, often kneeling and bending to weed and plant. He can get out of a chair easily and once warmed up after a few steps walks reasonably well. Here's what I say to him:

'You could well see a surgeon and get their perspective on your knee. Surgeons tend to do joint replacements for your sort of problem. My experience, with our local ones, is that they'd probably say, get a bit fitter, keep going and let's review it if you get to the stage where you're really starting to struggle.'

I 'm aware that some surgeons in private health might operate straight away though and I say this to Roy, 'If you were in Switzerland or the USA, they'd of probably operated on it already! But I'm going to give you my spin on this, from the angle of 'If I had what you have and with my knowledge what would I do?'

'Well, I know that if you had a knee replacement you'd lose range of movement, something that most patients don't realise, in fact they mostly expect that a 'new knee joint' will give them full range back. Your knee bending at the moment is pretty good and may even improve with some exercise. The vast majority of knee replacements end up with less than or around 90 degrees of knee bend.' (Note, this is a good 'follow-up' research project for someone?)

I show him on me what 90 degrees of bend is and get him to bend to the same.

'Do you see what I mean? When you lose what you have it makes kneeling and bending down a bit more difficult and most folks after they have had a knee replacement tend to avoid it. Some do manage but often not until a good year after the operation.'

'OK, that's one thing, the other is that your joint could be a lot fitter and so could you. As explained earlier, fitter people keep going with their grumpy joints very well – sometimes with awful osteoarthritis. A big thing about OA is that the symptoms tend to come and go. For example, it can be bad for several months then ease up for months and it can go on in this pattern for a number of years. Some find that the joint eventually stops doing this cycling from sore to OK and a bit stiff and it ends up being OK, just feeling stiff when they first move it.'

'Take a look at this fellow's knee (figure 4.8). He's an old rugby player, who had lots of ligament repair operations in his playing days. As you can see it's not only got a pile of scars it's also very arthritic. As a result the knee is a ghastly shape but he walks on it fine and it doesn't worry him.'

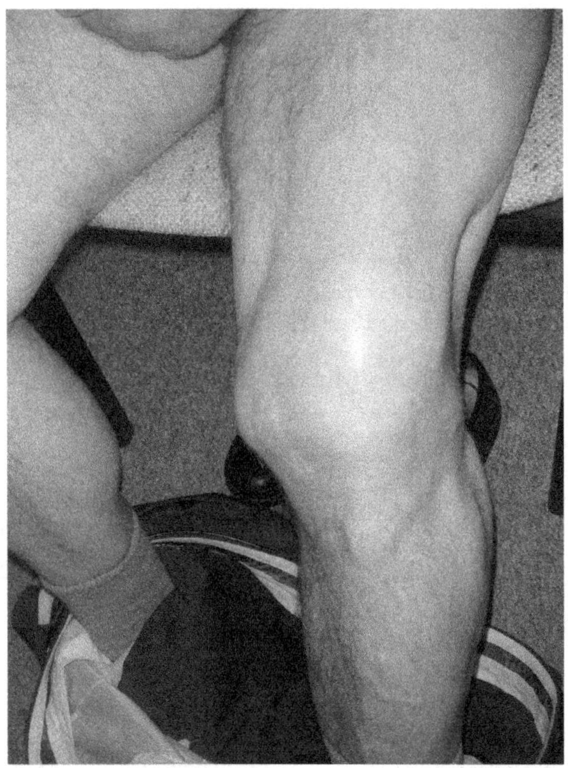

Figure GE 4.8 An 'old rugby knee'

'So, if I were you, come with me for a few treatments while I show you what you can do to help your knee. If you're keen, I'll get you going, monitor you for a while and see if you can't get a great deal better and fitter than you are now. Many do, but if you get fed up with it the consultant surgeon is always an option. But remember this, the fitter you are and your knee is when you go for an operation, the better the result and the more you will enjoy it afterwards.'

What about the questions about tissue mechanisms? The classic answer would be, tissue: possible chronic inflammation (maladaptive or adaptive?) and thoughts about contracted collagen and so forth... What about pain mechanisms? What's the classic answer? 'Nociception' but be careful, recall that in patients with arthritic joints, who subsequently have an amputation – subsequent phantom arthritic pains and stiffness exactly mimicking what they had before were commonplace.

A word about 'output' mechanisms – in case you're thinking I've forgotten them. The word is YES! (They are there in every pain problem, every time. What is there, is massively complicated and expressed by all the systems. The outputs to get a handle on are:

- movement patterns – pain behaviour

- thoughts and feelings about the situation

- levels of pain

- 'sympathetic' is far more difficult but has to be going on in all injuries, disorders and pain states of the musculoskeletal system
(CRPS is where some assumptions about the system can be made because we see changes in circulation and swelling for example. The best thing is to think about the optimal conditions required for recovery and healing and not to get tied up with such a reductionist perspective. See the appropriate chapters earlier in the book).

Chapter 4.5
Psychosocial compartment part 1: Introduction and overview

Must read book chapters:

Watson, P. (2013). Psychosocial predictors of outcome from low back pain. In Gifford L (Ed) Topical Issues in Pain 2. Biopsychosocial assessment and management. Relationships and pain. CNS Press, Falmouth: 85-109.

Watson, P. and N. Kendall (2013). Assessing psychosocial yellow flags. In Gifford L (Ed) Topical Issues in Pain 2. Biopsychosocial assessment and management. Relationships and pain. CNS Press, Falmouth: 111-129.

Kendall, N. and P. Watson (2013). Identifying psychosocial yellow flags and modifying management. In Gifford L (Ed) Topical Issues in Pain 2. Biopsychosocial assessment and management. Relationships and pain. CNS Press, Falmouth: 131-139.

Main, C.J. and P.J. Watson (2013). The distressed and angry low back pain patient. In: Gifford L (Ed) Topical Issues in Pain 3. Sympathetic nervous system and pain. Pain management. Clinical effectiveness. CNS Press, Falmouth: 177-204.

Main, C. J., C. C. Spanswick, et al. (2000). Wider applications of the principles of pain management in health-care settings. Pain Management. an interdisciplinary approach. C.J. Main and C. C. Spanswick. Edinburgh, Churchill Livingstone: 389-401.

Waddell, G. (2004). The Back Pain Revolution. 2nd Edition. Edinburgh, Churchill Livingstone.

Linton, S. J. (2005). Understanding pain for better clinical practice. A psychological perspective. Edinburgh, Elsevier.

Main, C. J. and C. C. Spanswick (2000). Pain Management. An interdisciplinary approach. Edinburgh, Churchill Livingstone.

Introduction

The evidence for the importance of psychosocial factors, in influencing the course of acute pain into chronic pain and pain related incapacity, is now so strong that if you are not aware of it or have not learnt how to incorporate it into practice, then unfortunately you'd fail my fit-to-practice exam! I hope you passed the 'Red Flag' exam earlier?

Powerfully, prediction of outcome is governed far more by psychosocial factors than any biomedical factors. That means a scan, with awful degenerative changes and disc bulges, does not predict that the patient who owns it will inevitably become disabled and in a wheelchair! We all know the patients who tell you, 'I saw the specialist, he took one look at my x-rays said I'd be in a wheelchair by the time I was fifty.' Pleasingly these days such harsh pronouncements are rare to hear but in the early 1980's, when I first qualified, they were commonplace. Even so, a great many patients remain confused, concerned and even unnecessarily disabled by what they have been told by clinicians.

Think about your own and your colleagues, current attitude to 'psychosocial' factors in dealing with patients as well as the goals of your practice:

With regards to 'pyschosocial': is it something like, 'I do all that anyway, I'm nice to my patients and I listen to them. I'm empathic. I explain about their problem and the therapy and try to motivate the patient?' Or maybe it's a bit more like this: 'I've been seeing patients for years and can tell a 'psychological overlay' type patient immediately.'

The first isn't too bad but the second is a ghastly example of the type of Cartesian reasoning and attitude that can be so ingrained when clinicians are schooled in a purely biomedical perspective. It's like the common belief that 'tissue and mechanical pain is true pain, other types of pain are psychological'. The therapist in effect blames the patient for their situation and for any non-compliance or non-responsiveness to treatment.

For many years, in my early manual therapy days, we all misinterpreted patient's pain-related distress, their on-going pain behaviour and high complaints about their pain, as physical signs of something bad and often something to be feared ourselves. Since the only tools we had were physical techniques we promptly went about finding clever ways of squeezing their presentations into some kind of joint problem, to which we could gently drive our fingers in to try and change it all. Regardless of any squealing from diehard manual therapists – the approach blatantly failed and continues to do so. Yes, the truth is that Geoff Maitland, brilliant manual therapist though he was, failed to help a great many of the chronic on-going pain patients in his clinic. I watched week in and week out for nearly two years. Remember my statement to Philippa, after coming home one day after work in Geoff's practice. I was disillusioned, dissatisfied and burnt-out. I said to her, *I reckon I've helped 5% of the patients 1% this month*. Why was that? Simple, the patients were complex chronic pain patients and manual therapy was a totally inappropriate form of management for them and I knew it. We know now from a great deal of research, that continuing to receive passive forms of therapy may actually be maintaining and reinforcing the problem.

The manual/musculoskeletal therapy gurus of the world annoy me for their lack of honesty in being open about their failing to help complex pain problems and more. They leave the audience thinking that the treatment they do helps, if not cures, every patient they see. It's just not true. I'll never forget seeing an Australian guru, on stage at a UK conference, telling a patient she'd just reviewed and treated on stage with a bit of tape across her back that she'd do well to come out to Australia to see her. I wished I'd stood up and shouted, 'Stay here love, it's safer, it's free and it's better.' My blood boiled and it still can if I let it! Why is it we worship 'treatment' based charisma that washes over us from overseas so much? I wonder that some of these invitees see us as some kind of therapy third world that's in need of educational development aid of some kind? *(Louis acknowledged that he was 'having a bit of a rant! Again! I hope the reader also remembers that Geoff Maitland was a huge influence, for his listening and communication genius. Something Louis respected and was thankful to have learnt from)*

Thankfully it was here in the UK in the mid to late 1990's that physiotherapy began to take on and grasp the multidimensionality of pain by instigating psychosocial yellow flag assessments. I'm going to be blunt. The UK is and has been ahead of the game for a number of years. I wish we'd stop inviting overseas celebrity physiotherapists here to tell us all about what we already know and actually started. We have the expertise here, quiet, confident and highly skilled; let us look under our own blankets and sniff them all out again, a good few are nicely matured now but a good few are young, highly experienced and perceptively brilliant clinicians and teachers. The pain revolution needs a practical and clinical revival.

Take a patient and send him or her to standard musculoskeletal therapists for assessment. Let's say we have three patients to send to our three favourite musculoskeletal therapies: the first one is sent to the Mckenzie therapist, the second to a Maitland and the third to a muscle imbalance therapist.

Then take the same three patients and send them to the high-street 'shopping basket' approach type therapists (kidding!). What I mean is to therapists who always do a thorough psychosocial appraisal as part of their work-up on the patient (like all good shopping basket therapists would!).

After the examination the patients are followed up and the therapists are given two questions. Here are the questions:

1. What criteria did/would you use to assess your outcomes?

2. Can you tell whether the patient you saw is going to recover quickly, get back to activity and return to work or become a chronic pain patient?

For the first question, the three guru/tissue based therapists in order are likely to go: 'The centralising and lessening of the pain with repeated movement; the lessening of the pain with x,y and z movements following the mobilisation technique; the improvement in muscle control over a certain range of movement that I taught them to do. And they all go: 'Also, the patient reporting they're feeling better and doing a bit more.' (Although my experience of Maitland is that we used to tell patients to avoid doing more in case they messed up what we'd achieved in treatment!)

Now like it or not, the dominant thing in the head of these first three approaches is a 'clinician-orientated' outcome; the clinician seeing better range and less pain or better quality of movement in relation to what they did to the patient in the treatment session.

Any therapist who incorporates a psychosocial appraisal will tend to have a broader based view of outcome – often being far more sided with a patient-orientated one. They'll have asked the patient what would be their goals from physiotherapy? Answer: getting a reduction in pain and also, a return to function and work. I never used to dream of asking what the patient wanted from me! But for the last fifteen years I have.

The second question now:
The Mckenzie therapist might say, 'They're going to do fine, the pain centralised very well.'
Maitland will go, 'I will be able to tell after seeing how they respond over the next one or two treatments.'
The muscle imbalance therapist might go: 'They're picking it up quickly, should be fine soon...'

Those with psychosocial yellow flag training will go:
'The first patient (who's already seen the McKenzie patient) has high levels of distress about their pain. They've become locked into a very anxious posture and movement pattern and are fearful of doing anything that will make the pain worse, particularly bending. They are actually scoring quite highly on pain/activity avoidance and there are some significantly low scores in relation to work satisfaction. Unfortunately, they're also scoring very highly on the catastophising question and they're not at all confident they'll be back to work in the next six months. So in answer to your question, this patient is at quite high risk of becoming chronically incapacitated. And of course, the second and third patients could well be similar without the slightest jot of awareness from the clinician involved.

The incredible thing is that we now have the tools to be able to predict whether a patient with acute and sub-acute pain—particularly those with low back pain—are going to have a bad or good outcome. Not only that, if the appropriate interventions are used early on with patients who are deemed 'at risk' of doing poorly – they can be prevented from doing so.

I want you to review the chapters and books above, but what follows is a very brief overview of the important 'predictors of poor outcome'. I'll then go through the ABCDEFW yellow flags and how to go about questioning in the clinical situation.

Factors predicting outcome:

See Paul Watson's chapter...

Watson, P. (2013). Psychosocial predictors of outcome from low back pain. In: Gifford LS (Ed) Topical Issues in Pain 2. Biopsychosocial assessment and management. Relationships and pain. CNS Press, Falmouth: 85-109.

What follows is a simple overview plus a bit of my spin and comments from Paul Watson's material. Thanks to Paul who was chairman of the UK Physiotherapy Pain Association from 1999 to around 2002.

Pain report: intensity of pain

If a patient reports high levels of pain in the acute stage of their condition and this is combined with high disability levels – this predicts a poor outcome and a likely delayed return to work. In the Gatchel et al (1995) study that revealed this they also found that physical examination variables did not help predict the rate of return to work. As Paul Watson points out though, not all studies support this. In other words, there are people who have high levels of pain who show marked pain behaviour at the time but who do get going and get back to work. For us, the main point is that if patients early on report very high levels of pain it's important to get them to understand why pain control can be helpful. Remember the 'pain killers only mask the problem' fallacy/misunderstanding that I argued in an earlier chapter 15.4? If it's safe to start loading, try to get the level of pain to a level where the patient is happy to get going! Pain control will be addressed at length in the 'Pain compartment' chapter.

Pain report: site and radiation of pain

Distribution of back pain, especially into the leg has been shown to relate to poor outcome. The greater the spread of the pain, if we think in terms of 'central mechanisms' and expanding receptive fields, makes this fit of course.

However, a thought and finding that brings caution. Paul Watson, in his research noted a slower return to work of patients given the diagnosis of 'sciatica', nerve pain, 'nerve root' pain or disc. So it may not so much be the extent of the pain but more the notion of what the pain means to the patient. 'Ah, nerve pain, that takes ages.'

Initial self report of disability:

Pretty obvious really: those who report the highest levels of disability have the furthest to go to recover. Self reported disability is one of the strongest predictors of a poor outcome, especially in the sub-acute/sub-chronic groups. The big thing is, if a patient comes to you who has had their problem for more than a few weeks and is still disabled and inactive – they are very likely to do less well. Shift the focus from the usual impairment based fiddling flim-flam to graded activity increases is the big message here.

It is paramount for the therapist to enquire about work – postures, positions, movements, mechanical stresses as well as the ability to have some control over how and what they do too. Concerns here can be addressed with appropriate (graded) practice in the clinical setting and at home.

Beliefs and coping as predictors:

As Paul says, everyone who has a pain or injury of some kind will have tried to make sense of it, labelling it and giving it a meaning. Tip: ask the patient what they understand is wrong and also what they've been told by others is wrong? And, what it all means to them too?

Paul sees three issues of importance here:

- specific beliefs about back pain and treatment e.g. 'My disc is out and needs putting back,' or 'A nerve is trapped and needs freeing' are common and often frustrating 'lay' beliefs

- fears regarding hurting and harming or 'fear-avoidance' beliefs

- coping styles/strategies

Clearly beliefs about the 'back' problem that are very structural and relate to 'out' or 'weakness' or 'wear and tear' can lead patients to avoidant type behaviours and passive coping styles. As discussed in earlier chapters this often leads to decreased activity, the preference for rest, leading to deconditioning etc.

Lets overview each of the three above:

Specific beliefs about back pain and treatment

Many patients develop pessimistic beliefs about the value of various treatments, about diagnoses, as well as about their outcome and their likely response to any treatment. These patients often let pain be their guide and some may link levels of pain to levels of harm. The reader should review Main, Watson and Spanswick's model in chapter GE 2.6.

Clinically, the main thing is that we need to know about the patient's beliefs here and we need to feel comfortable to be able to ask them.

Beliefs about the extent to which pain can be controlled appear to be a powerful determinant of the development of incapacity and *likely compliance with an activity based treatment programme.*

Recall from the locus of control discussion earlier, those with an 'external' locus of control are less willing to take responsibility in the management of their problem and often feel they are unable to have much/any influence on their own symptoms. These patients are often poor at compliance, give up easily, are not good at self-management and easily get frustrated. They need a lot of help to keep on track and have a tendency to 'need' therapy. While that may be fine for a while, what they really 'need' is to learn how to cope better and in so doing learn that they can manage and do well on their own. They 'need' to be guided to 'not-need' therapy. Clearly patients who may be easily labelled as having an external locus of control aren't doomed to stay there. With good management, a great many can be shifted to a more active coping style and to having a more 'internal' locus of control. Active, paced, goal orientated, self-management/CBT approaches are essential here.

Give a chronic pain-disabled patient a choice between going to an 'active' and self management orientated programme, or going to a 'therapist' for treatment are most likely to choose the therapist. Why? Because they 'do' something and the 'active' programme, they know will make them worse. They've tried to exercise. They've done all that and it's a waste of time.

As a clinician, who loves to help patients help themselves, a patient who has an internal locus of control is a joy. 'Hi Louis, what I want to know from you is... what's wrong with me... how long to get better... what do I do to help it...? And if there's anything you can do, is it worth it, or will it just get better anyway – no offence about the value of your fancy treatments?' Lovely, you're just like me!

What's been brilliant is that studies looking at beliefs about back pain have shown that when simple information pamphlets are given that challenge negative beliefs and support self management – there is less sick-leave, a reduction in negative beliefs about back pain and a positive shift in pain locus of control towards being internalised.

Paul Watson firmly states:

> *'People with back pain will do better if they believe that they have a role in managing their condition. Those who rely heavily on professional help risk becoming dependent on the physiotherapist. The over medicalisation of back pain, identification of spurious derangements and encouraging the patient to see the physiotherapists' 'hands on interventions' as the most powerful factor for improvement, all remove the sense of control from the patient. Empowerment of the patients' role in their own management would seem vital'.*

Fear avoidance beliefs

This has already been dealt with in the Fear-avoidance model chapter.

Patient's fears about pain and harm with movement and activity need assessing and then managing. As Paul puts it:

> *'By exposing the patient to the fear (exercise) in a graded and controlled way (a graded exercise programme) in a safe environment (the clinic) the therapist can help to desensitise the patient and then transfer these successes into the home and work environment. **This is potentially one of the most powerful effects of contact with a physiotherapist.***

People who are very fearful that activity is going to cause them pain and injury are likely to report more pain, be more disabled, have a history of prolonged work loss, and are more likely to remain off work and remain disabled.'

Paul and colleague Heather Muncey (Heather started the Physiotherapy Pain Association way back in 1994) noted strong correlations between patients with high scores of fear-avoidance beliefs and their levels of reported pain. Further, patients who still believed that activity was to be avoided or was structurally damaging had higher reports of pain after a pain management programme. Reduction in fear-avoidance led to reduced disability and was far more important than measures of depression or initial pain.

Pain Coping Styles and Strategies

This has been covered to some extent already. Psychologists often use the terms 'adaptive' and 'maladaptive' coping styles. Examples of 'adaptive' coping are being active, taking exercise, ignoring and functioning despite the pain and taking responsibility for pain management – in other words those with an 'internal' locus of control.

Paul quotes Jensen et al 1991:

'Patients who believe they can control their pain, who avoid catastrophising about their condition, and who believe they are not severely disabled appear to function better than those who do not. Such beliefs may mediate some of the relationship between pain severity and adjustment.'

'Maladaptive' styles of coping are 'passive' – the classic phrase that comes up is 'hoping and praying' it'll get better. 'Passive coping' includes the combination of avoidant/rest, high levels of medication and on-going use of supports, aids and therapists. All are predictive of a poor outcome.

A big deal in our clinic is 'optimism' about outcome; getting better and back to activity and work. Hence our 'BO', not body-odour but BELIEF AND OPTIMISM, little joke! What's in your head about the situation you are in can be a self-fulfilling prophesy.

Psychological Distress

The instinctive immediate emotions linked to pain are: anger, fear and anxiety/ concern. If you've ever bashed your head on a low door frame you'll know what I mean! Instant anger, pain doesn't do your mood state much good either, especially if someone laughs at you. Although soon seeing the funny side of it eventually helps a lot. Note that good therapists often have a great sense of 'appropriate' humour laced with infectious optimism. Have you ever noticed that when you're having an 'off' day everyone comes in worse? Someone should research that?

I've already discussed in the Vulnerable Organism chapter – about the sickness response and low mood, when you hurt it's a threat to homeostasis. Any threat to homeostasis drives appropriate energy saving behaviour and low mood is a useful way of making us not want to do anything! Also don't forget, the nice little phrase: 'when you're low you hurt more easily'. Or this: 'on-going pain runs your batteries down, depletes you're resources, your coping capacity bottoms out. Sometimes the stress graph (chapter GE 2.3 figure 2.3) can help.

Another way of looking at it is that anything unpleasant pisses most people off and if it goes on long enough dysphoric mood states, even clinical depression can result. Failed treatment doesn't help either.

So for psychological distress, think:

- exaggerated attention to bodily symptoms (boredom from doing nothing may be a factor worth considering here)

- anxiety

- anger

- the development of depression

Right: depression is not 'our' area, if you're a wannabe psychologist be careful. The best thing is to recognise when you're out of your depth and make an appropriate referral. Some therapists can't even deal with a patient bursting into tears. I guess we're all on a spectrum here. It doesn't bother me. I can understand it, especially those who are still angry. 'That bastard who hit me from behind yelled at me, went on about his f.....g Audi bumper and grill, didn't have the courtesy to say a little word called 'sorry'... Bastard..!'

Some of the common terms associated with low mood are: feelings of *hopelessness and helplessness*, or 'learned helplessness', the 'learned' habit of doing nothing and feeling useless, withdrawing from participation. Often feelings of 'What's the point?'...'I'm a burden to the family'...'I'm a sick person now I've come to accept it'...'I can see I'm dependent on those around me'... 'I can't be bothered anymore.'

Another term is '*somatic anxiety*' – the preoccupation with bodily symptoms. As discussed in earlier chapters, it's well worth spending a moment doing a slow scan round your body to see what's going on; feet pins and needly feeling, odd little pressure ache round the knee, achy sensation in my hips, funny lower abdominal tightness, shoulders feel weird, maybe a sniff of a headache, just a bit between the ears. Oh, heart's pounding.

Please read the 'Emotions' chapter 11 in Waddell's book. Make sure you read about the 'Distress and Risk Assessment Method (DRAM) – a combination of two questionnaires, the well-known Modified 'Zung' for depression and the 'Modified Somatic Perception Questionnaire (MSPQ). The combination was originally developed by the very affable psychologist Chris Main and is easy to administer and a good predictor of treatment interventions. I wished I'd used this when I was at Geoff Maitland's but that was a little too early. Chris Main actually published the MSPQ in 1983, but I was on a different planet then!

The two questionnaires categorise the patient into four: 'DD' – for distressed and depressed; 'DS' – for depressed and somatically anxious. 'R' for those who were classified as at risk and 'N' were those at low risk. (See footnote[1] for details of the classifications)

From the thorough research they did with back pain if a subject was classified DD/DS or R, they were 2.0 to 3.5 times more at risk of having the same or worse **pain** at follow up. In terms of **disability** the R group were nearly twice as likely to be at risk of remaining disabled or getting worse, and the DD/DS groups were over 5 times greater risk.

Paul highlights a study of 261 patients with chronic low back pain (greater than three months) referred to a McKenzie programme. The main outcomes were disability, pain report and receipt of wages compensation. The group were followed up one year after completion of the programme. The researchers looked at the DRAM categories and found DD/DS subjects were 3.3-8.1 times more likely to have a poor outcome. R patients were 2.4-5.0 times more likely to have a poor outcome. Clearly those who are psychologically distressed on the DRAM measurement are at increased risk of a poor outcome if managed by the McKenzie approach alone. This could probably just as easily apply to any other unidimensional treatment approach too. Note that while the Mckenzie approach is for the early part – hands-off-patient-does, with the exercises dictated and then prescribed by the pain response. If the patient doesn't respond to the exercises, the manual therapy hands then go on and the techniques that McKenzie taught were strong Cyriax type manipulations. One assumes that this could well have occurred with many of the difficult patients in the study. *Just a thought*! A big deal is again, to not get sucked in to believing that a strict guru driven tissue based approach is highly effective. It's/they are not.

Pain behaviour

I have already discussed this at length in an earlier chapter. Remember my 'patient from hell' Mr Grubb?

As Paul states, it is those that demonstrate the highest levels of pain behaviour, in the

---

1 - The Distress and Risk Assessment Method (DRAM)
      Normal (N) – Modified Zung <17
      At risk (R) – Modified Zung 17-33; MSPQ <13
      Distressed, somatic (DS) – Modified Zung 17-33; MSPQ >12
      Distressed, depressive (DD) – Modified Zung >33

simplest tasks, who are at the greatest risk of poor outcome.

He also quotes Waddell and Chris Main (1998) who emphasise that a wise way of looking at the Waddell signs and symptoms is to see them *'as an indication of the need for investigation of distress and fear* (of injury/pain/harm).

From the outcome research Paul quotes Gains and Hegmann (1999), whose study of fifty five acute back pain patients (pain of less than ten weeks) demonstrated that if there were one or more of the Waddell behavioural signs there was a much slower rate of return to work and that these patients used 'more physical therapy and more lumbar computed axial tomography'! Think about this result and it makes you wonder if the patients ordered their own therapy and scan? No they don't, it's actually a symptom of the medical Dr's behaviour whose tendency is to over-treat or over investigate those with overt pain behaviour. Just like we all did in Geoff Maitland's practice and beyond.

I have to emphasise that these patients, the Mr Grubb's of the world, are a huge challenge. For a great many, they're easy to get frustrated with. A plea here is to try to get to understand and observe good operant CBT skills in action with these types of patients. You're unlikely to change them with pain education or graded motor imagery! I will show you how I dealt with a 'Mr Grubb' in the case history section of the book.

Socio-economic factors

So for a great many this bit is all about: the patient is in it for some financial gain/ compensation pay out – they have to express this disability. In biological terms, as I've already discussed, remember the basic rule of survival: 'get as much as you can for as little effort as possible'. In the natural world this is a big deal and all about conservation of energy and resources.

Paul Watson reviews the evidence. It's great stuff. But as Paul says the evidence is complex and probably generates plenty of heat but not much light! I'll relate a few of his predictions and discussion points as a 'taster':

- *Long term back pain related incapacity rates will be higher in those social systems where there are more generous allowances for disability due to back pain.*
  Levels of back pain incapacity in Sweden have been linked to generous levels of wages compensation and the relative ease with which benefits can be claimed. Changes in Swedish benefit system have been accompanied by a fall in claims for incapacity. Study by Nachemson 1992.

- *Workers are more likely to be absent from work where wages compensation most closely approximate wages.*
  Paul did a study on the wages compensation on the island of Jersey, one of the Channel Islands. At the time of his study, 1998, the island State

paid wages compensation at a flat rate, which was low and unrelated to earnings. Return to work rates were comparable with findings on the UK mainland, where compensation rates were more generous. He points out the multiple factors operating and that any conclusion here is far from simple. For the most part workers are worse off on benefits than working. That was the 1990's. Now, 2013, the issue in this country is a current hot political topic again as the government tries to rein in their finances.

- *Those engaged in litigation or benefits appeals will remain off work longer.*
When I used to run the occasional course in Southern Ireland the physios there were adamant that the compensation system was a massive factor and many stated that they hated treating anyone involved in litigation. It's simple, as a compassionate developed country, 'we' like to do the good thing and support folk who are injured or disabled so that they can continue to live a decent life. On the other hand providing a 'reward' for being sick, ill or disabled is another way of reinforcing illness, disability and the all the other baggage of the 'compensation' culture many feel we're all wallowing in.

Paul cites Rohling et al 1995 study, they reviewed a large number of studies and concluded that there was indeed an effect for compensation in delaying recovery and increasing health care costs. However, Volinn et al 1991 and Hadler 1995 found no such associations. Gallagher et al 1995 found that compensation status was only significant in those with an external locus of control and who were more likely to consult healthcare practitioners. Waddell 1998 concluded that there is a relationship between wages compensation, increased work absence, poor surgical outcome and poor rehabilitation outcome. But he adds that most people on wages compensation get better and that it is only one of many social influences and must be seen in that context.
(Mick suggested that Louis add a bit more of what he thought here? Unfortunately he didn't. However, we did discuss 'being rewarded for getting better' as a way to maybe more effective rehabilitation. If appropriate, the perceived idea that you have to maintain your problem/ disability to gain the maximum reward was always discussed with the patient)

Now, last one…

- *The level of incapacity of claimants in litigation claims will improve on the completion of their case and receipt of compensation.*
Though we'd love this to be true, there's no evidence to support it. Greenough (1993): found that seeking lump sum compensation claims (medico-legal claims) was related to poor outcome from low back pain and psychological disturbance (greater distress). Settlement of these lump sum compensations did not influence employment status or resolution of the psychological disturbance at one year or five year follow-up.

Main and Watson (1995): found that engagement in litigation was a risk factor for poor outcome from rehabilitation in chronic pain patients with a history of prolonged unemployment.

Here's my thoughts and spin on this. First up, imagine having to pretend to be constantly be disabled? How do people do that?

I'm at a stage in my life where I have a spread of cancer to my pelvis and spine. It's not very nice and my legs are weak now, due to metastatic bone growth pressing and squashing the lumbo-sacral nerves. Yet I still play golf, walk the cliffs and I went snowboarding five months ago. I took a few painkillers and hey, bugger it. Well, OK, not everyone is like me perhaps. My point is that on most days I don't feel disabled. I'm not. The nasty pathology is still there and peeing could be better, but I can otherwise get on and be pretty normal. If I wanted to be disabled I'd have to take what I've got and make a big deal of it, constantly. I can't imagine how hard that would be to do.
(Louis was reflecting on his own situation here and acknowledging how disability is complex)

That's one thought. Here's another and it's a memory from the late 1960's, early 1970's TV series 'Colditz', that I used to watch with my Dad. Colditz was the name of a supposedly escape-proof castle used by the Germans for holding allied prisoners of war. The series is based around all the various escape attempts and relationships of the prisoners to each other as well as with their German captors.

Episode 10...'Tweedledum'... here's the summary from Wikepedia:

(Colonel Preston is the senior British commander in the prison. Ullmann is the German security officer)

'Wing Commander Marsh, an assistant to the British Medical Officer, decides to use his extensive knowledge of mental illness for an escape. (The Geneva convention states that if a prisoner is certified insane he should be repatriated). He proposes to 'go insane' and be repatriated. Colonel Preston agrees to let him, so long as he follows through with it to the bitter end. Marsh does a very thorough job: his bizarre, disruptive behaviour continually annoys the other allied officers, who remain unaware of the scheme. However, the Germans are not convinced, and Ulmann asks a Corporal to observe Marsh closely. The Corporal has a brother who is insane, so Ulmann believes he is a better judge of Marsh's condition than any doctor. The Kommandant initially refuses to allow the Swiss authority to examine Marsh, but relents when Marsh's evident madness embarrasses him in front of an important visitor. By the time the Germans are willing to consider repatriation, Marsh has done such a convincing job

*that even the Doctor is uncertain whether or not Marsh is simply pretend-
ing to be insane. After Marsh has been successfully repatriated to the UK,
it is revealed that his feigned psychosis has become genuine and irrevers-
ible, and that he has been committed to a mental hospital for long-term
care. Colonel Preston immediately forbids any further escape attempts
along the same lines.*

The whole point of this wonderfully powerful story, from my younger
black and white TV watching days, is that it powerfully represents how,
if you do something for long enough, it becomes ingrained and has
the potential to be permanent. Marsh feigned madness and kept up
the pretence until he was freed. But in feigning so wonderfully, the act
became a reality, he really became mad. Well, in the fiction of the series he
did. Ok, it was fiction, but it is my belief that there could be a great deal
in this. All good physios will know how hard it is to train out a long term
limp in a patient who has been doing it for a long time; and how patients
are often unaware of their odd movement patterns or postures.

I remember an elderly lady coming to see me who told me she'd started
getting neck pain. She sat opposite me and her head was in right side
flexion, probably about one third of range towards her right shoulder. I
didn't feel it appropriate to comment straight away, so listened to her
story and her roughly three month history. When she stood up to start the
physical examination I said,

'Do you feel straight?'

'Yes' she said.

'Show me what movements you can do with your head.' I demonstrated,
looking up, down, left, right, side to side and she followed. For her age
she had all the movements, even left side flexion.

Hmmm!

'Do you mind if I move your head to another position for a moment?'

'Go right ahead.'

I positioned her head square on to her shoulders.

'Can you keep it there OK?'

She did.

'How do you feel like that?'

'Really awkward, all lopsided and it's hard work to keep it there.'

'Now put it where you feel straight.'

Back she went to one-third right side flexion.

'When you look in the mirror do you notice that your head is to one side a bit? Does anyone comment?'

Amazingly she said 'No.'

'Would you mind sitting down a minute?'

Now, when she sat her head came straight, but that was because she sat twisted and shifted. It turned out the only mirror she had, or ever looked in at home was at her dressing table. A mirror above the sink in her bathroom was small and a little too tall for her, so she never looked in it. She had lost her husband and had lived quietly and happily alone in the country. All she mentioned was that her best friend, who came once a week for tea, had asked her if her neck was alright and it was that which had prompted her to seek help.

I guess everyone would like to know what happened to her. Well her problem could be classified as a simple low cervical spine flare up, that all normal humans get from time to time and most likely associated with spondylosis and degenerative joint changes. I used some simple exercises, some simple hands-on massage and also attempted graded posture retraining using a mirror standing.   The pain soon got better and she was grateful. I saw her three times over a two week period. The posture didn't change one bit. Now, I know her village and I knew a couple of other patients who knew her. Several months later one of them came to see me. I asked her about the lady with the 'wonky' neck and the patient went, 'Oh, we've got so used to her now, it's been like that for years!'

Now this is an example of an unconscious habit. Why it started I'll never know. What I am pretty sure about though is that a great many chronic pain movement patterns associated with 'pain behaviour', also become ingrained subconscious/unconscious habits and not just movements but also the grunts, tension and grimacing.

Early on in the management of injuries it's really important to focus on smooth, relaxed, thoughtless-fearless-movement.   I now tell patients that awkward movements, tense movements, grunting and tensing, holding of breath and so forth can easily become habits that are as hard to get rid of as biting your nails.

One last comment about this elderly lady with her wonky neck; you'll notice that I did pretty standard exercise/hands on treatment. You may be wondering after all this talking about the dangers of hands-on and passive therapy as to why I would be doing that? The reason is simple; this lady was perfectly active; she wasn't avoidant; she wasn't depressed; she was coping perfectly well and in a nutshell; she had not 'yellow-flag' issues of great concern. All she wanted was to see if I could give a bit of help with her pain. And like me or you or anyone, when something's hurting and someone can do some nice hands-on soft tissue massage to help, it can be great. But also give a little boost and some reassurance that all is well, is a natural and very helpful thing to do. Don't get the impression that hands-on are not allowed!

Back to litigation!

We don't actually say it directly to patients, but engaging a solicitor/lawyer is not a good move. In the clinic we sometimes use the cynical term: 'litigation maintained disability'. The point of all this is that if you're off-work because of pain, you're being compensated for loss of earnings and there's a possibility of a claim for what happened to you—it's very difficult to be normal in public, to be engaged in paced outdoor activities where you might be 'seen' and to look and try and move normally. I have had a great many patients openly admit to me that they got their compensation many years ago and since then have been unable to be seen to be normal and go out to try to get fit for fear of being seen and losing their disability status. What a tragedy.

So remember, as physios we can be coloured rather darkly, because we may quite often see those who remain in pain and are pain disabled who are in a compensation situation. Yet there are a great many others who go through the litigation process and recover well. We just don't see many of them. Regardless of what we might think, it is our duty to take every patient at face value and appreciate the difficulties and obstacles that sometimes present and that may make our work so much harder.

Work factors:

References:

Gifford, L. S., Ed. (2013). Topical Issues in Pain 5. Treatment. Communication. Return to work. Cognitive behavioural. Pathophysiology. CNS Press Falmouth.

Watson, P. (2013). Psychosocial predictors of outcome from low back pain. In: Gifford LS(Ed) Topical Issues in Pain 2. Biopsychosocial assessment and management. Relationships and pain. CNS Press Falmouth:85-109.

This isn't my area of expertise at all. See the fantastic chapters in the book above and read them, even if it's not your area. Why? Because of the fantastic changes and improvements that can be made by following the programmes and the improvements to ordinary practice that will occur just be understanding the work related barriers to recovery and return to work.

The main point to make here though is that work absence and rate of return to work is influenced by:

- satisfaction with work

- relationships with work colleagues and employer

- the workers perception of safety in the workplace

- the workers perception of workplace stress, perceived monotony and the physical demands of the workplace

- work satisfaction is a strong predictor too.

In addition, musculoskeletal pain has been shown to be more prevalent in those who perceived they had low job control and poor support from colleagues. I expect many of you have had patients that respond to the question:

'How is work reacting to your back problem and you being off? Any support or concern? Any communication going on with them?'

Often they respond with:

'I haven't heard a thing. I've worked my guts out for that firm for twenty years; never had a day sick leave and no one's phoned, been to see me, enquired how I'm getting on, asked when I might be back at work, or whether they can do anything to help when do I go back. I'm starting to feel quite upset really, even angry at times.'

In a study conducted in a nursing home, Wood (1987) found that a simple telephone call from a line manager to the absent worker inquiring after their welfare, offering support and expressing concern, significantly reduced the length of work absence. Think about it and it's pretty obvious, basic human communication and a bit of simple care makes the worker feel wanted and have worth.

So, return to work and the influence of work on the development of incapacity and long term absence are not just about the physical and ergonomic demands. It's also about how the individual perceives their work, their work stress, their level of control, their bosses and line managers and their job satisfaction.

So again the research is showing us that the obstacles to return to work, just like recovery, are predominantly psychosocial in nature – rather than due to the severity of pathology or impairment, those biomedical hard findings.

As Gail Sowden (2013) writes: 'Occupational obstacles to return to work are symbolised by 'blue' and 'black' flags. Blue flags are a sub-division of the yellow flags, having their origin in the occupational stress literature and are, 'Perceived features of work or social environment that are associated with rates of symptoms, ill health and work loss.' 'Black' flags relate to labour market and social security obstacles to coming off benefits and re entering work. It is the pervasive nature and detrimental effects of these obstacles that has lead to them being described as 'black' flags. Blue flags are about individual workers perceptions about their work whereas black flags affect all workers equally.

Examples of Blue flags:

- *high demand/low control* e.g. perceived physical/psychological demands of the job, physical and psychological capabilities and perceptions of control

- *unhelpful management style*

- *poor social support from colleagues*

- *perceived time pressures*

- *low job satisfaction.*

Examples of Black flags:

- *company policy on rehabilitation*
  e.g. absence of reporting system, lack of occupational health provision, minimal or no availability of selected duties or opportunities for graded return to work; an all or nothing return to work policy (sounds like the National Health Service!)...

- *threats to financial security*
  e.g. lack of financial incentive to return to work, or presence of financial disincentives to work! (like income protection policies, twelve months full pay, loan and mortgage protection policies, final salary pension schemes, benefits trap)...

- *litigation*

- *qualification criteria for compensation*
  e.g. having to prove that you are injured, disabled or unable to work and your ability to do this being rewarded; benefits system in which you are deemed either disabled or fit to work...

- *lack of contact with work.*

(Thanks to Gail Sowden, chapter 9 in Topical Issues in Pain 5. See also chapters 8, 10, 11, 12 and Nicky Hunter's chapter 13)

Gifford L S (Ed) (2013) Topical Issues in Pain 5. CNS Press, Falmouth.

Chapter 4.6
Psychosocial compartment part 2: The 'AB' of the 'ABCDEFW'

The ABCDEFW

Reading 'must' here:

Paul Watson's three chapters in Topical Issues in Pain 2 (two are with Nick Kendall) and the chapter in Topical Issues in Pain 3 – with Chris Main, 'The distressed and angry low back pain patient'.

If you're unaware of ABCDEFW it's a simple mnemonic:

A = Attitudes and beliefs about pain

B = Behaviours

C = Compensation and financial issues

D = Diagnosis and treatment issues

E = Emotions

F = Family

W = Work

Easy! Learn it off by heart and the stem and supplementary questions that follow. Thanks.

A = Attitudes and beliefs

1. Belief that pain is harmful or disabling results in fear avoidance behaviour. For example, the development of guarding and fear of movement.

2. Belief that all pain must be abolished before attempting to return to work or normal activity.

3. Expectation of increased pain with activity or work, lack of ability to predict capability.

4. Catastrophic thinking, fearing the worst, misinterpreting bodily symptoms.

5. Belief that pain is uncontrollable.

6. Passive attitude to rehabilitation. It is the health professional's role to fix the problem.

Questions to ask:

The basic Stem questions, labelled 'MW', all come from the Appendix, p193 of Chris Main and Paul Watson's chapter in Topical Issues in Pain 3.   I add my own follow-up comments too.

'Stem question' (MW)
*'If someone has had pain for a period of time, they usually have their own ideas of the cause. I know you're not a Doctor, but what do **you** think is the cause?*

Sometimes I find it quite OK to simply ask: 'What do you think is going on in your back, leg, knee, etc...? Often you'll get this for a neck problem say: 'Well the Dr told me that I had thin discs and wear and tear at the base of my neck'. This answer overlaps with the 'D' for 'Diagnosis' category and it's good to respond with another question like: 'What do you feel about that?' Or, 'Does that make sense to you?' Or, 'Some people find what the Dr's told them quite worrying, has it worried you?'

The whole point of this 'A' section is to find out what the patients' beliefs and attributions are about their pain problem and what it means to them. Their worries about it all are of particular importance and can often be easily allayed with straight forward information and simple discussion. Wading in and telling the patient what you think is wrong without knowing what the patient is thinking can cause a great deal of confusion. 'So you're saying I've got three joints out in my back and the Dr's saying I've got 'simple back pain'. Am I puzzled or what?' Or, 'The Dr read out my x-ray report and said it basically meant that my spine was arthritic now and that I should be a bit more sensible by being cautious and careful. Now you're telling me that I should start exercising more.' And then under his breath says/or thinks, 'I know who I'm going to believe!'

We also want to know how the patient's understanding of their pain relates to what they think they should be doing to get better (think fear-avoidance model helps). Here is a good time to enquire about any worry about the nature of the problem and their future as well as how it's affecting their attention.

Here are some supplementary questions to learn (MW):

1. *Do you believe that the pain itself is harming or disabling you?*

2. *Do you believe that you are going to have to get rid of all pain before you get back to work?*

3. *Do you think that increasing activity or getting back to work is going to make your pain worse?*

4. *Do you find yourself worrying in case your pain becomes progressively worse?*

5. *Do you find yourself becoming generally more aware or concerned about symptoms in your body?*

6. *Do you believe it is possible to control pain?*

7. *Do you believe you can do much yourself or it is just a matter of the passage of time or the help others can give you?*

I'm emphasising learning these questions because I did and I soon found that I started adapting them to the 'conversation' I was having with the patient. It allowed for a greater freedom and flow of information and in the end a better appreciation of the patient's knowledge about their problem and the impact it was having on them.

'So three weeks have gone by now and you said you haven't a clue what's gone wrong in your back. Before we go ahead and examine you, do you have any strong feelings about bringing the pain on or the possibility of causing more harm or more problems?'

'Well, it's interesting you should say that, because for the first four or five days I hardly moved for fear of putting it out again and bringing on the pain that floored me. I walked round like a penguin according to my wife. Then two days ago my neighbour came round and asked if I'd hold a bookshelf for him, while he leaned on it to sort out a fuse that had gone. I told him I'd hurt my back and I couldn't do much but in I went and leaned against it for him. It wasn't that simple and he ended up having to move it and I started helping him move all the books off the shelves. Well we finished the job and he suddenly went, 'Jim, are you OK, I forgot about your back?' and I said, 'Yes, I was, because I actually felt a lot freer in the back.'

...and another...

'You told me that you were an electrician just now and that you've been off work for five weeks. I'm wondering what your plans are for going back and what you feel about that?'

'Well, the Dr signed me off and everyone I talk to says don't go back until your back's completely sorted.'

A great many of these questions I often find it easier to ask after I've looked at the physical and got to know the patient and their movement confidence a bit better.

'I've had a thorough look at you now and I think you can see what I've found (shopping basket compartment summary – more later). Your back is really tight and stiff when you're standing but when I get you lying on your back and on 'all fours' your movements are pretty good. There's soreness in the centre of your back; all the nerve tests are normal. So how do you feel about starting to use a bit of exercise to get it going now?

'Fine, I'm feeling freer now and when I came in I was really fearful of you doing something that'd make it worse.'

'Some of the movements hurt a bit, was that OK?'

'I was a bit concerned at first but you telling me that joke took my mind of it and it actually got less now I think about it.'

'I'm hoping you're starting to think about your problem like I'm thinking about it?'

'What, stop being so careful and get it moving a bit more?'

I nod.

'So what about me going back to work then?'

'Well, think about the situations at work and whether they'd let you ease back in?'

'I'll give them a ring on Monday'

'Good, that gives you the weekend to get going with a few exercises and see how you get along.

(Before he goes... he has the 'Toblerone' recovery graph explained in parallel with 'what's needed for best healing' (graded increase in movement and return to fitness) and I tell him if he's anyway concerned to ring me and leave a message and I'll call him back. My strong emphasis is 'I don't want you sitting at home worrying. Ring me!' Now, you might think I'm mad, but over the years I've done this with nearly all my acute and sub-acute, even early chronic pain patients and because I've never had a call I must be doing something right! The key is the patient knowing they can phone and discuss things. (Complex chronic pain problems may be a different kettle of fish!)

The next time he comes in he's pleased with the Toblerone progress and spontaneously says

'You know, near the end of the session last time, when we were doing those 'all fours' arch and relax and curling up exercises you said something like 'think about the movement and being smooth and relaxed, try to stop expecting it to hurt. Go slowly and if it starts to hurt you easily stop and go back the other way. Then, when I got home I suddenly realised that my whole concentration was flipping to my back all the time!'

Now check question 5 above? All that's a bit round-about, but 'top-down-during-bottom-up' can be a big deal here.

Also though, it's quite OK to ask those questions out straight, but be aware that if they're out of context the patient can start thinking you're getting at them or you're making out that they're being a wimp in some way. Let's say you ask this out of the blue:

'Do you think that increasing activity or getting back to work is going to make your pain worse?'

You could get this:

'Do you think I'm wagging work, do you? You're starting to sound as dismissive as the Doctor. Look, it bloody hurts of course it's going to make it worse. You're starting to get on my nerves!'

So, a few key things with 'A' for Attitudes and beliefs:

a)   We don't want to add yet another diagnosis to the patient's understanding of their problem and create confusion. That means you have to know what the patient thinks is wrong.

b)   At this juncture it can often come out that the patient feels they haven't been investigated fully/seen a specialist. A good examination and reassuring discussion of the results can allay concerns here, plus a discussion of the value of x-rays and scans. As an aside, it amazes me what clinicians think can be picked up on a scan, let alone patients. It's as if you can get a scan and it'll reveal a Gray's Anatomy like definition and clarify every nook and cranny in the area.   Next time you see someone's scan of their spine take a good look and see what you can see. It's a rubbish picture. Gross at best. Big disc bulges and nerve compression, yes, well, just about. If clinicians think they reveal all – what on earth do patients think! Don't you get comments from patients like 'I had an x-ray/scan and they said it wasn't inflamed.' Eh? Or, 'I had an x-ray/scan and they didn't say anything about inflammation?' What? A scan is worse than a black and white picture from a 1960's TV. 'Can't see anything wrong with your back on the scan Mrs Evans but we can see a mass in your lower bowel, do you have trouble with constipation?'

c)   *The aim is to get the patient to air their fears and allay them once the 'depth' of the belief is ascertained (MW).*

d)   The 'A' questions also help you get a feel for the patient's 'locus of control' and whether they're willing to help themself or see that they have a role to play in their recovery. Whether they feel they have any 'control' in their own destination or whether they're 'avoiders' or 'confronters' and so forth.

Some further 'supplementary' type questions that I often use:

a) 'What are you expecting from me, from physiotherapy?'

If they answer, 'I hope you're going to fix me in one go' you should then go: 'Ok, how do feel about being involved in your own recovery, by that I mean getting going with a few exercises and starting to do more and more?

For the most part you'll get an 'Oh, yes, I was expecting all that, that's fine' type of reply. If you get, 'Well, I've got all the grandchildren to look after on Mondays, then on Tuesday my daughter comes for tea and Wednesday I've...' You may have a 'yes-but-er' type on your hands and self management life's now a little more difficult.

b) How do you feel about getting going – maybe even starting to think about going back to work in some capacity?

It's all about variations on a theme. The main thing is you've got to know why you're asking the questions and also be confident and know what you're going to do with the answers you might get. Sounds easy, sometimes it is, folk just listen, see your view point and get going. 'Wish I'd come here before' or 'Why didn't the Dr tell me all this' or 'The Dr didn't say that. No, nor that, no... and my husband said I shouldn't do that, no... I don't think that's a good idea at all. Can't you just do that machine thing?' And so forth!

As we sometimes say in our clinic 'Bloody hell, sometimes patients are just really hard!'

The 'A' category is, at the bottom line, often influenced by a good examination and simple education about the problem and it's recovery in terms that don't couch fear of structure. Think natural history, movement is best for best healing, pain 'Toblerones', gradual increases in movement and activity and gradually back to activities and work.

B = Behaviours

1. Use of extended rest of disproportionate 'downtime' (long periods of reclining/resting).

2. Reduced activity level and withdrawal from activities of daily living.

3. Irregular participation or poor compliance with physical exercise, tendency to be in a boom-bust cycle.

4. Avoidance of normal activity and progressive substitution of lifestyle away from productive activity.

5. Report of extremely high intensity of pain (always 10/10 on visual analogue scale (VAS)).

6. Excessive reliance on the use of aids or appliances.

7. Poor/reduced sleep quality since onset of back pain.

8. High intake of alcohol or other substances since onset of pain.

Questions to ask:

Stem question: (MW)
'What are you currently doing to relieve your pain?'

This question and the 'Behaviour' section is all about trying to find out what the patient is doing to deal with their pain – their 'coping strategy' and whether or not it is an active confronting style or one that is more passive and avoiding. As we've seen confronters tend to do much better than avoiders.

I've always liked the following way of putting it over to the patient in the 'Back Book' pamphlet produced by (Roland 2002). It's reproduced in full in 'The Back Book' by Gordon Waddell which everyone involved in back pain should have and studied. It's on page 335.

There are two types of sufferer:

One who avoids activity and one who copes:

- *the avoider gets frightened by the pain and worries about the future*

- *the avoider is afraid that hurting always means further damage – it doesn't*

- *the avoider rests a lot and just waits for the pain to get better*

- *the coper knows that the pain will get better and does not fear the future*

- *the coper carries on as normally as possible*

- *the coper deals with the pain by being positive, staying active and getting on with life.*

Who suffers the most?

Avoiders suffer the most. They have pain for longer, they have more time off work and they can become disabled.

Copers get better faster, enjoy life more and have less trouble in the long run.

The pamphlet then goes on to give some simple guidelines to follow. For example: keep up daily activities – they will not cause damage. Just avoid really heavy things. Start gradually and do a little more each day so you can see the progress you are making – be patient. It's normal to get aches or twinges for a time...

Main and Watson make some good points here:

Firstly, and aimed at you the therapist: is to not see pain behaviour – like lots of inactivity or complaints of high levels of reactive pain, as an indicator of the degree of pathophysiology.

Let me give an example: the 'Maitland' 'irritability' rule, which states that if the pain is highly reactive do a gentle technique. The implicit message for the therapist is 'back off and be careful'. An assumption from this is that highly reactive pain is a feature relating to the severity of the state of the tissues. (A big point is that the 'Biomedical' compartment of the shopping basket is there to reassure you that nothing is seriously wrong – that means red flags, a good neurological and listen to the history. For example, an elderly patient with a history of a minor fall or sudden movement reporting high levels of pain and lots of pain behaviour, may well have suffered a fracture. Never assume that the screaming ab-dab patient hasn't got anything physically wrong with them!)

Secondly, it is important to get a good handle on those who are trying to stay active but who actually may not be 'pacing' well. They may be over-doing it and then crashing out doing nothing for long periods due to big pain flare ups. Adequate pacing guidance is clearly required.

Thirdly, it is important we seek out those who are inappropriately resting and avoiding as a coping strategy as well as those who are becoming passive, for example simply relying on pain killers alone.

Fourthly, this is a chance for patients to be encouraged to identify what they are currently doing, what they find difficulty with and what they cannot do. Remember the PHODA? (Chapter GE 2.4). It's the Photographs of Daily Activity thermometer used to find out what chronic pain patients are fearful of doing. Clearly in the acute/sub acute situation doing the full PHODA is unnecessary. The key is getting the patient to identify the functions and activities that are being avoided and feared.

Fifthly, out of these enquiries we find out a great deal about what needs to be addressed in the 'activity participation/functional limitations' shopping-basket compartment. This information provided helps guide the patient onto an appropriate graded programme of relevance to their every-day activity. Try to overcome the 'pathobiologically' entrenched mindset that likes to list all the things that the patient can't do (i.e. what's wrong) and make a better list to include what they can do (positive reinforcement) and what they might like to start trying to do and how to go about it. Or, get *them to work out how they might go about starting to do it*, which is an opportunity to learn problem solving skills and how to come up with graded hierarchies.

Here are Main and Watson's *(MW)* 'Supplementary questions' (learn them and recite them before bed every night – only joking!). Note that some are more relevant to longer pain histories than shorter but the important thing is to adapt.

1. Do you find yourself having to lie down or take a lot of rest because of pain?

2. Have you found yourself doing much less?

3. Have you stopped doing most of your usual activities?

4. Have you found it difficult to practice the exercises you have been shown as regularly as you would like?

5. Have you found yourself overdoing it on a good day?

6. Have you found yourself becoming gradually less active and changing from your usual activities or ways of doing things?

7. How bad is your pain on a 10 point scale if '0' is no pain at all and '10' is the worst pain you could imagine?

8. Have you found yourself getting more and more reliant on aids such as walking sticks or other items to help you do things?

9. Has the quality of your sleep got much worse since you developed (back) pain?

10. Have you found yourself taking much more alcohol or recreational drugs since you developed (back) pain?

11. Have you started or significantly increased smoking since the onset of your (back) pain?

I find that I often ask patients to give me a run-down of a 'typical day' which quickly gives you an idea of up/down time and what they are doing. You can go on to compare it to a typical day before the problem started too. The 35 year old housewife, who gives you a typical day of being in bed until 10am; getting up takes thirty minutes; she rests after being up for thirty minutes; has lunch lying in front of the TV. When asked about her level of activity or physical confidence now compared to before the problem, she might go 'Hasn't changed much really' Or, it could have been 'Well, two months ago I used to get up at 6.30; jog for an hour; get the kids ready for school; walk the dogs; go to work until 3pm; meet the girls down the gym for a session three times a week and often we'd all go down the beach and surf after work if it was nice! Both answers tell you a whole lot about 'relative loss' of normal life and about their normal 'behaviour' and how it's changed.

The whole idea of 'behaviour' and 'behaviour change' may be quite novel for the therapist and even more so for the patient. Seeing someone limping, holding their back, resting a lot, not doing normal activities and talking about their pain all the time naturally makes us think that there's something wrong. And that something needs to be done to help. Once it's all put right, the limping, holding, complaining and lowered activity levels will all return to normal.   For the most part it doesn't seem right that we ignore the thing that's wrong and get on and treat what the sufferer is/isn't 'doing'! I had a neat conversation recently with Heather Muncey, the Physiotherapy Pain Association founder, and a highly skilled CBT physio. We were discussing the unique nature of physiotherapy. Heather said, 'We're the experts in analysing movement and changing movement behaviour.' I've always gone with our unique thing being 'rehabilitation' – getting people back to normal movement, normal activity and fitness. (As per my experiences on orthopaedic wards and in general physiotherapy hospital work) To get a better grasp on this in relation to the chronic pain sufferer I've always suggested that therapists need to be more like neuro physios. Take a moaning, groaning, limping, twisting, writhing, hobbling chronic pain patient and give them to a neuro physio! Tell the physio that even though the patient is going on a bit, there's nothing to worry about structure wise. Then sit back and watch how the neuro physio gets the patient moving better. Gradually working on functional movements, weight transfer, goal orientated tasks, encouragement of good movement, ignoring poor; repeating small steps at a time, putting it all together and so on. Quiet, guided and reassuring, rehabilitation in all its glory! Now what you are observing with the neuro physio is what we should all be good at – 'changing movement behaviour and movement patterns'! A massive problem is that the pain and our reflex biomedical feelings and thoughts about the source and mechanisms of the pain get in the way!

It's instinctive in a caring person to want to do something to help. Certainly watching CBT therapists deal with these presentations can leave the caring part of us in shock. Not that they're cruel to the patients, it's just that they're neutral or ignore pain behaviour – but it can look cruel for a while. However, stay observing and you'll start to notice how they subtly and positively encourage/reinforce more adaptive movements and behaviours.

It's well worth analysing where you sit and how your react with these types of patients – the 'Mr Grubb's' of the world, the heart-sink patients when you're time pressured, the ones who take five minutes to get out of the chair and into the cubicle with you. You may be ultra caring, 'soliciting', you help them with everything they do and in so doing reinforcing their maladaptive behaviour. On the other hand you may be the dead opposite, thinking they're amplifying, they're a waste of my time, they're pulling the wool over your eyes and taking the p..s. So you treat them with disdain, you don't help them, you're behaviour and attitude becomes punishing in itself. You don't even notice when they move a little better and if they do – you see it as evidence that they're inconsistent. Which proves your point about them being malingering time wasters and in so doing you reinforce their 'bad' behaviour even further.

If you want to get anywhere with these sorts of presentations try and see good behaviour-change technique as not requiring a 'soliciting/over-caring' approach or a 'punishing/non-caring' approach. The key is to extinguish the maladaptive behaviour via neutrality/no reaction but promoting or reinforcing the good/adaptive behaviour via appropriate praise and encouragement.

Good physios do sometimes do this naturally with less daunting and 'easier' patients. If you are learning or newly qualified I'd like to suggest you steer well clear of picking up the techniques of the punishing type physio. Oh, and the solicitous too!

Now another way of dealing with this is to link it to the patients' unhelpful beliefs about their problem and situation. And to then see that their current way of moving is likely to be unhelpful or have negative consequences. Information about 'disuse' and 'deconditioning' of the cardio-vascular and musculoskeletal system can be very helpful, if it's alongside, or follows information about pain and healing that reinforces the patient's tissue soundness and the hurt does not mean harm message.

As I've said before in the fear-avoidance section, we gain a great deal from finding out about activity-avoidance; it helps us formulate a relevant action plan to start graded confrontation and design appropriate behavioural experiments for them.

Chapter GE4.7
Psychosocial compartment part 3: The 'CDEFW' of the 'ABCDEFW'

C = Economic and Compensation issues

1. Lack of financial incentive to return to work.

2. Disputes over access to benefits.

3. History of claims due to other injuries.

4. History of back pain with previous receipt of sickness benefits.

5. Participation in medico-legal claim.

Questions to ask:

Stem question (MW): 'Is your back pain placing you in financial difficulties?'

This section is usually closely tied to the 'W' 'Work' section and questions there can overlap. For example you may ask simply, 'Are you off work because of the pain problem?' This reveals details of how long and any certification to be off work, but also eases the question/statement, 'Being off for XY weeks is quite long, are you coping financially?' This frequently further eases you into being able to find out more about their situation. Bear in mind the numbered points above so the conversation/questioning can be directed. For example the patient might offer that they've been off for so long that they have had to turn to benefits and you can then reply: 'So, is all that running smoothly, no problems or hassles with the benefits folk?'

Many physios report that they find it difficult to ask about 'compensation'. The term medico-legal is often easier to use. Physiotherapists are quite used to asking about being at work and finding out details of the historical background to a problem or incident that caused the problem. Clearly, if it involves some kind of accident, like road traffic or at work, then it's usually pretty natural to pitch in at some point with the question, 'So are you involved in some kind of claim or litigation?' If you suddenly find the patient looking at you rather quizzically and going, 'What do you want to know all this for anyway?' It's good to give an answer along these lines:

'Well, I'm interested in the impact the pain problem you're telling me about is having on your life. We know that things like litigation, financial difficulties and benefits hassles add a great deal of stress to the situation and research has shown that added stresses like these don't help the sufferer to recovery quickly. I'm only asking because of this and sometimes I help patients who are having a particularly hard time to get the right kind of help.'

A big tip with all this ABCDEFW material is know your questions· why you're asking them but also think about possible difficult situations and all possible responses you can give, especially when it might become awkward.

Here are the Main and Watson *(MW)* supplementary questions for the 'C' category:

1. *Have you been hit hard financially as a result of your pain?*

2. *Have you had a lot of trouble getting benefits etc. to which you think you are entitled?*

3. *Have you been dealt with incompetently or unpleasantly when trying to sort out benefits etc.?*

4. *Have you had to get involved in claims or litigation because of pain problems in the past or*

5. *(Have you previously had back trouble resulting in a claim or in significant time off work?)*

6. *Have you had to take significant amount of time off work because of pain in the past? If yes, approximately how long?*

Main and Watson emphasise that intervention as soon as possible in those who have history of previous work absence is vital. 'Leaving it until conventional treatment (analgesia and advice) has failed to improve the situation may be too late. Intervention should be geared to maintain activity levels and encourage early return to work even on modified duties if this is available'.

D = Diagnosis and treatment issues

1. Health professionals sanctioning disability. Not providing interventions geared towards improvement of function.

2. Experience of conflicting diagnoses of explanation for back pain, resulting in patient confusion.

3. Unfamiliar diagnostic language leading to catastrophisation (fearing inevitable poor outcome).

4. Continued receipt of passive treatment.

5. Expectations of quick and easy cure.

6. Lack of satisfaction with previous treatments for back pain.

7. Advice from professionals to change or withdraw from job.

Questions to ask:

Stem question (MW): 'You have been seen about your pain and been examined. Are you worried that anything might have been missed?

This section again refers back to patient misunderstanding about their problem covered in the 'A' section earlier. It also relates to the 'B' section too in that patients may be expecting to be 'passive' receivers of treatment.

I like the simple question:

'What have you been told is the cause of your problem and does what you've been told make sense to you?'

'Well, I've been given three things so far and I'm sure you'll give me yet another. First up, my pelvis was out and my right leg was longer than my left. Then, when I was told it was fixed, but the pain wasn't the consultant said I'd got a disc sitting on the nerve but that an operation was likely to make it worse. Recently I've been to some weird guy, that my neighbour recommended, who said that my liver and gall bladder were fighting each other. Does it make sense? Well it did to them. But I'm no better and from what that consultant said it looks like I'm going to have to live with it.'

'So what's made you seek me, a physiotherapist?'

'Good question, first up a mate at work said you'd shown him what to do and explained it in a way that made sense. Also that you'd said how long it would take to get better and you were right. Second, I'm fed up with not being able to do anything and I want to get going again.'

Top stuff, that was worth knowing about.

Here's a patient's answer to the 'Are you worried anything might have been missed' question:

'I'm glad you asked me that. The Dr said it was a muscle strain seven weeks ago and that it'd soon be better. Well it's got worse. I thought it might be a nerve problem so I went to the chiropractic pain clinic and they agreed and manipulated it quite hard. I was pleased and it felt better but after three days my foot started going numb and I've been limping since. Now, the chiropractor x-rayed it and showed me how the alignment was out as well. So, now I'm not only worried about the nerve, I'm thinking that the back is further out than it was before. You know, when you're lying awake at night in pain you start thinking frightening stuff and I've been thinking a lot recently that there's something far worse going on. Do you think I could have some kind of cancer or could it have broken?'

My response:
'I'm with you. It's good to know how you feel about what's going on. I'll do a full examination and I'll check for anything serious and if I think there's anything

serious going on I'll write to your Dr and we'll make sure you have it investigated fully. If it's any reassurance I've seen a great many patients like you over the years and it's only about once a year, if that, that I come across something that is really serious. That's one thing, the other is that research has shown that adequate listening to the patient combined with a thorough physical examination, that I'll do with you in a moment, will pick up serious things wrong far better than any scan or x-ray. The x-ray and scan are helpful to back up what's been revealed by our examination. If after the examination I do I'm concerned, I'll explain it to the Dr and request appropriate investigations...'

He nods and looks pleased.

I pause and then say.

'I'm surprised with all your worries that you haven't been back to the Dr to see what he thinks now?'

'Look you get four minutes in there. I did go back and he said that it was now a nerve and he gave me these tablets, they're useless.'

'It doesn't sound like he reassured you then?'

'He didn't even touch me or have me undress and have a look.'

In previous chapters there are many examples of how I deal with red flags, change the patients' understanding and attributions and reassure and move on. Please refer to them (chapter 4.2 and 4.3). The key is a full history/red flags and full examination. With the added ingredient of explain all the findings as you go. For example, any neurological signs need explaining and reassuring and all the various tests you might be doing too. I suggest you also review some of the earlier case histories, for example 'Kate' in section 17 which deals in detail with the ongoing communication and reassurance that I give during physical examination.

Please keep away from explanations that revolve around your favourite impairment focused examination like – muscle imbalance, accessory movements stuck, discs out or deranged. Please DONT DO IT!

If you do you're as bad and as unhelpful as what's gone before. (Remember the shopping basket approach – to ensure that you remain balanced and reasonable!)

Supplementary questions (MW):

> 1. *Have you been given different explanations about your pain?*
>
> 2. *Have you been anxious or confused about the explanations which you have been given?*
>
> 3. *Are you satisfied with the previous treatment you have had for back pain?*
>
> 4. *Have you been encouraged to limit your functioning and accept your limits?*

This last question is important – finding out what advice the patient has been given. Ask the patient also what they think about what they've been told. Does it make sense to them and have they been following the advice. A great many people do what they're told, especially if it's from a Dr or consultant and they often take far more heed of that advice than any far more appropriate and sensible given by a 'lower ranking' physiotherapist. Unfortunately this makes our work even harder than it already is, we sometimes have to work incredibly hard to convince patients, and even then can still be stymied by the consultant's quip to 'limit' what they do from now on, or something similar. Maddening!

When will the medical world realise that we are experts in movement dysfunction, deconditioning and some of us, in pain. When will physiotherapy realise this too?

E =Emotion

1. Fear of increased pain with increased activity.

2. Depression (especially long term low-mood), loss of enjoyment.

3. More irritable than usual.

4. Anxiety about and heightened awareness of body sensations.

5. Feeling under stress and unable to maintain sense of control.

6. Presence of social anxiety or disinterested in social activity.

7. Feeling useless and not needed.

Questions to ask....

Stem question (MW): 'Is there anything upsetting you or worrying you about your pain at the moment?

As I've already discussed pain is instinctively linked to emotions – notably anger, anxiety and fear. We tend to use words like annoyed, fed up with, upset about, worried and concerned; especially if the problem goes on and doesn't appear to get better, or it does a little, then comes back again. Emotions equate to stress and worry and as we've seen from a 'biological' as well as a behavioural perspective, these things don't help recovery and healing.

As Main and Watson emphasise for us:

'It is important to distinguish pain associated disability and distress from other life stresses. While it may be necessary to attend to both, they must be distinguished '

Unfortunately for those who don't feel comfortable in this area, high levels of distress are important factors in determining outcomes and it is vital that at least some areas of distress are addressed. Psychologists may be important, but distress related to pain and the situation that has resulted can be dealt with to some degree. Clearly the big problems lie with the more chronic end of the scale and this is where good CBT psychologists and medical intervention via psychiatry may be required. At the acute and sub-acute end of the spectrum reducing distress can be surprisingly easy at times.

Worriers stop worrying because you've spent time with them, explained the problem, the situation and the plan of action. They're grateful and often by the next treatment have made a great leap forward. Don't forget, reassurance is a pain killer here and the Toblerone recovery graph is so helpful in allaying fears when things take a turn for the worse.

A big thing here is time. Some patients just want the four questions answered: What's wrong? How long? What can I do? What can you do? And get out of your clinic empowered and free. Others want every little question and concern answered in detail and will come back with more and more. Questions need answering but if patients keep coming back with the same ones you mustn't just go over it again; it's so important to get them to review the knowledge you've given them and try and answer their own questions. If they can't do that, then it's your fault. You've been too complicated, too wordy, too over their head and you've failed to make it meaningful. Start again.

In the next section I deal in more detail with how I go about managing and assessing pain.

For now here are the supplementary questions (MW):

    1. Do you worry that daily activities or work will increase you pain?

    2. Are you getting demoralised or depressed about your pain?

    3. Are you becoming more irritable than usual?

    4. Have you become aware or concerned about other symptoms?

    5. Do you feel stressed or feel that things are getting a bit out of control?

    6. Have you lost interest in your social life or become a bit anxious about mixing with people?

    7. Have you been feeling useless and not needed?

(For further discussion see later chapter)

F = Family.

1. Over-protective partner/spouse, reinforcing fear of harm and encouraging catastrophisation.

2. Solicitous behaviour from spouse (taking over tasks).

3. Socially punitive responses from spouse (ignoring, expression of frustration).

4. Extent to which family members support return to work/normal activity.

5. Lack of person to talk to about problem.

Questions to ask...

Stem question (MW): 'How does your family react to your back pain?'

I'm sure most physios have found themselves in a cubicle with the patient and their partner and wondered who was more of the problem?

'So Mr Pecked, what's the problem?'

'He's hurt his back love, can't move, can't do anything round the house and I'm doing it all. Pain's from his back to his groins and down both legs. Spends most of the time watching the TV and in the shed, gone off his food and isn't interested in conversation, stopped work last Christmas and hasn't gone back. Well, it must be three years. Dr says he's got spondy-loss and we should move to a bungalow...' on and on.

That spouses and partners are part of the problem and the need to include them in some sessions has been clearly demonstrated. Watson and Kendall recommend that during assessment the spouse or families attitudes to the person's problem are important to know, especially if there's an obvious need to 're-educate' them about the nature of pain-associated disability.

As they say, *'The physiotherapist will have a very difficult time encouraging compliance with an activity based programme if the patient's spouse or significant other person continually reinforces the message that activity is potentially harmful and encourages the patient to seek passive treatment and rest.'*

Imagine the scene with the patient doing his new exercises in the front room:

'Hey love, look at this, come and see what I'm managing to do now!'

'If you ask me, you're going to end up in the back of the ambulance again if you keep doing that. Remember what happened the last time you got all enthusiastic and started jumping around, two nights in the hospital and about a month to get back to where you were. If you keep doing that I'm going over to stay at Cissies.'

What better way to shift processing back into the 'threat' processing centres!

The whole idea is to get the family onside and involved. CBT therapists may even train partners of chronic pain patients in techniques of appropriate reinforcement. It's always great when partners take on the any new programme with enthusiasm and even do the various exercises as well, or help with planning the day and the pacing.

Supplementary questions (MW):

> *1. Do members of your family undermine your confidence and keep reminding you to be careful what you do?*
>
> *2. Are members of your family trying to stop you doing things for yourself?*
>
> *3. Do members of your family make negative comments or ignore you when they see you are in pain?*
>
> *4. Are members of your family encouraging you to try to get back to work?*
>
> *5. Is there anyone you can talk to about your pain and its effects?*

As you can see, the questions try to ascertain whether the spouse is being on the one hand: over-protective, doing everything for the patient and not allowing them to do anything,

'You sit there dear the less you do the better you'll be, just ring the little bell and I'll come running, anything at all.'

That's the classic 'solicitous' spouse who is a danger to life and brain – leaving the chair-bound to wallow in boredom, uselessness, hopelessness and depression!

On the other hand, the other extreme, is the 'punishing' spouse. As we mentioned for the punishing therapist earlier, there's that nasty element of cruelty that often drives the already maladaptive behaviour to even greater extremes.

W = Work

I have already outlined the blue (how the individual perceives their work) and black (features that do not relate to perception) flags.

'Return to work' issues related to musculoskeletal pain, especially for those of long duration are a specialist area. However, they're still important in our normal day to day input with less pain disabled patients and in our interactions with them, where a major aim is to speed return to work if not keep patients at work.

Here are the main features of important predictive value for consideration with the 'yellow flag' assessment:

- history of manual work (forestry, farming, construction, truck driving, labouring, nursing)

- repetitive boring work

- previous work history, frequent job changes, experiencing stress at work, job dissatisfaction, and poor relationships with peers or supervisors

- belief that work is harmful, that to do it will cause damage or be dangerous

- unsupportive or unhappy current work environment

- low educational background, low socioeconomic status

- job involves significant biomechanical demands, such as heavy or frequent lifting, manually handling heavy items, extended period in static postures (sitting or standing, driving), whole body vibration, constrained postures, inflexible work schedules preventing appropriate breaks

- minimal availability of selected duties to facilitate graded return to work

- negative experience of workplace management of back pain (e.g. absence of reporting system, discouragement to report, punitive responses from supervisors and management)

- absence of interest from employer

Questions to ask...

Stem question (MW): 'How is your ability to work being affected by your pain?'

The important feature is for us to focus on the pain associated limitations perceived by the patient to be of importance regarding their return to work. For example, a patient may indicate that there is no way they could lift anything; yet during the treatment, when simple lifting tests are offered to see what they'd be prepared to do (for example lifting a 5lb weight from a chair onto a plinth) they were actually quite willing to. As part of this patient's programme a simple lifting task was undertaken after general movement exercises and simple stretches. The patient soon increased their confidence, lifting progressively greater loads in ergonomically sensible patterns that suited their physique. Patients often respond that they've never been taught how to lift, or if they had, they'd found it really awkward. The important thing is practice and increasing appropriate muscle tolerance and strength by 'getting used to' the new patterns of movement. My experience, on the courses I taught, is that a great many physiotherapists aren't capable of using 'correct' lifting technique too. Often their legs aren't strong enough and they haven't the co-ordination capability of keeping their back in a neutral position while doing the lift. We need to practice what we preach, and don't just tell the patient how to do it; spend time practicing in every session, check and re-check the patient to see if they are getting it and improving. A common issue is often being over-tense.

A 'W' factor of great significance is that many employers will not consider workers for return until they are 100% – a factor shown to have a detrimental effect. Quite often 'light duties' are considered a waste of time and frequently don't even exist in some working environments.

Rehabilitation must include, from the very start if at all possible, graded and modified work activity movements and loading, so as to maintain and then improve on the previous level of fitness.

Supplementary questions (MW):

1. *What do you think are the major problems for you in staying at/getting back to work?*

2. *Is work stressful?*

3. *Do you get satisfaction from your work?*

4. *Do you believe that your work is harmful for you?*

5. *Is your job physically demanding in terms of heavy lifting, extended standing, difficult postures or inflexible schedules preventing appropriate breaks?*

6. *Is it a pleasant place to work? Are your workmates sympathetic to people who have pain problems?*

7. *Are restricted duties or graded return to work possible for you?*

8. *Do you think that the way back pain is managed at work is satisfactory?*

9. *Do you think your employer is interested in employees who have pain problems?*

Some wisdom from Chris Main and Paul Watson to finish off here:

> *'You need to try to identify if the person is afraid that their work is damaging them. You need to analyse what they do and how they do it. You need to try and find out what they can currently do now, what they cannot do and also ways that they may be able to get round these, as well as who they need to speak to at work to enable an early return to work. Finding out if changes are possible is a good first step – changes not only to what is done, but the time it's done too – hence adequate pacing!'*

Main and Watson warn to avoid blaming work as the cause of the pain. The best thing is to help the patient be more prepared and fit for the work they do.

Chapter GE4.8
Psychosocial compartment part 4: A bit more on 'Emotion'

Essential reading again:

Main, C. J. and P. J. Watson (2013). The distressed and angry low back pain patient. Topical Issues in Pain 3. Sympathetic nervous system and pain. Pain management. Clinical effectiveness. L. S. Gifford.(Ed) CNS Press Falmouth: 177-204.

With regard to emotions; getting information is one thing, dealing with it is another. Sometimes though it's fine to just listen, acknowledge and get on with more mundane physical issues. We know that simple disclosure of our feelings can often go a long way to making us feel better, at least for a while. Think about the patient who has been in pain for several weeks, who has had difficulty controlling their pain, loss of sleep, isn't pacing well, can't manage at home and isn't getting much help. No one they've been to see has taken time with them and no one has helped. They're naturally emotional about it all, they express this, have a little tear, express their frustration which is acknowledged and then the voyage into their problem continues. By the end of the session – given a good amount of time, a clear rationale to the problem and a logical pathway for recovery/management, the patient often leaves a great deal happier and significantly relieved that someone 'at-last' has got on their case and is making things happen.

Getting into emotions may not be your scene, as I think I said rather flippantly somewhere else, if it's not your scene maybe think about re-training as a dentist! Sorry couldn't resist it, but whatever you do, if you don't like emotional patients, the more difficult and chronic end of the spectrum is probably going to be a no-go area for you. Even the more acute side of things has a considerable emotional component if you really take care and listen. I really doubt if you can get away from the emotional side of pain and be effective, remember the three dimensions of pain are, sensory-discriminative, emotional-motivational and cognitive-evaluative – in every pain, every time. If you block out one or two of these dimensions you're not dealing with reality of pain.

I've already mentioned some of the stem and supplementary questions for 'E' emotions. Here are a few more that I slip in at an appropriate time.

1. Are you coping OK with this, or are you at the end of your tether?

2. You sound pretty fed up with the whole thing?

3. Are you worried about what might be wrong, or that something's been missed?

4. Have you got any concerns or worries about your problem or the effect it has had on you recently?

5. Is there anything worrying or frustrating you?

6. I'm interested in the impact this has had on you?

With some patients these issues can be harder to approach and it's worth having a sense of 'I don't think I'll go there – not appropriate right now.' Or you may just be thinking, 'I haven't got time for that stuff, I'd never get finished if I got into that.'

I want to emphasise that the first session with the patient, the taking time with the 'impact' on the patient and finding out about the whole problem, in all its dimensions, is so massively worthwhile – in all classifications of pain presentations. It sets the scene and makes later management so much easier and more efficient. Take your time. If you haven't got time, stop the patient when times up, book them in again as soon as you can (I often say come back at the end of the day) and finish it all off to your and the patient's satisfaction. After a lengthy first session the follow-ups usually become much more efficient and far less time-expensive.

(I often got asked on my courses, 'How long are your appointment times, because we only have twenty minutes?' My standard first session was forty five minutes and subsequent appointments forty five minutes too. For a patient who needed it, a double first session usually worked well, an hour and a half.)

Early in my career I worked in hospitals and private clinics where there were huge time restriction pressures – not good for the patient or therapist. Now in our clinic, the restriction is often the total number of sessions the patient can afford! So you have to get good at 'sorting' out the patient's problems quickly and get them convinced to get involved with their recovery from the start – we work hard to do this.

If you feel the 'emotions/distress' area is important and can't think how to broach it, try the 'third person' approach:

'Many patients with your sort of problem get quite fed-up. For example, they get anxious about the pain and its possible cause; they get frustrated and cross about the way the problem is limiting their activity. They're fed up with not sleeping; they're getting low mood, or even depressed or stressed about the quality of life and other things. They're fed up with work and their colleagues' reactions. They're fed up with the Dr and some of the therapists they've seen and the treatments that haven't worked. I'm interested to know what are your feelings and thoughts'

Now if the answer is, 'Why, what's that got to do with you?' – you've misread the situation. They may feel you're being inappropriately intrusive. This is the time when you need a good answer otherwise you could lose the patient and feel a sense of terrible unease and foreboding.

Try this...

'Well, it's been shown that patient's with pain problems, who have a lot of distress, like anger, frustration, depression, anxiety and fear don't actually do as well in their recovery as those who are coping and managing OK. We find that if we can understand how a patient is coping with their problem and find out what is upsetting them we can try and help them deal with it. For example, two days ago I had a fellow in who had an odd chest pain – he was frightened of going to the Drs and it turned out he was worried sick about a heart problem. After a thorough examination it turned out that he had a problem between his shoulder blades. I was able to reassure him and also persuaded him to go and get checked by the Dr. He soon got better and was massively relieved. Other patients report huge frustrations with their pain impacting home life, but once they get calmer and see they can get going they soon work out how to carry on and manage better. We have a little saying here that stress slows the healing process up. The reason is that stress diverts all your resources and energy to the worry and nerves rather than to the recovery process. It is well known that people who are distressed can heal up to 60% more slowly. Also, when you're fed up you don't feel like doing exercises and getting involved in your own recovery. Calmer is better, you get going again, you heal and you use energy more wisely.

Here are a few more examples to use:

'We often use waking up at night because of pain and being upset/cross about it – and then not being able to get back to sleep. It's all about *'Adrenaline'* – if you get wound-up your body makes masses of adrenaline. Think about a sudden noise in the night, you're on your own in the house. How do you feel?'

'Scared'

'Quite and what's going on in your body?'

'Heart's thumping and mouth's dry. I get all tense.'

'Exactly. Soon you find out that it was a window banging and you go down and close it. What's it like trying to get back to sleep again?'

'Impossible, usually it takes ages – you're wide awake and the heart doesn't seem to want to stop thumping.'

'That's adrenaline: it gets you wound-up and ready for physical action; it comes on very quickly and stays for a long time, just in case that thing that frightened you is still around – think like a hunter-gatherer.' 'Was that a lion I just heard or was it just a rustle of the bushes in the wind? Not sure? Best stay alert just in case, only the slothful dumb-head goes straight back to sleep.'

'So if you wake in the night with pain and you then get mad with it – you get?'

'Adrenaline'

'Yes and that stays about and you then can't get back to sleep. You get even madder because you're tired and you've got heaps to do in the day and everything just winds you up even more. So, if you understand what I'm saying and you wake in the night with the pain, try not to go all 'adrenaline' and mad and wound up. Stop, think, try and chill, get up, do something, accept the pain does this and then when you're ready go back to bed and see what happens. Getting back off to sleep is never easy but getting adrenaline into the system doesn't help. Adrenaline stops you relaxing and in turn stops productive resting and sleep. Remember most of the body's healing takes place overnight when the body has nothing else to do; your mind and consciousness turn off but you're body is off doing the mending and repairing without any disturbance from anywhere else!'

Some patients can quickly accept that stress puts healing on hold or slows it up. Review the stress chapters for all those healing and stress examples – you can use these to illustrate. The big deal is that energy is diverted to 'escape and tension' mechanisms at the expense of recovery, repair and healing mechanisms.

The other major side of the coin, as hinted at, is that when you're low you don't feel like helping yourself – you can't be bothered. When you do less, you get less fit, you become deconditioned and the body is then perceived as 'vulnerable' and as a result becomes more sensitised and more likely to produce new pains. See the Vulnerable Organism chapter (GE 2.3) and use the diagrams there with patients when appropriate. Case histories later will review this.

When people are low, their 'tolerance' is far less, minor things upset them and the system reflects this – just like when you have the flu, small knocks and bangs hurt a lot more than when you're well and full of life and energy.

If it turns out that a patient's worries relate to something being seriously wrong it's vital to take your time, and do a good red flag assessment and a good physical examination/neurological (not just reflexes, power and sensation but Babinski, proprioception, balance and coordination too). Above all make the examination a focus on the positive and normal findings, don't go being 'smart-ass' and finding little things that are irrelevant but that you think might impress the patient! The deal here is to reduce any source of worry and concern.

With distressed patients, the focus should be on a realistic examination, looking for positives for the patient and explaining them in non-threatening terms – which is very much a non-intuitive way of going about things to those schooled in a biomedical or biomechanical model of pain. See it as a new skill to learn.

What I am not saying is that I ignore fundamental and important findings. If a patient has lost a reflex or has significant muscle weakness of wasting due to neuropathy I tell them and explain it, but realistically and positively. If a patient has been told they have spondylosis I don't deny it. I review it, show them x-rays of others, I discuss what degeneration of the spine means – realistically, but also positively too. If pathology is there that is considered 'normal for their age' I explain it and 'normalise' it with the patient.

The back is incredibly strong, but you wouldn't think so if you listened to a great many clinicians way of explaining things. And look it's not what you told the patient, it's ***WHAT THE PATIENT HEARD AND INTERPRETED!***

(See the Pink Flags chapter after this)

'BO' is not for 'body odour' but for 'Belief and Optimism' and sometimes it can be a part of this section and the discussions that arise from patients. It's all about helping the patient see that by changing their attitude to a more hopeful one and using more adaptive coping strategies things will improve. That's 'telling' the patient though. Alongside this is the patient starting to feel and witness their own progress through their own, initially guided efforts. The proof-is-in-the-pudding, 'try it and see' is a vital statement.

To rather dramatically help back you up – remember, patients who go into operations believing they'll do well, do! Those who believe they might die are more likely to!

I often find myself saying to patients:

 'You must feel that everything I suggest to you or do with you makes sense/seems reasonable. If there's anything I say or suggest during our sessions together that you are not happy with, doesn't makes sense, or worries you – you need to tell me. I need to know. I want you to feel comfortable enough with me to say, Louis, that's a load of crap.'

Here's an example. I give a patient a bending exercise to do and they're thinking that what I've asked them to do will make their pain a whole lot worse and put them back a week. They need to tell me they're not at all keen and very wary. I had a patient once who said, 'Look Louis, I'm not doing that. I haven't bent forward for two years.' I realised I'd totally misread the patient, the situation and their thoughts and beliefs. It's moments like that which make you realise how poor communication can be sometimes.

Star charts

With more on-going pain patients I sometimes have little ten minute 'star-chart' sessions if I think they might be helpful. Figure 4.9 illustrates a 'fears and concerns' star-chart that I did early on with a complex chronic pain patient. I simply drew a circle in the middle of a piece of A4 paper and wrote 'Fears and Concerns' in it.

I decided to do this after about ten minutes of talking to the patient. I said, 'You seem really concerned and worried.' To which the patient, a middle aged man who'd recently lost his job, said with a rather heavy sigh and look of desperation 'I've no idea where to start.'

I drew the circle and off we went, getting his 'list' of things.

He had on-going back pain of about eight months and had pretty much withdrawn from his normal life. He was feeling very negative about getting better and was particularly upset with the lack of any progress.

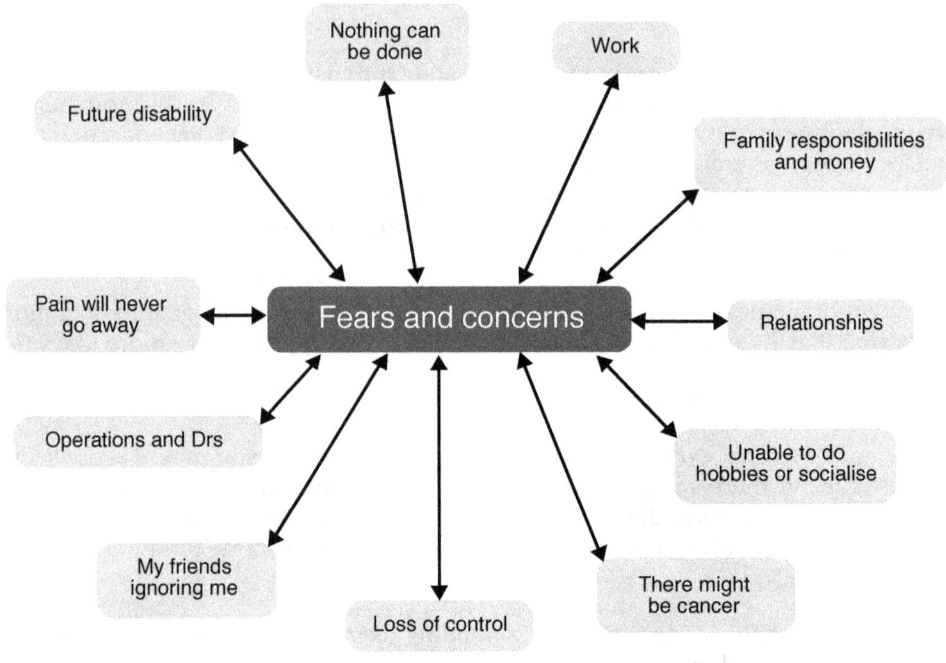

Figure GE 4.9 'Fears and concerns'

I photocopied the chart. I kept a copy and I gave one to him. Every so often through the rehab process I got it out again and he commented on each one. One of the most useful things in his recovery was the use of the 'recovery-graph', figure GE 2.4. It was the key thing in getting him to shift from thinking that he needed a better diagnosis, then it would just be appropriate treatment and he would be better, to a perspective that required him to be a big part of the process. Start easy, build slowly was vital. His progress was easily monitored, via various physical goals and occasional reflection on his attitude, his focus and his understanding of what was going on. Within a month of starting a graded programme we were able to put big crosses through; 'Operations and Drs'; 'Pain will never go away'; 'Nothing can be done'; 'Future disability'; 'Unable to do hobbies or socialise'; 'There might be cancer'; 'Loss of control' and he was a great deal more confident about the family and work related worries improving too. By unmasking and revealing what the patient's concerns are it means they can be dealt with directly – good examination, explanation, reassurance for example. Less stress and distress deals a massive benefit to anyone trying to get better.

Distress we may be able to deal with

Main and Watson suggest we get distressed/angry patients to:

- identify when they are beginning to think negatively

- identify when they are becoming tense and angry

- take steps to stop such thoughts and being positive relaxation (see later, but simple smooth floppy relaxy movements can be helpful in some)

- pace physical activities (see later)

- pick achievable goals (see later, but note that these patients often madly over do an exercise, then suffer later, and then get distressed/angry all over again)

- look at what they've managed to achieve, (see function compartment of shopping basket)

- reward themselves when they achieve even small targets.

Distress we cannot influence easily

This relates to distress created by other issues going on in patient's lives. For example, home life, relationships, some work issues, the patient's past...

Hear, acknowledge and realise that there are yet more barriers and obstacles to your patient's recovery and, be very careful.

My experience dealing with chronic pain disability, when it's combined with complex chronic low mood, is that it can be almost impossible to deal with as an individual and non-psychology trained therapist. Even then I imagine it would be hard. Having the luxury of a local CBT /pain management unit where multidisciplinary teams work together in helping the patient has to be a wonderful thing. We need to be able to recognise when our inputs are unlikely to help and when alternative inputs are appropriate.

On the other hand, I have found that being open with some of these difficult and emotionally complex patients and clearly stating what I can do and cannot do, has often surprised me over the years. I have helped a good many patients through difficult phases in their lives, who, despite having complex psychopathology have been able to make good progress. This is because our focus remained on clear physical goals, good pacing, the use of relaxation, lots of reinforcement and often their great appreciation for time being taken to explain things, in a much more palatable and positive way than they'd ever heard before.

Main and Watson suggest:

* physiotherapists must learn to distinguish between pain and disability related distress and more general distress

* you must decide what you can deal with and what requires someone else

* learn to be open and honest with patients (brilliant – easy to say, for some it takes years to be good at and a bit of age, open mindedness and a big pinch of wisdom are sometimes required – be humble)

* get help from others, distressed patients are very hard work – you are not a failure, don't feel bad

* have a departmental policy for referrals of high risk patients.

To finish here: there are questionnaires and all the relevant ones and how to use them are in Gordon Waddell's book 'The Back Pain Revolution' and Main and Spanswick's: Pain Management an Interdisciplinary Approach.

For me the main ones I've used over the years are:

The DRAM which is the modified Zung and the Modified Somatic Perception Questionnaire (MSPQ)

The FABQ (Fear Avoidance Beliefs Questionnaire)

The TSK (Tampa Scale of Kinesiophobia)

The Linton and Hallden 'Yellow flags' questionnaire (for skilled practical use of this see Kendal and Watson, chapter 4 in Topical Issues in Pain 2. They go through a typical patient, the results of the questionnaire and how to deal with the results). See also chapter 12 of Steven Linton's book 'Understanding pain for better clinical practice. He calls it the 'Orebro Musculoskeletal Pain Screening Questionnaire' but it's the same thing. There's lots of great practical advice too.

Don't forget to think about Waddell's 'behavioural' signs and symptoms too. To me the signs can easily be included in a normal physical assessment. But note that a 'normal physical assessment' is generally not appropriate to a chronic pain disabled and highly distressed patient.

Chapter GE4.9
Psychosocial compartment part 5: Pink Flags!

This essay is a slightly revised version of an editorial I did for the Physiotherapy Pain Association Newsletter, Issue 20, Dec 2005.

Why is it we know far more about how things go wrong, i.e. pathology, than we know about how things go right, i.e. healing, recovery and how pain goes away?

In pain science for example, we know a great deal about inflammation and how peripheral nociceptors become sensitised and we also know a great deal about how the afferent nociceptive barrage causes central changes.

We know about pathology of tissues. For example how they degenerate and fall apart, but most of us would be hard pressed to say a great deal about how the tissues/body copes, adapts and is still able to manage and get on its way following injury or as it ages.

Ask any group of physiotherapists or Drs and consultants for that matter how long the various stages of healing go on; how they overlap and how strong the tissues are at the various stages, for skin, for ligament, for tendon, for disc, for muscle, for bone and nerve? And I wager you won't get a very confident answer for any of them? The medical model of pathology associated with disability prevails and with it the notion that if we know how a problem happened, we can intervene to prevent it. (And intervene – with some doubtful, but profit making intervention too. Stay sceptical it's important)

Shame on us! Here we all are, dealing with recovery day in and day out and we don't know enough about how we heal and adapt; how the body controls central sensitivity or peripheral inflammation; how the nervous system monitors and controls inflammation and healing; how pain mechanisms are dampened down; how discs degenerate, adapt and cope, how joints adapt to ageing, how muscles, tendons and ligaments adapt and change in response to activity and inactivity. And how the way we think and feel might influence the process – how it all happens and how long it takes and so on.

Surely, if we knew more about how we recover naturally, the best conditions for recovery and how the body copes with adverse conditions we would be able to intervene more positively alongside these natural processes? Yes, I know we do, but it could be much better. I would argue that most of the time our attention is given to the bad, not the good. To what's wrong and not what's right? To 'find' something rather than trying not to find anything! This focus of 'bad', of 'pathology', or of some kind of 'impairment' also applies to the biopsychosocial model and CBT approaches, just as much as it does to the more traditional approaches as far as I can see. Take yellow flags (psychosocial predictors of a BAD outcome), blue flags and black flags (work related psychosocial predictors of a BAD outcome). They're all negatives predicting negativity, in a world that seems to thrive on criticism, blame, litigation and wrong-doing. Agreed, we need to know the bad to get to the good, but if you get too much bad you get negative. You lose hope and you fulfil your own prophecy, 'This patient has a high yellow flag score. What's the point of trying? Next patient please...'

In our practice Philippa and I have been emphasising the positive side of everything more and more. We check for the bad (red flags), reassure the patient and then (or in parallel) – look for the good! In a moment of simple, almost childish inspiration 'the good' can now be called 'PINK FLAGS'.   Here I'd like to thank the participants on the Cardiff 'Graded Exposure' course, December 1st/2nd 2005. To whom I put the 'positive flag' proposal to – suggesting either pink or a traffic-light inspired green for the colour. I would like to acknowledge Richard Rudling-Smith, one of the participants, who had also been thinking this way for some time and confirmed that although green is for go, pink is fun, happy and sort of rhymes with positive!

So, here we are: the new 'PINK FLAGS – ABCDEFW initiative'. The 'positive' flags that predict you are going to do well, the ones that lift optimism, the ones that we should find, whittle-out and talk about more with our patients. And I would predict that they are the ones that promote healing, recovery and pain cessation too.

I always think of the 'shift' or antalgic posture, often adopted by patients with acute low back pain, as the body's clever response to aid recovery – a positive pink flag! Tell the patient that the shifted posture is usually temporary, show the patient how it corrects when they lie down and reassure them it's part of getting better (the 'limp' of the back!)

It's easy, take the yellow flags and paint them PINK. If they come in yellow with the patient – work out how to make them shift to pink. Good rehabilitation, good management, good explanation, reaching targets, helping the pain, better pain management, keeping going, positive coping strategies, still at work, adaptive levels of pain behaviour etc.

Here's an example for the 'A' in the ABCDEFW.

Pink flag A = Attitudes and Beliefs

1. Low fear, low concern about pain.

2. Belief that to keep going at work and normal activities helps recovery.

3. Expectation that being active will eventually lead to quicker recovery even though exacerbations may occur.

4. Believing that you're going to get better and that you will get back to all previous activities.

5. Belief that pain is quite manageable and controllable.

6. Desire to be involved in one's own recovery and not reliant on medical management – that one's own biology will do the job far better in the end and that there is no such thing as a magic fix.

7. Belief that pain does not mean harm.

Why not be far more explicit here with patients?

During physical examination, try saying to the patient when you start looking at standard movements, something like this; 'What we are going to do now is look at some movements of your back/neck/shoulder. When you do the movements I am interested in any responses from you about what happens, but I want you to tell me just as much about any movements that feel good and OK, as those that may feel bad. I am just as interested in the **positives** as the negatives!'

So we tune the patients in to looking for what they can do, as well as what they are having difficulty with. It's far more balanced and all part of the shopping basket approach's aim of helping the patient to see for themselves their situation and, that it's not necessarily as bad as they thought it was.

Put this book on your Christmas wish list:

Seligman, Martin(2002). Authentic Happiness. Using the new positive psychology to realize your potential for deep fulfilment. Nicholas Brealey Publishing, London.

This book is all about psychology starting to look at and investigate positive mood and happiness and applying it to patients. It's the exact opposite of pathologising mood. It's new 'pink' psychology.

I'm going to take one more category for 'pinking' up and later I'll illustrate it in relationship to physical findings, movement rehab and with explanations.

The Pink Flags B = Behaviours (and a bit of D too!) that predict a good outcome:

1. Staying active and avoiding extended rest periods/reclining...

2. Attempting to maintain normal activities, accepting they may have to be modified/slowed down/worked into smaller 'building blocks' if necessary... i.e. lifting one bag of shopping at a time, using more bags... adjusting how you lift to make it easier.

3. Good compliance with exercises and good pacing, avoiding boom and bust.

4. Accepting the level of pain and going with it as far as possible but finding and using the best strategies for keeping it at an acceptable and functional level. Not talking about it all the time and trying to stay relaxed.

5. Keeping going without being too reliant on sticks and supports... though quite acceptable for a short time if they enable you to stay functioning (more later).

6. Try to maintain a good sleep pattern, staying relaxed when woken by pain and using active coping strategies to try and help.

7. Keeping a balanced diet going and avoiding any toxicity via drugs, smoking and alcohol.

8. Seeking help that doesn't insist on regular treatment but helps you manage it yourself.

9. Keeping relaxed movements and function going. Using appropriate relaxation.

10. Seek reassurance and guidance, not cure. Avoid those who can't explain the advice to 'don't do' that they give out... and give the impression that you must have regular treatment and regular check ups... and who also indicate you spine is weak or wrong in some way...

The list could go on. Think about the 'E' for emotions yellow flag too and do your own conversion!   I'm starting to wonder if skedaddling out of the relationship or the boring crummy work situation isn't a tad pink? Up the rebels!

Chapter GE4.10
The Disability and functional limitations/ activity and movement restrictions compartment

My simple definition here is:

This is what the patient reports they can no longer do or have difficulty doing as a result of their problem.

In the late 1990's, when Dave Butler and I were very much engaged in the pain revolution, we called this hypothesis category (the term being used by Mark Jones, the clinical reasoning expert) 'General Physical Dysfunction'. Now I feel the terms, disability and activity limitation or restriction better describe it, and are more in line with the general literature on disability and handicap.

Think:

- disability/restrictions related to **Activity**: like walking normally, walking distance limited, housework, gardening, socialising, hobbies; think general and specific activities, for example, gardening and bending, lifting, crouching, kneeling, being on all fours, getting in and out of a chair, up and down stairs, driving the car, cycling, rowing, sailing, fishing...

- disability/restrictions related to **Inactivity:** many pain sufferers are on the move all the time and find it difficult to sit, stand still, lie down, sleep, do their yoga poses...

Note also:

- **the Activity related Disability/activity restrictions are closely linked to the 'B' for Behaviour and 'A' for Attitudes and Beliefs in the yellow flags.** For example, the belief that activity, or movement is likely to be harmful and withdrawal from normal activities. The tendency to avoid, rather than confront movements and activities deemed likely to hurt or harm is another example. Think in terms of 'fear-avoidance' can be helpful, but sometimes the patient just doesn't know whether they should move or rest and want your advice. Simple? Or it should be

- often a key issue is 'confidence'.

Some key questions at an appropriate time during assessment:

1. *Since the problem started are you still doing all your normal activities or have you been restricted in some way?* See what you get. Here's an answer: 'The Dr said I'd just sprained my back and it was best to quietly carry on the best I could and to keep going at work too. Well, I struggled on for about two weeks and finally had to give in. It was agony, so he's now given me a sick note for two weeks and I've been resting.

   'Has that helped then?'
   'Well I'm due back to see him the day after tomorrow for another note. To be

honest it's really much the same, that's why I've come to see you.'

You now go on to find out what his current activity levels are. The 'typical day' process can be helpful here but asking about common activities is often essential. Importantly, you need to get a list of the activities he was doing before the back pain and what he's doing now for comparison. One gives you the activity goals, the other the starting point.

2. Are you still able to move around freely and easily or has the problem caused some difficulties with movements and activities?

3. Has the problem stopped you doing anything or made you change the way you do things? Important from this question is that you may find out that the patient is carrying on with a lot of activities, but has adopted different patterns of movement in order to do this.

'Oh yes, I'm still gardening, but I'm doing the weeding and planting lying down. My Mrs. keeps getting cross with me for coming in soaking wet and covered in mud all the time.'

Or...

'I'm still walking but everyone's telling me I'm walking sideways like a crab. I haven't noticed mind.'

An important part of our input is to observe movement and when appropriate restore normal movement patterns. A great many patients have adopted 'clever' new ways of doing things, that are maybe all right for a short while to keep them functioning, but are not the best habits to get into given longer periods of time.

Most physios will find what I am about to say rather 'wrong'. When I get an acute (recently happened and nasty painful) problem in and they're struggling to function and do things 'normally' I often spend five minutes or so going through different ways of moving to overcome the pain. I actually teach them 'antalgic' movements and postures if it helps! Sacred normal movement where art thou?

Here are some typical examples: an acute low back pain patient with radiating leg pain... who walks in bent forwards to ease the pain and who can't come upright without shooting leg pain – give him crutches and encourage him to relax in the stooped posture while walking and standing. It's OK for a short time. It's so common, it has to be seen as an 'adaptive' posture and anyway he will also be doing some kind of comfortable extension or 'to-neutral' exercises, for example on all fours and lying down. As time goes on the crutches will go and more normal postures resumed. That's graded exposure, start-easy-build-slowly; fire-apart-depart.

Forget the pressure of achieving: 'I walked into the physio doubled up and went out straight.' I'm sorry, I've learnt over many years that sudden changes in things is 'risk taking' and often a recipe for a big flare-up or even spells of worsening neurological signs.

Next example: the calf strain and the twisted ankle – turn your foot out, walk flat footed when you're in a hurry. But when you have a few quiet moments, walk normally and slowly with small easy steps so as to remind the system of normal movement patterns.

The rule is: ***Fiddle with posture and movement in any way you like but keep the 'hunter-gatherer' (patient!) functioning.***

Rest is intermittent, or if at the start of a problem a max of a day or two. 'Doing nothing' is far more 'dangerous' than walking around like a stuffed penguin.

4. *Are you at all anxious about doing any of your usual activities (if struggling give examples), 'Would you for example, lift normally?'...* Note that this question gives you information not only about activity capability/ restriction, but also about the patient's levels of concern too.

5. *Are you having problems with being still, like sitting, lying, standing and sleeping?* We have to be balanced and not be thinking that the 'yellow flags' are dictators to the cause of movement. A vast number of patients with spinal pain have huge difficulties getting comfortable. They are often almost constantly restless being still and this all needs addressing and strategies put in place.

I'd just like to underline again here that this section is placed before the 'Impairment' section for a very good reason and that is because function is far more important to the patient's life. It is also shown to be more important when it comes to outcome.

The majority of patients need to leave your session with clear instruction about some aspect of returning to function. For example, it might mean practice walking, pacing up walking time and distance; practicing normal stair climbing, practising sit to stand, if that is a problem, a lifting programme etc. (All graded with start-easy-build-slowly rules)

I also like this question (which is a variation on a theme from a question earlier):

Has this problem stopped you doing anything, or are you carrying on as normal?

If it's say a back pain patient and the answer is, 'No it hasn't stopped me doing anything. It just keeps on hurting no matter what I do.' I might follow this up with 'So you'd be happy to lift the couch here with me now, or help me unload a ton of sand?' (I'm cheekily smiling by the way!) 'Well, ah, that sort of thing hasn't cropped up, but I think I'd probably be a bit careful with that.' OK, you told me you run and garden just now, you're carrying on with that happily?' 'I am indeed.' Etc.

Now, disability is often what the patient 'tells us' they are struggling with or cannot do. That's fine, but it's related to this 'self report' issue and it's been shown that patients actually tend to *underestimate* their actual activity levels. Yes they do! A simple example is the patient who says they can't bend, but when you observe them getting their shoes and socks off, or sitting unsupported on the treatment couch you can see that their back is fully flexed. Careful, that's a bit 'impairmenty' Louis! That's just to get the ball rolling though, so you can see what I mean and start to understand that we all move around and do things all day long without thinking about it much. Studies that actually record patient's up time and down time, using electronic movement detectors, often indicate that patients may for example be on their feet and moving for longer than they report.

What all this boils down to is the *need for objective assessment of function* – especially in the sub-chronic and chronic groups of patients who report significant activity restrictions.

Canadian based therapist Maureen Simmonds, an important name in the world of pain and movement along with UK based Heather Muncey (who I've mentioned before), use the following standardised tests. These are mainly used for spinal problems but can be used whatever the area of complaint (patients with on-going pain, even if it's in their upper quadrant are often functionally moribund..!). I want you to have in mind a patient like Mr Grubb and see that these tests give a wonderful baseline from which to work and later reflect for positive reinforcement. Here they are:

- repeated sit to stand – 5 repetitions done twice and average time recorded

- repeated trunk flexion – 5 reps times two, average time recorded

- loaded reach test – subjects stand next to a wall on which a meter rule is mounted horizontally at the shoulder height. They hold 4.5Kg weight with both hands at shoulder height and close to the body and then reach forward with the weight. The maximum distance they go is recorded

- 50 foot walk test – walk 25 feet, turn and walk back as fast as possible – record time

- 5 minute walk – walk as far as possible for 5 minutes, record distance. This is usually done in a corridor or somewhere appropriate and the patient asked to walk up and down for 5 minutes. A chair is placed at either end and the patient is told they're free to rest if they want to. (A typical recording for Mr Grubb type patient might be 2 laps of the 25 foot corridor taking over a minute and for the rest of the time he was seated). Try and remain neutral and impassive. The recording should be in a 'reinforcement free' environment. The patient gets their base line and it's an easy process to start grading up at home – in the right context.

- 360 degree roll-over. Lying supine the patient is asked to roll over and all the way back, first going round to the right, the time is recorded, and then they are asked to repeat but this time going to the left, and time recorded.

(Mr Grubb recording would be something like – 20 seconds only got half way onto left shoulder, failed to the right and gave up)

- the 'Sorensen' fatigue test (for patients with minimal dysfunction). The patient lies prone with thighs and calves stabilised. They are then asked to lift the upper body and hold for as long as possible, the time to fatigue is recorded.

(This would be inappropriate for a Mr Grubb. I often do the same thing for a half 'sit-up' or half 'sit-back'. For example, with Mr Grubb I could do this: get him to sit sideways on an armless chair, feet on the floor but tucked under the bottom of the treatment plinth or some kind of bar for support, then ask him to lean back to about half way and hold it for as long as they feel they can and record time it takes. For more able patients, I might get them to do a partial sit-up (feet firmly supported) say, to the point of head and shoulders just off, then hold and record time to fatigue).

Reference here:

Simmonds, M. (1999). Physical function and physical performance in patients with pain: What are the measures and what do they mean? Pain 1999 - an updated review. Refresher course syllabus. M. Max. Seattle, IASP Press: 127-136.

Two big **key points...**

- physical **capacity** is determined by physiological factors

- physical **performance** is determined by physical and psychological factors.

You are unlikely to lift an object off the floor if you feel that:

- bending will injure your back or your nerve

- bending may exacerbate your pain.

Ref: *Watson, P. J. (1999). Non-physiological determinants of physical performance in musculoskeletal pain. Pain 1999 - an updated review. Refresher course syllabus. M. Max. Seattle, IASP Press: 153-158.*

An important thing to note is that by doing the above kind of activities during assessment you are already drawing the patient's attention to function and getting going rather than to a fix. The 'impairment' compartment focused assessment draws the patient towards finding something wrong that needs addressing and may well leave the practitioner struggling to back track towards function. Critically, the approach is really that 'the more chronic pain disabled the patient, the more one should steer clear of looking for impairments'. It really means there's little need for doing a standard musculoskeletal examination and a great need for looking at and getting baseline measures for physical function capabilities.

Eyes and hands-off the nitty-gritty, fiddly-de-diddly little bits and pieces now... Remember these patients have usually been viewed and reviewed by a great many other Drs and specialists. There's even no need for a neuro examination unless the history taking is telling you that something may have been missed. For these types of patients this is definitely, 'a let's see what you can do' approach rather than, 'finding all the things' wrong approach.

With the more acute and sub-acute patients standard basic examinations are required (but make them 'Pink' and therefore shift the emphasis more to function – especially where the yellow flag assessment is indicating a high level of 'A' 'B' and 'E' factors (avoidance, resting and a passive attitude to recovery associated with concern, anxiety and fear related to pain and movement).

Chapter GE4.11
The Physical Impairment compartment part 1

I define physical impairments as those things that we find on our physical examination and include the following:

- sensitive tissues – tissues that hurt when palpated or touched

- sensitive movements

- altered movement patterns – gross movements and specific movement

- altered biomechanics, altered alignment and asymmetry

- loss or range of movement – in joint, nerve, muscle etc.

- altered muscle strength – power and endurance

- alterations in muscle bulk

- problems with co-ordination – gross and specific

- neurological abnormality

Sensitive tissues

Tissues that hurt when palpated or touched. In pain mechanism terms this is an exploration that reveals the extent of mechanical/touch related allodynia. Don't forget to think about hyperalgesia too, via the definition 'an exaggerated response to an input that would normally be uncomfortable or hurt in some way'. But also, that the definition slips up somewhat when considering 'primary' and 'secondary' hyperalgesia. Primary being a 'true' positive for tenderness, the tissues that are tender are abnormal in some way and secondary being a 'false' positive for tender tissues – the tissues that are tender and sore have nothing wrong with them. It is my strong opinion that a great many pain patients, from acute right through to the more chronic, have a high degree of secondary hyperalgesia/allodynia, or 'sensitivity that is out of all proportion to the damage done, or sensitivity that has no meaning in terms of damage.

Finding and almost 'mapping' the extent of a patient's sore-to-touch tissues not only tells you a great deal about the degree and spread of sensitivity, it also informs the patient that you've examined them and actually found something.

Remember, widespread tenderness to palpation is one of the 'behavioural' signs. I can think of a great many back pain patients, whose actual physical movements are not at all bad, but when it comes to palpation they tense up and can get quite jumpy even with the slightest of pressures to the skin. Think like this: compare this type of sensitivity to that of a nasty skin burn? Here the amount of sensitivity fits. But, when the skin of the back pain patient looks perfectly normal anatomically/tissue wise this amount of sensitivity has to be viewed as not a reflection of the tissue status, but as 'allodynia' or 'secondary hyperalgesia.' In other words the sensitivity is due to a 'processing' problem. That a tissue problem elsewhere might be responsible for setting up this degree of sensitivity does need consideration.

My advice is to think:

1. How long has this been going on? Sensitivity as high as this is only usual in the very first day or two of tissue injury and even then it's rather too high on 'volume'. If the pain and sensitivity have been around for a long time, and they often have, then the clinician should be thinking 'maladaptive' processing problem here.

2. High levels of sensitivity like this may be associated, in the 'peripheral' sense, with nerve injury/nerve related supersensitivity – see the Nerve Root section for full explanations.

3. It's just maladaptive, maybe just a 'cost' of the initial cause of the problem and if you feel you want to tackle this finding think 'touch desensitisation' programme.

4. Don't go, 'This is nuts, it can't be real, the patient is over-egging it.' Blaming is a complete waste of time when dealing with pain sufferers. This type of response or finding if very common and we now have a good understanding of its mechanisms, certainly enough to give a good explanation to the patient and a pathway to help deal with it (desensitisation).

So, excessive sensitivity to palpation is a great example of pain out of proportion to the damage done. It is maladaptive and it simply goes in the shopping basket as something that could be addressed in management, just like any other palpation finding. I was pondering Geoff Maitland when I was writing this and thinking, you know he would have loved to understood and known about all this stuff when I was with him back in the late 1980's.

> *If you find increased tissue sensitivity to palpation and touch, pop it in the impairment compartment of the shopping basket and it may be something worth addressing at some point (desensitisation?)*

Sensitive movements

Think movement allodynia/hyperalgesia. Again, as with touch sensitivity try to think:

- 'primary', the pain on movement/mechanical testing relates to tissue abnormality, but even so, thanks to maladaptive processing, can still be excessive and inappropriate

- 'secondary', where the pain on movement or 'mechanical testing' relates to processing and not to tissue abnormality. Again pain response may be excessive or inappropriate and therefore placed well up at the maladaptive end of the spectrum.

In the very early acute injury situation; movement related primary and secondary hyperalgesia may well be very helpful in relation to protective responses and creating good early safe conditions for the first phases of healing. But, think about the *type* of tissue that may be injured and how long it might require being 'looked after' before getting to a 'stronger' phase, or 'you'll cope fine on your own' phase? As we've already seen, ligaments, tendons, discs and all collagenous tissues for that matter are very slow to heal and strengthen. Could it be argued that maintaining sensitivity to movement for a long time is of value, since these tissues require such lengthy recovery? I think so. The key question is whether the movement (and tissue) sensitivity is 'reasonable' or 'adaptive' for the actual tissue situation. I'm thinking of the classic medial or lateral collateral knee ligament strains, which not only remain very sensitive for a long time (months to a year or more) but also maintain a 'sharp' pain protective response when under certain loads. Like knee rotation, and with valgus or varus forces, as when running and suddenly changing direction. Clinically the common finding is that the response in many patients is more than it needs to be. So I 'think of a spectrum' of presentations: at one end are those two to eight months or more, ligament injuries that 'tweak' occasionally when they do an awkward or sudden movement, as well as at end of range positions. Yet, at the other extreme are those with the same injury who continue to report difficulty moving; are still limping, get a great deal of sharp pain with the smallest movement and are very reluctant to move the joint very far into range and certainly not to the end of range. The joint may continue to ache as well. This second presentation I would consider to be maladaptive, out of proportion to the tissue situation and capability and one where 'better loading' is needed as an adequate healing stimulus. This patient needs a graded programme for their range of movement and plenty of desensitising and even appropriate help with pain control.

It is also worth considering that it may still be safe to gradually start loading anyway, for example because other tissues can provide adequate support and protection. That just one tissue may want rest is sometimes just too selfish for the well-being of the whole organism! I'm particularly thinking spine related injury/pain states here. Remember 'Why should the disc bother to hurt?' The outcome is the same whether an injured disc is loaded and moved or immobilised – it degenerates further! So the owner of the disc might just as well get on with life. The only proviso from me is that the nervous system may be vulnerable due to the changes in the disc. As long as recovery of movement range and function is done in a graded way the patient and we are safe

> *If you find increased sensitivity to movements, pop it in the impairment compartment of the shopping basket and it may be something worth addressing at some point.*

Altered movement patterns

It seems to me that physios have gone crazy on this topic over the last ten to fifteen years. ***The muscle imbalance/kinetic control/core stability thing, is to my mind, a misguided passion of many and for the great majority of patients***

more a hindrance than a help! It's a brilliant example of impairment 'ultra-focus' causing the clinician to miss the bigger picture as far as I am concerned. The problem is that its advocates and acolytes have their reasoning heads buried, strangled and stifled by its philosophical high commandments and commanders. I urge all those involved to read those who have looked at the literature in detail (like Eyal Lederman) and folk like me who can step back and see the bigger picture.

Right now I'm thinking of a young marathon runner with a withered left leg and a terribly unstable left knee joint, who ran over the Paris marathon finish line right next to me in four hours and forty five minutes. For the last four or five miles I had been spell-bound by her incredibly lopsided gait. As she pitched on the withered leg, the knee buckled about 20 degrees into adduction, yet on she went, quietly running and quietly chatting away to her companion. After the race I went up to her, 'Sorry to trouble you, but I'm a physio and I have been fascinated by your left leg and knee, tell me does that trouble you when you run?' She smiled and responded, 'It's part of me, I never even think about it!' Amazing, because of the fantastic 'imbalance' with no repercussions. Compare this to the analysis of a young athletic patient who came with back pain, thoracic pain and headaches. She saw me after not getting anywhere with her last physiotherapist who told her she had an over pronated foot resulting in a torsioned tibia and a complex kinetic chain problem going right up her spine. I naughtily wondered if I could transplant that young 'disabled' marathon runners' 'unstable' left leg onto her. Almost daily we look at the incredible feats of athleticism of paralympians with deformed and withered limbs, in the pool, wheelchair and on the track.

OK, a big part of good physical therapy is to restore good quality, relaxed normal thoughtless-fearless-movement and range of movement. I have no problems here. When it is appropriate I do look at movement quality and range and pain response and it largely it is hugely amenable to a *simple* graded exposure type of approach and it is always in the bigger functional picture. More examples later...

> *If you find altered movement patterns, pop them in the impairment compartment of the shopping basket and they may be something worth addressing at some point.*

Altered biomechanics, altered alignment and asymmetry

The same argument as above. Big question is: 'In the bigger picture is what you're finding relevant? Could you be creating more of a problem by highlighting this for the patient, when little is going to change or help?' I can't think of any patient I have ever seen with 'altered biomechanics' that I have thought: 'Go and see a surgeon to sort that out.' Here I'm thinking of things like 'patella tracking'. I have seen a great many who have been to surgeons and on closer questioning have found that the patients say things like 'Well, I guess if I hadn't had it done it would have ended up a lot worse than it is now.' Or, 'The knee was never very good and while the operation was good for a while, overall I sometimes wonder if it was worth it.'

The one situation where altered biomechanics may be helped by operation is when it is part of a bigger degenerative joint presentation and the sufferer is given a new joint. But even here the results may be good or bad; the patient can end up with a bigger leg length discrepancy than before! Plus a further loss of range! How many 'hips' have you followed through that still complain one year later that they used to be able to get their socks on but no longer can. Most accept it can get on. But improving biomechanics as a way of helping pain has to be taken with great caution I feel.

> *If you find altered biomechanics, altered alignment or asymmetry, pop the findings in the impairment compartment of the shopping basket and they may be something worth addressing at some point.*

As an entertaining aside, here is a commentary from my blog: It is slightly abridged to cut out the unnecessary...and involves a question from a contributor called Anoop... The title of the blog piece is:

Sex and leg length discrepancy

From Anoop...

Hello.

I've just heard about your blog. I have read your articles in 'Peak Performance' online, about treatment of chronic pain in athletes and a couple of book chapters. In there you write about checking the patient for leg length discrepancy, asymmetry, hamstring length and ROM. My question is what do these measures tell us about the person's pain or tissue condition? If a person has leg length inequality, what could it tell us?

Thank you so much, Anoop.

My first reply:

Right, that leg length mention was almost in there by reflex I feel. I have to credit my colleague, good friend and co-author Steve Robson with it perhaps? No, we both did it together and it was his fault!

You ask about the relevance of leg length? Well, it's absolutely no big deal and what could be done about it anyway? Tell the patient/sportsman and make them worry about it unnecessarily? Tell them it's because of an SI joint up-slip or something. Sorry, not my scene; it creates fear of structure and unnecessary notions of weakness in the very people who want to feel invincible and it's, well, bull-s**t!

A great many patients come in and say that the chiropractor /osteo/physio told them their leg length was out. So, if they say this I always check it and 90% or more of the time it's fine. The patient lies flat. I ask them to wiggle the hips and back and get as straight as they possibly can. They bring their legs together at the ankles, both medial malleoli hit each other exactly. I get the patient to take a look and they usually go 'Ah, it's OK!' And then I usually say 'They must have fixed it!' and smile (if appropriate). Or, if it is slightly different I say 'If we took fifty people off the street with no problems at all, we'd find a large number of them had small differences like yours. Having a leg length difference is 'normal', is very common and is of no consequence. Anyway I can lengthen or shorten whichever leg you want, watch'...

I shift the patient's pelvis slightly to one side and hey presto – the legs are the same length. Or, bring both legs marginally off to one side, or push one of the legs back through the heel. All with the effect of slightly side flexing the back/pelvis and hence creating an apparent shortening of one and lengthening of the other leg.

'Hey, I can make your longer leg even longer and your shorter leg even shorter! Here's a good party trick, show your kids. Get them to watch your feet and tell them one leg's going to grow shorter. Just subtly and very slowly pull your hip up from the pelvis/back – little by little. Do it sitting with your legs stretched out on a chair, do a bit of chanting at the same time – even turn the lights down a bit to create atmosphere!

Chiropractors and others charge for this flim-flam and faith healers make gullible worshippers think that a miracle has happened. Check out James Randi on faith healers,

http://www.youtube.com/watch?v=wsKBP1TOdYI. Randi discusses and shows how they do it without the help of the Lord. Swing the legs to the side and pull the shoe off a little – maybe even surreptitiously create a fearful trance-like atmosphere, to distract the sufferer and the audience too and while this is going on, push the leg so the knee bends a bit too. Look these guys are seriously taking the p..s! Making a load of money and they don't pay any taxes. They have massive multi-million dollar homes and cars, all from the donations of the poor and gullible who they continuously hassle for money. These people are worse than shocking in my opinion. Randi and his group of sceptics have been exposing them and showing the public the shams that they really are for many years now. It's unbelievable frankly.

Do chiropractors really think they're lengthening/shortening the leg? Is there a chiropractor out there who wants to be whistleblower and afterwards go hide in an embassy somewhere? (*Julian Assange, the Australian hacker, computer programmer and Wikileaks founder and director has been holed up in the Ecuadorian embassy in London. Fearful of arrest, over the leaking of classified US security information given to him by whistleblower Bradley Manning – who yesterday was given a thirty five year sentence for his crime! At the time of writing, 'he' – 'Bradley', has just changed to 'her' – 'Chelsea'!*)

This next bit is where the sex comes in!

Symmetry in nature is amazingly difficult to achieve. I'd like to quote Matt Ridley, author of 'The Red Queen: Sex and the evolution of human nature'.

'It's a well known developmental accident that animal bodies are more symmetrical if they were in good condition when growing up, and they are less symmetrical if they were stressed while growing. For example, scorpion flies develop more symmetrically when fathered by well-fed fathers that could afford to feed their wives. Making something symmetrical is not easy. If things go wrong, the chances are it will come out asymmetrical.'

Consider that most biological molecules, large as they are, twist and contort into the most fantastic shapes that are usually far from symmetrical (a process called 'protein folding'). That we are all made of asymmetrical protein molecules makes it quite fantastic that, at least for the most part, we do end up looking pretty much symmetrical; it has to be an incredible biological challenge, but one which is necessary when you think of say movement efficiency and fitness to operate.

I know this is rather politically incorrect, (please try to stay planted at the biological level) but have you noted how attractive symmetry is? (Faces in particular) And how unattractive asymmetry is? In nature, if you want to be reproductively successful, don't have a short leg and look lopsided, or walk with a sway and a dip. If you happen to be an organism that flies for a living it's not going to be pretty to have asymmetry of your wings. Not only don't you look to cool, you're also going to have a struggle getting airborne and no potential partner in their right mind is going to want to pass their genes on to the next generation with yours.

So, cruel thought it may seem, sexual evolutionary selection has worked its wonders to produce a strong link between good genes and good looks – a big part of that might just be symmetry!

Back to Matt Ridley again and his discussion of Møller's study of swallows' tail streamers (not the swallows we see in the UK). Møller noted that swallows with the longest tails were the most successful at securing mates. He also noted that the *longer the tails the more symmetrical they were too. So, Møller cut or elongated the tail feathers of certain males and at the same time enhanced or reduced the symmetry of the tails. Those with longer tails got mates sooner and reared more offspring, but within each class of length, those with enhanced symmetry did better than those with reduced symmetry...*

What girls make the boys do for a good time! But biologically it all boils down to advertising your good genes – plus your good upbringing (well fed, stress free, and as a result, well developed) and therefore your fitness to sire the young lady swallow and be a good provider for the subsequent offspring. Girls go for symmetrical fit and strong boys who've had a good up-bringing and vice versa too. Plus, well, what about that human stallion driving a Rolls Royce and controlling the Formula 1 Racing Empire, or that strangely symmetrical guy who won Wimbledon this year

(2013)? Oh, not for you?

So the moral of the story is to put that heel raise in, not only are you a tad taller, you are a tad more symmetrical too. It might feel really weird to start with but you're much more likely to score!

It works, I've just tried it!

Thanks for listening and sincere apologies to any who may be offended.

Now do I ever use a heel raise to correct it? If it changes processing it may be worth it. You try going round all day with a small heel cushion in your foot. Yes, try it. Novel feeling? So use any trick in the book to change processing. Go for it. But in doing so for goodness sake, don't make the patient leg-length obsessed, they might just go see an orthopod for an osteotomy!

Reply from Anoop...

Louis,

Some interesting thoughts from Lederman's article 'The fall of the postural-structural-biomechanical model in manual and physical therapies: Exemplified by lower back pain' (see ref given below, for more references to the statements given here).   In the part of his article about leg length and pain: leg length differences as a cause for back pain has been debated for the last three decades. It is estimated that about 90% of the population has a leg length inequality, with a mean of 5.2 mm. The evidence suggests that for most people, anatomic leg length inequality is not clinically significant, until the magnitude reaches approximately 20 mm. Although some earlier studies, comparing people experiencing back pain with asymptomatic controls suggest a correlation, more relevant are prospective studies in which no correlation was found between leg length inequality and LBP.

Patients who have acquired their leg length differences later in life, as a consequence of disease or surgery, may also help to shed light on the relationship between pathomechanics and LBP. Individuals who developed a shorter leg due to Perthe's disease had a poor correlation between leg length inequality, lumbar scoliosis and low-back disorders, assessed several decades after the onset of the condition. In studies of patients who had marked changes in leg length due to hip fractures or replacement, such changes were not associated with back pain assessed several years after surgery.

One of the arguments in favour of an association between leg length differences and LBP is the supposed success of heel lifts in reducing back pain (list of refs). However, all these studies failed to include controls or sham heel lift (such as inefficient soft foam lift).

Eyal Lederman's two articles are must reads:

Lederman E. (2010). The fall of the postural-structural-biomechanical model in manual and physical therapies: Exemplified by lower back pain. CPDO online journal March p1-14 (www.cpdo.net)

Lederman E. (2007). The myth of core stability. CPDO online journal June p1-17. (www.cpdo.net)

My response…

Thanks Anoop.

It's always gratifying to find no support for something stupid, but it's also necessary to balance this by trying to find support for the stupidity too (and weighing it up fairly, like good scientists should). The task is then to analyse the quality of the support for the stupid thing – whereupon you often find you get a double gratification-buzz-whammy because the quality of the stupid support is also stupid.

The big deal here is *interpretation* when a heel raise does indeed help the back pain; which I'm sure it has done in a great many who've otherwise suffered for years, they've been quickly helped by this simple, but surprisingly costly (therapist expert fees plus a bit of choice rubbery-plastic – when packing sponge works just as well) and who are now enthusiastic neophytes.

The assumption that it was their leg length all along is what should be called into question. The belief that it was 'out' and is now fixed, plus, the new sexy symmetrical feel and that amazingly good novelty feeling, add to the over-all wellbeing feeling of the positive experience.

That processing might have changed is rarely entertained and for me, should be the first port of call.

Let's take another example which seeks the truth near the end by actually interviewing the pain and getting its opinion! Wow, this is cutting edge.

The subject is normally very healthy but has a new back pain and on the first occasion seeks the help of a 'cranio' who holds his head very gently and makes immovable joints swagger back to their correct place of rest at the same time rebalancing some juice in the CNS that flowed incorrectly somehow. It's a weird but very relaxing experience that afterwards feels really like nothing much happened. Anyway, all corrected, our happy patient, free of pain, now goes bungee jumping and never feels better. Consideration for the careful work of the cranio and that fluid imbalance disregarded, hey ho!

Anyway all goes well until the 'unfortunate' returns a year later with the exact same pain to find the 'cranio' therapist has been replaced by a reflexologist who now ignores the skull for some reason and makes a diagnosis via some thickened skin in the foot. It soon becomes clear to the 'reflexo' that it's this guy's pancreas and the back pain will be fixed once the pancreas is sorted. Ten easy and pleasant treatments later (the same number as the 'cranio' did by the way) and the said bungee jumper feels better and decides to follow up with another jump to positively reinforce the therapy like the last time. He strangely seems to disregard all the careful work done on the foot reflex zones as the bungee cord gets strapped firmly to the feet and several times G force happily prevents our patient from almost smashing his face into the ravine below. Feeling pleased, he then follows this up with some wing-suit-free-fall-off-a-cliff that luckily finishes with a parachute drop. And even though he has quite a hard landing on his pancreatic foot zone, everything is completely tickety-boo for months afterwards. Said patient wonders if it was his foot, his head, his fluid or his pancreas but totally disregards his back as a possible cause of his back pain. Cool!

Anyway, what helped? To the first therapist it was the displaced cranial suture and the 'cranio' fluid and for the second it was the thick skin on the foot and therefore the pancreas. For the bloke it was exactly the same back pain every time.

When the back pain was later interviewed it gave a shockingly honest appraisal of the real situation. According to our reporter who was there, the pain said:

'It was processing that changed and a whole bunch of novelty chemicals were released, thanks to all the various environments it had been exposed to.'

The pain also added, as an aside that 'Time and a very determined healing process also helped him.'

The final headline quote by the pain was, 'Yes, I've always been gullible'.

The press listened and so did the original therapists but none of them believed the pain was telling the truth and so it never got any publicity!

So (I like morals) the moral of this story is that just because a pain improves with a technique to a particular structure does not mean that that structure was the cause of the pain, or that what the therapist thinks they did to that structure cured it. I would particularly like to point this out to all those who get sucked into the sacroiliac joint. It's yet another version of the leg-length joke.

Oh, and the pain said it was happy to be interviewed again if there was any trouble caused – or if anyone didn't quite get what it was trying to explain.

Thanks for revving me up again. I eventually had to chuck the heels out they drove me mad... I'm now asymmetrical and lonely!

Louis

Chapter GE 4.12
Impairment Compartment part 2

Loss of range of movement: joint, nerve, muscle etc.

This is pretty self explanatory and an area that many physios love and excel in. Loss of range of movement is a significant part of many degenerative joint problems and may be an adaptive process. On the other hand loss of range in degenerative joint disease doesn't always occur and sometimes an awful joint can be virtually full range.

I'll never forget Harry's knee. Harry came to see me about twenty years after my father had last seen him (back in about 1975). He explained that my Dad had told him that he'd ruptured the knee ligaments in the middle and sides of his knee and that Dad had given him some exercises to do to keep his quads strong. My Dad apparently said 'If you keep those quads strong and active you'll help keep the joint stable and you'll be fine.' Harry did what he was told, but two years later re-visited Dad concerned about it making a noise like sandpaper when he moved it.

'I told him the noise made the kids want to puke (be sick!) when I came down the stairs!' Apparently Dad then told him the joint cartilage was thinning and if he wanted to he could have an x-ray and see an orthopaedic consultant. Remember this was at a time when knee replacements were not at all common and not at all good compared to the Charnley hip replacements that were gathering in popularity.

Harry told me he'd said to Dad, 'What's the point?' and Dad had agreed.

'Think of 'the noise' as a party trick but make sure you keep the range of movement full and don't stop using it' were apparently Dad's very words. So Harry carried on running his hotel and sailing as often as he could.

'I carried on scrambling around the boat, squeezing myself down the bilges and doing the engine – kneeling, squatting, everything. But now it's just started to stiffen when I straighten it and for some reason I can't stop it.'

Harry was 75 years old and sprightly, he could still kneel and squat and even get up without holding on from a full squat. Brilliant! Lots of knee noise though! I reviewed his exercises and made some suggestions for helping extension on a bit. This was helped by me doing some nice end range manual therapy, on and off into extension for about fifteen minutes – the joint would regain its range. He was pleased that it would still get there and he could see that a little longer and a bit more pressure was all that was needed. Luckily Harry had good tolerance and low pain reactivity. I saw him a couple of years later on his boat – he did a pretend 'Can-Can' and a full squat on the deck for my amusement.

The other good example that I rather like was related to me by fellow physiotherapist and ex- chair of the Physiotherapy Pain Association Vicki Harding. Over the years Vicki had spent some time living with families in Japan. Kneeling is a big part of life in traditional households and requires full knee bend of course! Vicki mentioned that even in those with severe knee arthroses, be it related to OA, or RA the sufferers rarely lost the ability to squat and maintained full range of movement.

What's fascinating is that if you type 'squatting and arthritis' into 'Google' and do a search you'll get back a whole pile of sites telling you that squatting is bad for your knees and a definite cause of arthritis! Now if you type in 'squatting is good for knee arthritis' you'll find things like: 'My knees hurt for years until I started doing squats.' I love this sort of thing. Whatever you do never say 'Don't do' or 'You must not do' or even 'You must do' a specific activity. There's never going to be support for such a dogmatic stance. Knee squats may be achievable and beneficial for one person but a disaster for another. Think graded exposure and that everyone's different; there's no harm in doing a little part of a squat and building from there. Everyone has some kind of limit and we're all very different.

> *If you find a loss of range of movement, pop it in the impairment compartment of the shopping basket and it may be something worth addressing at some point.*

Increased range of movement: joint, muscle, nerve, ligament, tendon, collagen fibril etc.

Yep, we can pick this up too. I've always found 'genu recurvatum' or knee hyperextension a bit sick-making, but I've never said that to anyone who's got it. In fact it's incredibly common and seems to pose no problem. Physical therapists and the like seem to find fault with excessive movement and the go on to pathologise it, when in actual fact it's just one end of a spectrum of mobility.

We have the Cornish farmer at one end, who can't touch his toes or cut his own toe nails to save his life and at the other, the folk who can fold themselves up into a small box. My pet hate is the designation of 'hypermobility' and 'instability' especially in the spine. I once had a 'chronic headache' patient who was told she had 'hypermobiltity and instability of her upper two neck vertebrae' by a physiotherapist! For five years following that she had hardly moved her neck for fear of injuring her spinal cord and spending the rest of her days paralysed, wheelchair bound and dependent. Over a period of six months with plenty of reassurance and a graded exposure approach she regained a good normal range for her age.

In order to understand 'hypermobility' properly it is important to study and have clinical experience of handling two conditions: Ehlers-Danlos and Marfans syndromes. Both are heritable diseases associated with abnormal elastin in connective tissues. If you can think of people who can do a full splits, have 'double-joints' or have extreme flexibility; and also have skin that easily pulls a long way away from the body – you are viewing someone with a good deal higher percentage of elastin in their connective tissues than most. Perhaps at the extreme end of the spectrum are the disease states but for most it's just a weird quirk of our variability, which for most is of little consequence. I have not reviewed the literature on hypermobility but it is often said that it's associated with increased joint pain and even osteoarthritis. I'd like to acknowledge that like everything you care to observe there's a great variability; a long spectrum from dwarf to tall, to giant; from diseases like Ehlers-Danlos and Marfans to hypermobility; to normal, to stiff, to hypomobile; to diseases of joint and musculosketal stiffness – like OA and ankylosing spondylitis. It's worth remembering that connective tissue is everywhere in the body, not just the joints and muscles. So it's hardly surprising that Ehlers-Danlos sufferers have super-elastic and hence 'fragile' blood vessels with tendencies towards aneurysm, potential for rupture of blood vessels, valvular heart disease and postural orthostatic tachycardia syndrome (POTS!).

'Orthostatic intolerance' (OI) is intolerance of standing still. The theory is that excessive distension of veins in the lower limbs while standing causes blood 'pooling', hence a decrease in cerebral blood flow. This sign is more common in females (ratio of 4:1) who are on the whole more flexible than men under the age of 35 (we all stiffen as we age). And interestingly is found in up to 97% of those who have 'chronic fatigue syndrome'. It may be worth asking patients about orthostatic symptoms. That is symptoms associated with standing still especially in warm temperatures or hot indoor environments.

Symptoms like:

- light-headedness

- dizziness

- nausea

- fatigue

- tremors

- breathing and swallowing difficulties

- visual disturbances

- sweating and pallor.

Some patients develop swollen bluish legs, providing evidence of blood pooling. In 'POTS' there's a rapid increase in heart rate by more than thirty beats per minute during the first ten minutes of standing. Another form of 'OI' is NMH or 'neurally mediated hypotension, where there's a precipitous drop (20-30mm Hg) in systolic blood pressure when standing.

I find this stuff interesting – what I call 'end of spectrum' stuff, where we can learn a lot about the everyday middle of the spectrum; the snippets of signs and symptoms we pick up in day to day listening and looking at patients that relate to the more pathological presentation but are not the full-on thing at all. I can think of a host of 'on-going pain' patients who've volunteered problems with standing still, who get light-headed, are very fatigued, complain of swollen legs, are hypermobile, or have some other combination that touches on 'OI' but certainly wouldn't be diagnosed with it.

'Spectrum' thinking is thinking about 'variability' and accepting we're all hugely different, yet all very much alike. I've found over the years that many physios are unable to accept people who are naturally stiff. They feel that everyone should be able to touch their toes and do the lotus position like they can. They're always telling them that they should do lots of stretches, that it's bad for their joints to be stiff etc. The problem is of course that it isn't true – for pain states stiffness seems to be more of a factor than being supple and mobile. Some stiff people are painful, some aren't; just as some super-flexible people are painful and some are not.

To me it stands to reason that our 'sampling' system should detect a situation of vulnerability as per Ehlers-Danlos, where it may detect abnormal connective tissue and therefore be more inclined to induce increased sensitivity and even pain. The same logic applies to stiffness too. What fascinates me is that when a joint is causing chronic pain, the orthopaedic response (if it can't replace the joint) is to immobilise it, fuse it and stop it working by some means. This is exactly what naturally happens to many joints and stiffening and ankylosing may well be a good 'ageing-led' end result after many years of back pain. There cannot be any set rules. We have to deal with the presentation in front of us. The best option is of course the one that works. Some get great joy out of keeping moving and getting more movement; witness the popularity of stretch and yoga type classes with many people. For others it's the exact opposite.

> *If you find markedly increased ranges of movement, pop it in the impairment compartment of the shopping basket and it may be something worth addressing at some point.*

Altered muscle strength, power, endurance

I haven't much to say here except that I like muscles because they're really amenable to change. Give a muscle a bit of extra work to do and it soon adapts, gets on with it and gets used to it. Physios traditionally do simple static testing and that's it. Functional testing and muscle testing that repeats soon shows up the fitness of the muscle in terms of endurance capability and makes the patient aware that they've got work to do.

For example, the classic sciatica with loss of calf reflex that actually *can* walk on tip toes. One could jump to the conclusion that the calf is therefore fine and no further testing is necessary. On the other hand and having a strong 'impairment' hat on, but being mindful of the weaknesses of over focusing in this 'burrow', one could look a little closer and get the patient to do repeat calf raises and more than the standard five or six repetitions.

What I do is show the patient what I want them to do. I go up and down on one leg emphasising the knee straight and the rising up using the calf muscle. I always say to start on the good leg and that the objective is to work the muscle to a feeling of 'just getting tired' in the muscle. The patient counts every repetition. So on the good leg, off they go – often reaching fifteen or more repetitions before starting to get the muscle-feels-tired feeling. The instruction now is to do exactly the same on the other leg, to the point where they get the exact same tired feeling. And this time, to their surprise, they find that the tired feeling comes on after nine or ten repetitions and they're struggling.

It's now obvious what they've got to do and I say 'That's another one for your shopping basket homework. I'll make a list at the end.'

I also add that the best way to work it is in more natural and functional ways – like tip-toeing around the house and up and down the stairs at any opportunity, that way it's easier and you actually do more and it doesn't hassle too much. But I also ask them to every now and then do the calf raise exercise and count it to test how it's going. When muscle weakness involves mild neuropathy as here I always say to the patient:

'If you work the muscle, you work the nerve. Your nerve isn't functioning as well as it should but working it sends little biological messages called 'trophic-stimulators' that encourage the nerve to re-grow, re-connect and get fit again. Just like muscle needs exercise to recover and get stronger so does nerve... use it or lose it!' – or words to that effect.

As I am sure you've gathered I am definitely not a fan of all this focused 'individual' muscle type exercise and having to 'localise' it to just the lateral, upper internal cuff segmentally functional lumbrical muscle or something ridiculous. The worst one is the 'transversus abdominus' localisation exercises that seem to be all the rage. Oh, groan, get a life will you guys.

So, my exam first question: 'What's the most important function of the abdominal muscles in life?'

Usual answer:

'Back stabilisation'...fail...

'Abdominal bracing during lifting to prevent back injury'...fail...

Out of repeated classes of anything up to fifty or more participants on the aches and pains lectures I did no one gets the answer I like and gets a pass!

Someone sometime says coughing, occasionally there's a 'pushing' and straining, child birth, constipation, peeing – but very rarely is there someone who immediately pipes up 'breathing'.

Why's that? Well, is it because we're so friggin lazy that we've become almost 99% reliant on silent quiet diaphragmatic breathing? We so rarely get out of breath and realise that getting air quickly out of the lungs, to get more in, is all about the abdominals. Look at four- legged animals in the wild, or even fit domesticated ones, no sign of a gravity sagging gut – they breathe fast and hard to survive and they use their abdominals to do that. You don't see dogs doing sit-ups or core stability exercises; they just get out there and move and breathe.

So for me the most important abdominal exercise is out of breath stuff – not tummy tensing in a specific way to localise transversus.

I remember once being told by a course participant that there is no way I should be giving or doing sit-up exercises, or even partial sit-up exercises with patients because it involved hip flexors! What? It's a normal movement when you get up out of bed? But this person says you shouldn't do that? You should turn onto your side first and get up that way. What, oh, in case you injure your back? No wonder we live in the great 'fear-avoidance' phase of human existence! When I hear this sort of stuff I get grumpy and slightly despair and wonder if there is rationality out there?

If you find altered muscle strength, power or endurance, pop it in the impairment compartment of the shopping basket and it may be something worth addressing at some point.

Alterations in muscle bulk and other observed impairments...

Physios are generally very good at observation; picking up changes in symmetry, in muscle bulk, in spinal posture, scoliosis, kyphosis and lordosis. I have no problems with this so long as it's relevant to the bigger picture. Often it's not, as argued with leg length.

If you find alterations in muscle bulk or other observable tissue impairment, pop it in the impairment compartment of the shopping basket and it may be something worth addressing at some point.

Problems with movement co-ordination, gross and local

This is good stuff on the one hand, but my pet hate when it becomes 'muscle-imbalance', on the other. Reserve the minutiae for perfection.

I've now got a patient in my head with an eight month old sore shoulder problem and when he lifted his arm into flexion he did an odd skip-up with the shoulder girdle. It was fine coming down. No movements or tests that I had done to that point reproduced or had got anywhere near the problem. His shoulder pain was simply a noticeable ache after cycling or swimming that lasted for several hours, occasionally bothered him at night and went on into the next day. Repeating the cycling or swimming just re-engaged the pain reaction again. He admitted to being careful with reaching up and loading the shoulder.

I got him to repeat the movement a few times to confirm what I was seeing.

'Do you know what I'm looking at and finding interesting?' I say to the patient.

'Is it the little jerk I do?'

'Yes, it's quite unusual, tell me about it.'

'I think I began doing it soon after the problem started and it came without much thought but it seemed to make it easier to lift the shoulder.'

'Right, so can you now do the movement and stop yourself from doing it?'

He tried again and had to go very slowly, when he reached about 100 degrees flexion he stopped and said.'

'It's starting to hurt right now.'

Doing it fast didn't hurt but the skip was still there.

I then got him to repeat the slow arm raising movement trying to do it without the jerk but this time a little more out towards abduction, the result was pain again. I got him to keep repeating the movement but going further and further out, a little every time, until he could do a smooth normal movement without the pain or the desire to jerk. He soon found it after going out about 30 degrees. We then went on to use the 'fire-apart-depart' rule to reinstate normal pain-free movement. He practised it for 5 to 10 to 15 reps anytime through the day with the proviso that the movement should be as smooth, as thoughtless and as pain-free and comfortable as possible for the first few days. After that he was to start drifting the movement in a bit. I also got him to go up freely out to the side but to come back down in the forward flexion plane which I knew didn't hurt.

During the treatment session I had found that if I did the – no pain/jerk, up out to side, then down through the 'zone' – then very quickly stop half way down and quickly go right back up through the 'zone' again there was no pain and no jerk. Speed had conquered it for a few reps but had started to make it sore. So we kept that one on hold for the shopping basket task homework later stages!

I explained the nature of the problem as a 'habit' of movement combined with a 'habit' of the pain system and that our goal was to 'trick' the habit and pain response out of the system. I explained fire-apart-depart too. He quickly got the idea, understood what he was trying to do and worked through the various movements. Surprisingly, that one treatment was enough. He rang two weeks later to say the problem had completely gone and he was doing things without thinking about them and he'd been swimming and cycling again without any problems. He said he'd be back onto me if it came back and he couldn't get rid of it himself and I never heard from him again. Let's party! Explain it? Sorry, what I told him was the best I can do and these sorts of odd presentations aren't at all uncommon. Habits of pain and habits of movement make sense to me.

The moral of the story: impairments in the right context have an important place, they're not banned!

If you find alterations of movement patterns and co-ordination, pop what you find in the impairment compartment of the shopping basket and it may be something worth addressing at some point.

Neurological abnormality

This is not only important in biomedical terms but also reveals some things that may be able to be put in the shopping basket and addressed, or at least kept an eye on. Weakness related to nerve loss of function I've already discussed above. It always amazes me how practitioners go about treating nerve root and neuropathy related problems, focusing on symptoms and techniques to treat and ignoring the rehabilitation of the weakness. The number of patients with power loss in biceps, triceps, muscle girdle (remember serratus anterior is largely supplied by C7 – a commonly injured nerve root), calf, hamstring, foot evertor/invertors, toe extensors and flexors, hip abductors and extensors etc. – who haven't been given any form of rehabilitative exercise to get them going astonishes me. That is so basic; such bad practice and frankly negligent!

Sensory recovery following nerve injury is often very good. Touch, massage, or any of a great variety of inputs can only help to do the same to sensory nerve recovery as we do for motor nerve recovery; which is work the sensory nerve and the sensory system and it may just work harder to get you back in touch with the lost bit of body again. So long as touching the numb area isn't reminding the patient how bad it all is and creates a negative mind-set. Check!

Other!

I'm sure I'll have missed your special thing...visceral palpitations, pelvic alignment, skin health – whatever. I don't really mind, so long as it's not attached to some weird and whacky pseudo-scientific therapy that costs a fortune and worries the patient. Look, we now have much better explanations for most presentations than we've ever had in the history of our species – so much better than those who still side with models that derive from the nineteenth century or even long before! There's no need for them anymore, we have far more rational explanations now. We just need to adjust our mode operation and explanation to fit with them. For a great many, this unfortunately is a massive and far too painful shift.

In overview, the assessment of physical impairments in the right context can be important as it:

1. Helps us to understand the extent of hypersensitivity – in relation to movement and touch/palpation and can provide a focus for 'desensitising' inputs in management.

2. Some findings help us to biomedically categorise a patient's disorder e.g. a nerve root.

3. Reveals some signs that are relevant 'Red flags' – neurological weakness, altered sensation, reflex abnormalities but also any anatomical/biomechanical/structural abnormalities that may be of concern.

I'm thinking of a patient who came to me unable to stand on his right leg and who's mid to upper quads looked very odd. His leg was incredibly painful above the knee and round the knee cap. After a thorough examination it turned out that he'd completely severed his quadriceps tendon. I've only seen one of those in over thirty years of clinical work. The Dr had diagnosed a 'muscle sprain.' He had surgery and recovered very well after quite a long rehabilitation (a year to full confidence).

4. Reveals a list of physical impairments that can be focused on in management in a positive way – especially when they clearly relate to functional difficulties.

5. Gives the patient confidence that a thorough investigation has been done (especially if it's explained well and in understandable terms as you did the examination).

The patient is then more inclined to listen to you and believe you as well as feel a sense of relief if the findings are not dramatised.

6. Note: there may be dangers of doing a too thorough examination! The patient might leave thinking. 'Blimey, I thought I'd only got a small knee problem, maybe a ligament or something. But this guy's found I've got a leg length problem; that my pelvis is out, that my spine's curved, one shoulder is higher than the other, that there's something called a 'sub-what-do-ya-call-it-lux-it or whatever in my neck and that I should be left handed! I went in feeling fairly OK but now I'm stunned and worried sick and I'm also sick about the cost of the ten treatments he says it's going to take to put me right.'

7. So, not too much but be aware of the reasoning behind what you may have left out, that you could come back to later and also it may pay to not make a big deal of some findings.

For example, patients often do have a low thoracic scoliosis, they've probably had it for years, why worry them by pointing it out now? I guess many clinicians want to point it out to either show how smart they are, or maybe in case the patient sees someone else and they point it out and then the patient would then think they were hopeless. Fear of being rumbled eh?

Leaving physical tests out rather than doing them is all a function of what you need to know in the light of what you feel needs to be done. For example, a long term bilateral upper limb problem relating to whiplash or office work.

The bigger picture tells you that if they're good neurologically then the best start to make is in getting them moving again, getting them fitter with pacing and simple goal setting. In this instance doing multiple fiddly upper limb tension tests to them and finding all sorts of pulls, zings and pins and needles may do more harm than good. Doing a quick active form of the upper limb tension test (see nerve root section) may be helpful just to give some kind of baseline but even then it may be largely irrelevant.

Say the patient was raising the arms very tensely and only of limited range – everything hurt, well it's more than likely that the upper limb tension test would hurt too. If, by focusing on normal smooth movement, you find within three or four weeks the patient is able to swing their arms full range – then clearly there was no need for exploring upper limb tension tests. Those who hold them dear will of course argue that they need to be treated. My purpose of pointing the 'no-need' out is one of the keys to the whole ethos of this big pain story I'm writing!

The arguments could go on and on. If you're a new physio you may need to examine these things in these patients, just to see how complicated the pain response can be from things like the upper limb tension tests and also, how provocative sometimes too! The point is to learn to be able to limit what you do, but do what you do really well!

8. When we do a physical examination we observe 'willingness' to move, we observe quality of movement and we observe pain behaviour. When I first graduated and looked at patients' movements my whole focus was on the movement and getting the range to pain response – the 'Maitland' movement diagram, for every single movement I looked at. What a 'groan' process that was! Soon I started to realise that I was much better watching the patient's face, while at the same time keeping an eye on what they were actually doing.

So for example, I rarely stand immediately behind a patient when they're doing forward lumbar flexion. I'm round to the side, watching the sides of their eyes as well as seeing their whole body reaction. After that, if I'm interested, I can always get them to repeat the movement and watch with intent at the intervertebral action – but as experience gathers, you get old and smarter and a whole pile of information arrives very quickly and that information is often more than enough. The point I'm trying to emphasise here is to think beyond the anatomy and mechanics to realise you're watching pain behaviour and possibly the level of fear-avoidance/confidence in the form of tension, slow and cautious speed of movement and the range of movement willing to be done.

Sometimes the patient might bend forward just reaching their knees and they have gone very slowly and cautiously. I might say to the patient, 'You don't look happy going forward – it all looks rather cautious and fearful, is it?' Then you might get. 'Oh, I was just going slowly so you could see and I

wasn't sure how far you wanted me to go!' I respond: 'Show me what you're happy to do?' The patient then does a normal speed bend forward and touches the floor. 'Hurts a bit, at the end.' 'Ah, right.'
Careful not to be too intense!

I hope the reader is with me on my 'shopping basket' approach so far? I hope you can see that I often tell the patient that I have a shopping basket with various compartments? And that, as I find out more and more from the patient, I explicitly put things I find in it – rather like you do as you wander up and down the supermarket aisles choosing items and putting them in the trolley.

The patients often find this helpful and by the end of the examination they can tell me what I've put in their basket, or what we've put in there together. Quite often the patient can see what they have to do to get better. So the shopping basket provides a list of things that the patient can work on, that I can work on and also what we can work on together.

Let's take a patient with classic sciatica, who's called 'Bern'. He's had it for six weeks now and been off work.

'Right Bern, I've had a good look at you now and we've got some stuff in your shopping basket. Let's go through it, you start...'

'That calf raise and poor balance on the right leg wasn't so good.'

'Yes, but that's quite common and I can show you how to work on that. Good – anything else?'

'I can't bend forward or back very well but my twisting was pretty good. What also surprised me was how well I bent when you got me on all fours. Oh, is that useless reflex something I should worry about?'

'Remember, I said the reflex often 'goes' with 'sciatica' and that it's a good basic test for just one part of the many nerves that go to your leg muscles. It tells us that the nerve isn't quite working like it was and it fits with the muscle weakness we found, your calf and also a bit when you pulled your foot up and the area of pins and needles. The real big message here is that while one part of one nerve isn't quite working properly, most of it is. In fact most patients with this sort problem, if they work hard at it, get back good strength – often better than they had before. I'll explain more about recovery and the natural history of sciatica in a minute but for now we've got some stiff and sore movements in our basket and some weakness, anything else we could put in there from earlier?'

'You mean when you were saying about putting my level of walking and activity in the basket. Oh, and you also said you'd put my thoughts about what was wrong in the basket, what was that all about?'

'Well, you said the Dr told you it was 'sciatica' and that there wasn't anything anyone could do, that it would get better on its own, to take it easy and stop work and that you'd probably have grumbles with it for a long time.'

'That's right and that's reminded me you also said you put the pain in the basket!'

On it goes. With some patients I even find I can get them to put their own yellow flags in the shopping basket, as here with Bern. We had his low activity levels in it, not that I said anything about it being wrong, it just went in; in the context of things to do at some stage, things to eventually get back or things to start working on soon.

It turned out that Bern was just doing as he was told. 'Dr knows best' and was actually very willing to get going with guidance. Having a better handle on the situation and the cause hugely helped. Also, the understanding that graded/gradual was always safe, plus the understanding that 'Tobleroning' of the pain was normal; that his back was strong; that nerves play havoc with the amount of pain they cause (we used shingles as an example of pain out of all proportion to the damage done) and that for nerves to recover they need to be worked. All this helped him speed his recovery and confidently engage with appropriate treatment inputs and suggestions.

This 'In Parallel' management as I like to call it is a far cry from the 'in-series' approach of Maitland that I was schooled in from the early days. ('In series' refers to doing only one 'technique' at a time, assessing response and only go to next technique when first is deemed unhelpful – this may take weeks!)

Is it possible, once you've done your physical examination, to be able to give the patient a 'take home' diagnosis? Yep, it's 'Biomedical'! Straight out of the 'Biomedical' compartment! But don't you get the comment from patients, 'What do I tell the Mrs is wrong with me then?' Or, you imagine when they get home the spouse is going 'Well, what did he say? What's the matter? Was what I said right?'

The last thing you want for the patient is, when they get home, having to explain some complex list of 'things to do' from some airy-fairy shopping basket – or even worse, some esoteric 'pain mechanism' explanation.! When dealing with patients I like to give them a diagnosis based on the findings and history and I do it like this.

Let's take a 65 year old patient who has a very limited and sore shoulder joint. He's called Reg. After doing all the 'shopping basket', near the end I say something like this:

'Right Reg, you're probably wondering what the diagnosis is? From my point of view I hope you can see what we've found and what we need to get on with? You've got all the exercises we've worked out and practiced for example. However most patients want to have some kind of diagnosis for what's wrong and especially so they can tell those at home who may want to know. For your problem, if you were to go and see a good Dr or a consultant they would tell you that you've got a 'frozen shoulder' or more technically they sometimes use the term 'capsulitis'. Both mean that the shoulder is stiff and painful and as I've explained, has a natural history that gets better.' I then write the words in bold at the top of their 'home' sheet in case they forget.

So that means that words like 'sciatica', spondylosis, hip arthroses and so forth may go down. CARE though. The huge emphasis is on the positives from the shopping basket, the things to do and that can be done to help, speed up, make better or whatever is appropriate. These diagnostic words need to be used with great caution as they can be terribly labelling and are associated with thoughts like: 'There's nothing that can be done, I've got arthritis, I have to be careful for the rest of my life,' type thinking.

An important question to the patient is this: 'Is there anything I've done or found or said that you want me to explain further? The last thing I want you doing is taking something away from here that you've half heard and then worrying about it. I want you to feel you can ask absolutely anything, especially anything about an issue that's of concern?'

Chapter 4.13
The General Health compartment

General Health and fitness

I'm absolutely no 'expert' here in the research sense or having had any training in fitness and health studies. However, I am a human expert and know how to get fit just like I know how to rest, to eat and go shopping. The fundamentals are pretty straight forward. In the same way as 'eat less' is to slimming, so 'do more' is to getting fitter. That is cruelly easy to communicate but as always – given the biological laziness rule that we are all imbued with: 'get as much as you can for as little effort as possible' – it can be very hard to do.

A great many of you who read this won't remember having to get out of the chair to switch on the telly or to change channels. Man has perfected the 'get as much as you can' rule and invested trillions in helping us do the one thing biology craves – doing nothing in order to conserve energy, taking the easy option. For the first time in man's history, that's approximately the last hundred years or so and ever more rapidly recently in my lifetime we've found that food arrives ready to eat in a shop. With a deft few strokes of the keyboard and a fiddle with an ergonomically designed mouse that barely uses a calorie of energy for every years real-time use, I could order up a pizza and be eating it in thirty minutes. All I have to do is walk to the front door and take it off the delivery man, unpack it (just don't get frustrated with the packing, don't even go there while we're on this topic) and eat it – about thirty five steps at most. Now think about gathering all the pizza ingredients from scratch!

Let's have a look at the features of Walter Bortz's 'Disuse syndrome' – plus a sprinkling from me and a few others.

*Bortz W. M. (1984). The disuse syndrome. Western Journal of Medicine **141**: 691-694.*

The following is a summary of the detrimental effects of immobilisation and inactivity that may be relevant to the establishment and maintenance of pain and pain related disability states:

- muscle wasting, weakening and loss of endurance

- degeneration and atrophy of all components of musculoskeletal tissues, hence loss of strength and elasticity

- reduced motor control and proprioceptive efficiency, hence reduced balance, slower reaction times and impaired protective mechanisms

- stiffer joints, slower movements and abnormal accessory movements

- decreased ability to use energy substrates efficiently

- decreased neuromuscular transmission and decreased efficiency in muscle fibre recruitment

- autonomic changes similar to those found in chronic regional pain syndrome 1 (CRPS 1) e.g. sweating changes, swelling, changes in skin temperature and colour and increased sensitivity

* pain and increases in sensitivity to touch and movement (allodynia)

* cognitive dysfunction

* mood changes

* decreased self-efficacy

* reduced coping capacity

* loss of vitality and loss of energy

* circadian (24 hour) rhythms de-synchronise

* increased risk of injury at work

* increased costs of compensation claims

* higher frequency of back pain

* less efficient metabolism – may include healing

* cardiovascular deconditioning.

I'd like to quote Paul Watson from his chapter in Main and Spanswick's book:

Watson P. (2000). Physical activities programme content. Pain Management. an interdisciplinary approach. C. J. Main and C. C. Spanswick. Edinburgh, Churchill Livingstone: 285-301.

> *'Physical activity is perhaps the most powerful component in pain management programmes. Increasing fitness is important not only in reversing the disuse syndrome, but in giving a powerful signal to patients that they are beginning to regain a degree of control over their musculoskeletal system. It is therefore extremely important from both the physical and the psychological point of view.'*

There are huge benefits of exercise, most notable a massive increase in sense of well-being – all the opposites in fact to the 'Bortz' list given above. Think 'PINK' of the disuse list!

Here are some tips from my experience:

1. Exercise regularly and enjoy it, try to make exercise a normal part of life, not, absolutely not a chore. There must be a massive physiological difference between doing exercise you enjoy and exercise you despise.

2. Avoid boring exercise.

3. Walking is fantastic – but doing the same walk every day doesn't do it for me. I like variation and above all novelty and exploring. In the UK we get the Ordinance Survey maps out and plan a new route. I don't do 'Apps' sorry.

4. Don't be conned by those who say five minutes a day is all you need, well five minutes is better than nothing I guess. Try to find one hour or at least thirty minutes if you can

5. You don't need to kill yourself, just do it regularly and enjoyably.

6. It's good to push a little and get to what Dave Butler used to call 'GOOB – 'gently out of breath'. The level of exertion that allows a conversation while continuing to exercise.

7. Time goes quicker when you're outside doing it: like cycling, jogging, running, walking, rowing, or being involved in some activity/sport with others – tennis, golf and gardening.

8. We call gym exercise 'pointless exercise' because it is so mind-numbingly boring. And hard to motivate yourself to do while looking at yourself in a mirror! I go bonkers. There are some though who love it. That's cool, gyms are fine then. Just do it and enjoy it.

9. It's good to do it with others and make it social, you don't notice it then.

10. Start easy build slowly, pace, goal-set etc.

11. Unfortunately exercising is a much harder solution than having a physical therapy 'treatment' done to you, taking a pill or having an operation, though it's a great many times better for you in all dimensions. When medical input is necessary, combining it with some form of exercise seems vital.

If you're a novice, training for a half or full marathon my suggestions are, first, realise that if you decided right now you wanted to do a full or a half marathon you could! Just step out of your front door and start walking. Even in this terribly 'physically' (and mentally?) unfit age we live in the vast majority of people, even though they may not believe it, are perfectly capable of walking the thirteen miles and a hundred and forty two yards for the half and even the twenty six miles two hundred and eighty five yards of the full marathon. Or secondly, follow a tried and tested running schedule and graded programme if that gives them more confidence to succeed. Whatever fits with your thinking.

I often say to my patients to reassure them about their structures, that if I could make the pain go away right now with a magic wand they could walk from here to John O'Groats (that's from here in the most SW tip to the northern most tip of the UK mainland i.e. several hundred miles).

I have a certain great fondness for the comedian Eddie Izzard. In fact he has to be on my list of heroes. One reason is this: in 2009, at the age of 47, untrained, unfit, a bit overweight and never a runner, Eddie set out to do forty three marathons in fifty one days for 'Sport Relief'. That's over a thousand miles on the roads of the UK. It was like I said just now, he just stepped out of his front door and off he went, day in day out running his marathons. Granted he had support but this is where the bit that really 'irked' me comes in. He had some kind of therapist travelling with him. I think she was called Jo? At the end of every marathon she would tend to his body and particularly his blistered and infected feet. Every night she seemed to be telling him to 'Not to run tomorrow or you'll have permanent damage' – or words to that effect. I just wanted her to shut-up; have faith in human determination, to stop trying to be so controlling and just do her best to make him as comfortable as possible and encourage him for the next days' endeavours. She's what I would view as a 'typical bad therapist' I'm afraid. Doom-laden! Thankfully Eddie ignored her and carried on to finish what he set out to do. Remarkable! But I think, given appropriate support and determination, a great many quite ordinary people just like Eddie are capable of one hell of a lot more than they think they can!

Now my final piece of advice, about marathon running or any form of endurance activity, you don't have to do what the therapists or magazines tell you; be confident with your own judgement and just go out and find your natural comfortable 'keep-going' pace and stick to it. You'll actually find that it varies from one session to the next and that as you do more and more you may get a little faster. One of the worst things for me was to go running with a friend and find that their pace was too much for me, the pressure of keeping up with them was awful. If you're an unskilled novice, just do your own thing and ignore others urges to push harder or get the pace up. Running socially is great but let others come to your pace, at least to start with. If you like to really push yourself that's fine but I'm not talking about those types, I'm talking about the simple capability of the ordinary person and most of all the patients I see every day.

Here's a short piece I wrote in one of my PPA News editorials: PPA News May 2002, Issue 13: 3-4. (Please note that it was written over ten years ago)

Quite a pill eh?

This piece was stimulated by two things. First, was a comment Mitch Noon made recently while giving a talk on the placebo and the therapeutic alliance. Mitch is a clinical psychologist down here in Cornwall. He outlined some 1980's research that investigated the effect of weekly psychological group therapy for metastatic breast cancer sufferers. In the study of 86 women there were two experimental groups. One group received the psychological therapy for ninety minutes a week for one year while a 'control' group had 'usual medical care'. After twelve months the therapy group used less psychotropic and analgesic medication and demonstrated significant improvements in mood/anxiety and depression compared to the control group. Further, at ten years the intervention group had an average of eighteen months increased survival time.

Then Mitch made the comment that struck me…'eighteen *months increased survival, if that was achieved by a drug there would be quite a reaction to it, quite a bit of publicity, it would be heralded as a major breakthrough in the treatment of breast cancer.'* Or, as per the title of this piece, 'Quite a pill, eh?'

Group psychological therapy – what does that do? Well it gives people knowledge, it makes them aware, it empowers them to understand their condition better, it teaches them to deal with the ups and downs of their predicament, it teaches them how to gain a better sense of control, it helps them get on with their lives and stay productive and positive.   It helps and teaches patients to self-manage their own quality of life, even with a life threatening disorder.

It so happened that in this study there was the added spin-off of increased survival too. We all like the idea of something that lengthens life but, as the saying goes, 'it's not how long you live, it's the quality of life while you live'. Sadly, there aren't any pills that lengthen life without some awful side effects!

A major point is that patients learn skills of coping, reasoning and managing – they are empowered, they can improve the quality of their own lives, they gain a better sense of control and they continue to use the skills for the rest of their lives; they don't need the Dr, they are not passive recipients, they learn to help themselves. The great untapped pill that is within us!

Are there any other interventions that rely on patient effort and skill and that would, if they were pills – have the public clamouring for them, earn shareholders millions and be headline news?

Yes, the right sort of exercise for you!

So the second thing that stimulated this piece was a book which came my way.   For years I have been looking for a user friendly book that:

- tells me how to measure patient fitness

- gives some good basic exercise physiology

- gives a good background to the benefits of exercise that I can pass on to patients

- shows me how to start someone off who is unfit, sets simple baselines and gets them involved in getting a bit more active and fitter.

I've found it!   The slight irony is that the book belonged to Trish Mace, a local 'exceptional' physiotherapist/person who very sadly died of breast cancer fairly recently. Her husband gave me her collection of physiotherapy books and this one was among them. Some of you may have come across it already but I'd like to give a warm welcome to:

'Exercise on prescription. Cardiovascular activity for health, by John Buckley, Jane Holmes and Gareth Mapp. Publishers are Butterworth Heinemann.

This book is multidimensional. It sees all aspects of the benefits of exercise that fits the PPA supported approach to health. There is no lip-service to the psychosocial benefits here – in fact there is a whole excellent chapter, early in the book, on psychological aspects of physical activity and exercise. In my opinion, this chapter in itself would be a great starting point for anyone wanting to understand how psychosocial issues impact people and patients and how they can be put into practice.

A major message of the book is that inactivity is dangerous but that activity and fitness is hugely beneficial. There is a nice little cartoon on page 13 of a sofa with two rounded unfit looking individuals standing next to it. On the sofa is a placard that reads: 'Government Health Warning, The US Surgeon General reports that purchasing this item and using it can be dangerous to health'.

Here are a couple of gems from the book:

1. *The Earl of Derby once stated that 'those who cannot find time for bodily exercise will sooner or later have to find time for illness'*

2. *The Allied Dunbar National Fitness Survey investigated 6000 adults in England, aged 16-74 years. A six-point rating scale from 0 –5 (0 being the lowest) was used to determine the amount and intensity of activity performed and the number of bouts of exercise in these categories undertaken in the previous 4 weeks. The useful and astonishing results were:*

   - *80% of people surveyed believed that exercise was beneficial*

   - *61% of men and 69% of women in activity level zero actually believed themselves to be fit*

   - *47% of men and 57% of women in activity level zero actually believed themselves to be active*

   - *70% of men and 91% of women were not active enough to gain a health benefit.*

Inactivity and unhealthy lifestyles, that individuals have and could do a great deal about, relate to life threatening conditions like:

- *Heart disease* – but 'there is a 50% reduction in coronary heart disease in middle-aged to elderly men who have regularly participated in exercise all their lives (**quite a pill eh?**)

- *Stroke* – a sedentary individual is three times as likely to die early from CVA than a regularly active person.

- *Diabetes* – a study of 5990 men found that between the years of 1962 and

1976, 2020 men developed non-insulin dependent diabetes mellitus (or NIDDM – the one you 'acquire' when you get old).   Those men who had higher reported leisure-time activity levels were less likely to develop NIDDM. For each increase in energy expenditure of 2000 kcal per week, there was a reduction in the incidence NIDDM by 24%. This equates to a daily half hour bout of vigorous activity such as jogging or tennis, or one hour per day of a more moderate activity such as walking. In those men who had the higher risk for developing NIDDM, exercise showed a greater protective effect in preventing its onset (**quite a pill eh?)**

- Also, risk factors for the above that include – obesity, high blood pressure, increased blood fibrinogen and cholesterol levels, can all be improved significantly with activity.

What I liked about this book was the way it dealt with exercise on two levels:

1. Exercise for health benefits and
2. Exercise for fitness....

You don't need to sweat and hurt and feel terrible to acquire significant health gains. All that is required is for individuals to build up to a 'moderate amount of physical activity'.

'It is now known that even low but regular levels of increased physical activity can help improve health with benefits to blood pressure, cholesterol, weight and mental state.' (p 4)

Chris, a patient of mine had high blood pressure – he went on a diet and regularly goes to the local GP surgery to be checked by the practice nurse. The nurse always asks him about his exercise and insists that he has to do minimum of twenty minutes exercise three times per week. Apparently she does not consider a three hour round of golf as 'exercise' – she wants him grinding away on a static bike as per the formula we all know so well. But, according to 'Exercise on Prescription'

'Simple regular activity (not necessarily sport) equivalent to a daily 20-30 minute brisk walk can be beneficial to health. If the duration is greater than 30 minutes per day and the intensity of the exercise undertaken increases to a range of 40-70% of an individual's aerobic capacity, the protection against Coronary Heart Disease(C HD) is further increased...

After a heart attack it has been shown that for the next 2-3 years there is a reduced risk of further myocardial infarct and 20-25% reduction in all causes of death if patients had participated in an exercise rehabilitation programme.'(p 14)

(Exercise is quite a pill!)

That many people do not consider walking a sufficient exercise for fitness is really unfortunate, because it is probably the most pleasant, most useful and easiest exercise to start easily and to build up. The Stroke Association in the UK has produced a great booklet called *The Reluctant Exerciser's Guide…'Incorporating the eight-week fitness challenge.'* My one was given to me by Catherine McBride, a local senior NHS Physio. It's basically geared to getting couch potatoes (cartoon on the cover) off that dangerous couch! There are walking, swimming and cycling programmes. To give you an example, level 1 – week one of the walking programme reads: 'In your first week, walk from your starting point at your normal pace and continue for five minutes. Then turn round and step-up the pace slightly. Try to do the return journey in four minutes – but don't expect to judge it exactly right first time. Week 2, is eight minutes out trying to return in seven and so on up to eight weeks where fifteen minutes out and thirteen minute returns are the goals. Level 2 follows and builds up to a thirty minute brisk walk where you try and reach the same spot on the following days but in less and less time.

That's enough on it – read the books if you're interested – I think you'll enjoy them and it'll be good for you and good for your patients and I believe there are plenty of brilliant 'Apps' to help you along too.

Conclusion: the right kind of exercise, meaning exercise that the patient can fit into day to day life, that is actually enjoyable to do, and that people want to do has impressive benefits. If it was a pill then it would be quite something and quite a headline in the Western world's press. Combine feeling good and fit with the issues relating to the psychological skills discussed earlier and you are likely to be doing far more than any pill or surgery or fancy treatment ever will.

At the time of writing and editing this (November 2013) the popular press has been awash with listing all the health benefits of exercise. Maybe we don't hear them because we also have the 'fix-it' systems in place – therapists, Drs, pills and hospitals!

There are three problems:

- changing patients/peoples beliefs and behaviour

- changing Drs and therapists thinking, beliefs and behaviour and

- the training of Drs and therapists outside the medical model.

Good things are happening all the time though. Mitch, who I mentioned earlier, sent me a copy of a Department of Health document called: *The Expert Patient: A new approach to chronic disease management for the 21st Century.* It had been produced by a multidisciplinary task force looking into self management issues for chronic illnesses. The 'expert patient' is one who is empowered via self management strategies to achieve a good quality of life and minimise the life impact of the chronic disease or condition that they have.

Evidence of the efficacy of self management plans are presented in the document. For example in asthma self management approaches:

- reduce asthma symptoms

- improve lung function

- reduce attack frequency

- reduce the requirement for reliever and steroid treatment

- reduce inappropriate use of antibiotics

- improve compliance

- improve the quality of life.

Self management of diabetes has been shown to:

- reduce blood glucose levels, with no increase in severe hypoglycaemic attacks

- markedly improve quality of life and

- produce a significant increase in satisfaction with treatment.

Good quality self management, fitness, or simply increased activity and a bit of control –

QUITE A PILL eh?

Chapter GE 4.14
The Pain compartment

This is a separate compartment because it is so important and usually the primary reason patients come to see us. As I said earlier I've purposely put it last because it so easily goes first and their takes a stranglehold on therapist-reasoning, whose instinct is to focus on and try and relieve the pain and not see the many other issues that surround the patient and their situation. That usually means applying some form of therapy in the context of something found to be at fault during examination. Therapists usually waffle on about inflammation and stuck joints to suit whatever therapy they're doing. Yes, if you want a pain treatment to work, you have to invoke as much top-down as you reasonably can; if that's 'bullshit' so be it, so long as it doesn't create maladaptive constructs for the patient leading to maladaptive coping strategies – like becoming dependent on the treatment! As I will demonstrate in the patient sections that follow I try to create a sound and logical context in which a pain treatment is applied.

Clinically, pain and the patients' description of their pain are often one of the first things that we listen to, record and get details of. For the most part, like well-conditioned laboratory mice, we get our body charts out and dutifully fill them in. In my lectures I always used to note that the 'body-chart' represents only one dimension of the so-called three dimensions of pain. Let me remind you.

The three dimensions are:

- sensory-discriminative

- cognitive-evaluative

- emotional-motivational.

Sensory-discriminative refers to the 'location of the pain', the 'intensity', the 'quality' and the 'behaviour' of pain over time. So on your body charts the location is obvious, but you also need descriptions of the type of pain and its behaviour – like 'constant deep ache,' or 'sharp only at end of range/often with movement'. Intensity of pain uses descriptors like 'nasty' or 'background' or 'nagging' and the use of simple 0-10 numerical rating scales. Getting aggravating and easing factors further fulfils the 'behaviour' compartment details.

It looks simple but sadly is often hurried and given inadequate time. Please note that the words the patient uses to describe their pain are important, and like it or not express a degree of the emotional dimensions of their problem and situation. Think of words like 'ripping, knife-in, draining, stabbing' and you should be able see what I mean.

I sometimes find myself saying to the patient after filling in a body chart: 'How would you sum all this pain up' and get some very interesting responses...

> 'One minute my life was normal and then the lights went out'
> 'I've been frightened to really tell anyone because it seems so unbelievable'
> 'The god that came up with this was sick in the head'

> 'If I could just get one hours relief I could die happy'
> 'I am overwhelmed and I cannot operate as a human being'

All these examples came from patients with pain of less than six weeks duration. My point is that pain just cannot be considered as isolated from the thinking, feeling human that is attached to it.

Spending time getting the details of pain from the patient is a giant step in the therapeutic encounter. You have to listen, you have to take your time and you have to make sure that nothing is missed.

But sometimes there are exceptions and as I will illustrate in the clinical examples section this is usually with chronic maladaptive pain problems.

In order to reason pain I find myself thinking about what I might be able to do to help, or whether I should be thinking, I should be trying to help with the pain. So here is a list of all the possible ways I can think of, relevant to my practice, which may be able to help pain.

The pain-off-list, a possible 'toolkit':

- drugs

- movement, activity, function, exercises, stretches, floppy movements etc.

- various forms of rest

- supports, crutches, collars, binders, tapes, compression bandages and Tubigrip, orthotics and many other bits and pieces

- avoidance!

- standard physiotherapy 'modalities' I'm happy with:

    a) heat and cold

    b) TENS and other currents

    c) ultrasound plus or minus currents at the same time

- hands on – manual therapy, massage (in a multitude of contexts)

- relaxation

- reassurance, decreased concern, a better understanding – lessening the threat value

- acceptance and adjustment

- attention and focus changes

- distraction

- de-sensitising

- fire-apart-depart
- novelty, excitement and fear
- going away, holidays etc. – relates to novelty
- socialising
- hobbies
- work
- recreational drugs and alcohol, even some foods
- anything that can 'trick' the pain off
- achieving goals
- working on well-being
- family relationships, love and sex or no sex
- resolving personal problems
- improving confidence
- feeling free
- feeling in control
- knowing about pain and its meaning
- feeling physically fit
- feeling mentally fit and well, 'balanced'
- laughter and fun
- music and entertainment.

It could go on and on but I think you'll agree that this list is a little different to what you might find in a standard text book. The point is that I hope you can see, from what has gone before in this book, how all these things may help or influence pain.

In the clinical examples sections some of these will crop up and be discussed, for now I'm going to tell you how I give and explain a TENS machine to a patient. What follows is an expansion of an editorial I did for the PPA News called 'Tricking Pain.' (see Gifford L.S. (2007) Editorial: Tricking Pain PPA News 23:3-8)

Editorial : 'Tricking pain'

Re-activating patients with pain, getting them going again, pacing up their activity and exercise levels is all very well until they hit the dreaded pain flare-up and setback 'wall'. Who in their right mind is happy when things go pain pear-shaped? It's hardly surprising that many patients stop coming, stop complying and give up their programmes when a flare-up hits – especially when a good flare-up strategy is not in place. Loss of confidence and yet another failure can be devastating.

Early on in management I frequently try to find as many ways of calming pain down (and the patient!) as possible. The goal being to make the patient confident that if they do hit a pain flare up, they know that they have an active and effective strategy to quickly bring it back down again. I reason with the patient the simple idea that if they are good at bringing pain under control fairly rapidly then they will be less fearful of a flare-up happening and hence more confident with their graded physical programme.

Things I use to help formulate a flare up strategy I often get from careful enquiry with the patient. The 'pink' question is therefore to ask them what makes their pain better (in my manual therapy training I always had to ask what makes it worse). I might get the following:

- the drugs they have that work well

- heat, cold

- various forms of rest, stretching and other exercises

- massage and movement

- calmness, relaxation and re-evaluating the situation as logically as possible (don't panic!)

- anything else? Ask!

I make sure I write the agreed strategy down for them clearly and almost forcefully. Shut it up, turn the pain circuit/cell assembly off – if it keeps going it keeps installing itself, the 'pain-habit' gets further entrenched in your system the sooner it's turned off the better, etc. are some of the phrases I sometimes use.

One of the best things, if you can achieve it, is for patients to come in with a flare-up and to get the pain down there and then.

1. It shows them that the pain can be stopped quickly – that their system has the ability to stop the pain given the right circumstances or inputs and that if they practice they can get more efficient at doing it. Further, if they do get better at doing it they will be helping to rewire and re-install their own, very much out of condition, natural 'pain-killing system'—their 'endorphin' system—their pain-off system (which you will have adequately and simply explained to them!).

2. Quick pain relief, however long it works for, also helps to reinforce (even prove to the patient?) the notion that:

a) Their pain is the result of continuous high levels of 'electrical activity in a nerve circuit' – their 'annoying tune' is playing full volume and not more tissue damage (because if there has been an injury it doesn't suddenly heal in a few minutes).

b) That hurt doesn't mean harm and that the goal of increased fitness and better function is quite possible and actually, quite safe.

What better way to help patients understand that their pain is the result of totally unhelpful 'electrical activity in nerve circuits' and that they have the means to stop it and that if they keep practicing and experimenting they may well be able to get better and better at stopping it rather than getting better and better at starting it!

3. If you know you can control your pain well, you are much more confident about physically getting going and keeping going.

Ongoing pain problem, Dave...

Dave has a huge healed scar on his left knee. He worked in a local scrap yard until two years ago, when a fall at work resulted in a chunk of flesh being gouged out of the soft tissue on the upper medial aspect of his left knee.

The story was complex but familiar to anyone who regularly sees chronic pain patients:

- off work and poor relations with work

- lawyers involved

- huge financial issues

- sitting at home doing nothing

- falling out with family

- spending long periods in bed

- fed up, angry, emotional etc.

- negative about the future

- fed up with health professions and complete lack of progress

- lots of pain behaviour – holds knee all the time, leans away from the left side, walks in a protective way   'The last time the Dr examined it I was in bed for a week...'

- a reasonable standard physical knee examination was impossible (jumps and says it hurts if any hands move within 5cms range. Yet quite capable of full weight bearing. So, 'pain-behaviour' issues to be addressed)

• pain all over the leg

• he's had standard physio/Drs consultants with lots of tissue based diagnoses and still on waiting lists for further orthopaedic type investigations. He was well and truly 'caught' in the medical model 'net'.

Dave did well with all my explanations of on-going pain mechanisms, the normal healing process and its timing and all the orthopaedic diagnoses he'd been given. I did not deny any of the diagnoses he had been given, but focused instead on a model of explanation that focused on an 'even-if-damaged/or worn – it's still capable of being a great deal better/fitter; plus, a very careful emphasis on the notion that (like many other similar patients) the pain was out of proportion to the amount of damage done. From there the explanations shifted to 'circuitry' and 'processing' 'volume to high' type ones and he seemed to grasp them reasonably well.

Dave started a simple reactivation programme with enthusiasm and within 2-3 weeks was walking 20 minutes, 3 times a day; he could touch his own knee with confidence and had learnt to correct his antalgic/habitual postures and movement patterns. He was doing generally very well. I was actually able to touch and do a full examination of his knee – cruciates, stability, collateral ligaments, range of movement, patello-femoral, palpation of the scar etc.   And then discuss all the positive 'pink' findings. Then he said…

'Louis, you know, you're the first person who has listened to me, explained anything properly and done and explained the findings. What you're saying is a huge relief and makes me quite hopeful.'

I smiled (and like I do, I cynically thought that he could well have said this to his last therapist!). But I was pleased too and went on to reinforce his enthusiasm and determination but re-capped on the fluctuating nature of on-going pain (Toblerone). I slightly wondered if he heard me in his almost euphoric state.

I gave him two more simple exercises to start to 'grade-up'. The first was sit to stand from an easy height – with the goal of increasing numbers and then to gradually go to a lower height as his confidence allowed. The other exercise was very low step-ups with a view to increasing height and ultimately being able to go up and down stairs with a normal reciprocal gait. We decided to leave it a fortnight.

Two weeks later Dave limped in, he looked like death.

'I've been in bed for the last five days. It's agony. I can't go on like this Louis, I did four of those stand up exercises and the pain was the worst it's ever been. I'm really giving up on the idea of doing them and of going back to work. I've resigned myself to being happy just to do a bit of walking occasionally.'

(I hope you are thinking blue and black flag issues here – Psychosocial compartment?)

We talked more. He wanted to have his leg amputated he was so upset with it.

I moved back to the pain explanations, the circuits, the triggers, the habit of pain, he was almost too angry and distressed to listen or hear what I was saying.

'Your endorphin system needs a kick up the ass and it won't work if you're miserable like this. I'm going to try and cheer you up with a TENS machine. Have you heard or been given one of these in the past?'

No he hadn't, surprisingly? Or not surprisingly – after all, they're no better than placebo, so they're not 'evidence-based'... hmmm!

(NOTE: *While the following may seem rather patronising from time to time, appreciate that my tone, which is obviously hard to convey, and the wording I used was carefully chosen and highly appropriate for the patient and the situation*)

I went on...

'Dave, this pain can go down. It will scttlc, this sort of thing that's happened is what pain experts call a pain flare up – remember I talked to you about this, remember the Toblerone, it happens with all patients who have long term pain like yours and if we manage it well you can get on again. Calm down and let's do something positive. Listen to the story I'm going to tell you.'

We made eye contact and he nodded frowning.

'Thirty years ago two pain scientists discovered why rubbing and squeezing where it hurts helps relieve pain. They found that the rubbing stimulates little nerve endings in the skin and causes them to release very powerful pain killing chemicals – they're called endorphins, you may havc hcard of them?'

He nodded that he had.

'Endorphin means natural morphine and it is at least ten times more effective than any pain killer a chemist can make. Our bodies can kill pain, especially when it really matters. You may have experienced quite nasty cuts and bruises without realising it when playing rugby or gardening, and you may have heard of people reporting no pain at all in nasty accidents where quite awful injuries occurred. This pain relief is down to those endorphins.'

'If you pour endorphins over nerves in a pain circuit and the circuit dramatically stops – no pain, it goes instantly. One of the problems with people who have on-going pain like you have, is that their endorphin systems don't work so well, so the pain circuits get to play too easily and can go on and on for a long time. It's as if the endorphin system has gone to sleep or forgotten how to work.'

Dave was listening to me now. He looked calmer and was gripping his knee less frantically.

I went on…

'Now, endorphins, as I said, come when you rub where it hurts, they also come when you are frightened for your life or under some kind of awful physical threat. If right now you were out in the bush in Africa somewhere and you came across a buffalo, lion, or a rhino even and they started to run towards you – even with your knee as it is, you would run for your life and not feel a thing in your knee. Yes?'

He smiled, 'You're right'

'So, what I'm going to do right now is give you ten seconds start while I get my hand-gun.'

'Got the point' Dave said, smiling even more.

He was looking more relaxed still, he'd stopped rubbing his knee, but it wasn't appropriate to point this out to him.

On with the story…

'I can't do that of course, I'd love to cure your pain by shooting you, but I'd lose my job! But, there are other important things that bring on the release of endorphins. For example, endorphins are massively released when we feel good about ourselves, when we are happy, when we are having a laugh, when we achieve a goal, when we are highly focused on one thing; even pain somewhere else in our body can cause the release of endorphins and stop pain.   You may have heard the old saying that pain relieves pain? So, any intense sensation or stimulus can cause the release of endorphins, cold, heat, massage, manipulation, loud music, and also, less intense 'nice' things can too – like soft music, relaxation, mind-altering drugs, alcohol, even chocolate. Combine things and the effectiveness can get even better—soft music and a nice massage from someone you like or feel comfortable with—you feel good, your aches and pains get better.'

Dave looked a great deal better. There was a pause.

'Go on', I said.

'I've just realised that what you've just been telling me about is happening to me now – just by listening and being interested and stopping thinking about the damn pain has made the pain get a lot less.'

'That's a great connection to make Dave. Circuits winding down, needle is coming off the record and remember all that stuff from when we first met up?' I quizzed…

'Your pain killing system still knows how to work; it's not gone completely! More practice required and it should get better at it!'

'Let's get back to this TENS machine for a minute – you're getting the idea, which is great. Right, TENS stimulates the nerve endings in your skin that release the endorphins. Two things about endorphins: they are anti-pain and they are anti-inflammatory – they are your big friends here.'

I then showed him the TENS machine.

'This machine has sticky pads that go on the skin and when you turn it on and turn the volume up you feel a tingling sensation. Most people find it very pleasant. For it to help we'll need the following:

1. It must feel OK – no tension, quietly comfortable, not frightened.

2. It's best if it feels nice/good/you like it – remember endorphins also come with good feelings. I want you to really appreciate, as you already have started to very well, that to make this endorphin system work there are two parts to it. Firstly, you (I point at his head) and your reaction to the sensation. This part I call 'top-down' and means that your brain, if it likes it, will send endorphin loaded signals down to the spinal cord and to all the pain circuits coming and going around your knee. On the other hand, if you don't like it, can't see the point of it, don't believe in it – it won't work half so well. That's the first thing, feeling positive about it if possible. The second is the bottom-up effect, (I point to his knee and gesture upwards) – the simple input from the machine into the nerves of your skin and on into your spinal cord and nervous system – that also stimulate endorphin release.

3. I also need you to feel comfortable with the idea that we are actually 'masking' the pain, or better, 'tricking' the pain to go off. Many patients feel that this is a crazy thing to do because they understand the situation as: pain means something is wrong, getting rid of the pain does not fix the problem, in fact it may make it worse as not feeling pain means that they may do something and injure or upset it even more. I hope, that from all that we have discussed over the weeks I've been seeing you, you can understand that the problem with your pain problem is that the pain circuit is having too free a reign, it plays itself too easily and for far too long and what it's telling you is of little help as far as your knee structure is concerned. Your anatomy and mechanics are good enough for you to be able to run but the pain circuit just won't allow you to.'

Dave nodded.

'I'm with you.'

'Right, let's try it. I'm going to do it on your good knee first so you get to know what it's like and feel comfortable with it and all the controls – then we do it on your painful knee, but only if you're keen and confident.'

I paused and looked at him, he nodded, slightly emotional.

'You realise we're trying to trick the pain away?' I said.

'I never would have believed this a month ago, but it makes so much sense now'.

We laughed. Crazy world!

We both knew it was going to work.

On went the pads to his good knee, up went the volume and we worked through all the settings until he felt comfortable with 'rough' current, 'smooth' current, modulated and bursting current.

'Start with the one you like the best, but feel free when you get confident to get nicely nasty with it – burst, high volume etcetera' I said.

'Ready to try on the bad knee now?'

Off we went around the scar, up went the volume, he played with it and we both relaxed.

The session had gone from high intense, high emotion to calm and back in control.

'How are you doing now?'

Dave was looking down, relaxed, smiling and quietly said,

'That's amazing, that's the first time in the last four months that I can't feel any pain at all.'

'Tricked the bastard' I said.

We laughed again.

I'd just like to note, that with many patients we spend time finding the best placement for the electrodes too. It's well worth trying TENS yourself, say on your own back and move the electrodes around, some places it feels really sharp and burning, others it's far more diffuse and comforting. The patient must understand that they play with it until it feels nice/good and not nasty and annoying.

Dave soon got back on the physical programme. The TENS helped his confidence a lot. He decorated his house, starting cycling and also began speeding up the walking. He also tentatively paced up the sit-to-stand exercise that kicked the flare-up off – I did a little 'behavioural experiment' with him for that one. He also started a graded kneeling programme (cushion on chair putting knee on it and taking some weight through) and with my help (a letter explaining his programme) sorted out a meeting with the local job centre.

When I last saw him it was a little bit of a case of 'so far so good', but you can bet there's bound to be another set-back coming at some point.

The message here may be that physiotherapy is very much still a communication 'art' preformed with the aid of simple props like TENS – which can just as easily work or fail depending on the way their 'action' is explained and set-up by the therapist and understood by the patient. Surely then, it's a little of what you do, and a lot of the way you do it. CONTEXT is everything. You have to make quite an effort with a big 'sell' spiel sometimes!

The outcome? Isn't it a product of two people working together, two brains working together and therefore two nervous systems working together towards a beneficial change?

In the clinic I have the following TENS handout I give to patients to back up what I explained. If you photocopy and use it, it would be really nice if you could simply acknowledge where it came from, thanks, Louis.

Understanding and getting the best from the **TENS** machine

TENS stands for 'trans-cutaneous-electrical-nerve stimulator'!

It was invented back in the late 1960's as a result of early pioneering work by two very famous pain researchers – Ronald Melzack and Patrick Wall.

They discovered that there are nerves in the skin that when simulated by rubbing, squeezing or electrical stimulation, send electrical impulses into the spinal cord which then release 'endorphins'. Endorphin stands for endogenous (made inside the body) morphine. In other words they are the body's natural 'morphines' and they work very powerfully to stimulate tiny nerve fibres in the spinal cord that then act to stop pain messages from penetrating further into the nervous system to cause pain.

We naturally rub, squeeze, massage or put heat on pain to try to ease it – think of times when you bump your shin or knock into something hard.

TENS enhances and uses nature's way of relieving pain and like morphine for pain control – can be very powerful. The good thing about its production with TENS rather taking it in pill form is that its action is kept at the place where it is needed rather than spreading throughout the system. High levels of morphine in the brain are clearly not going to let you feel normal!

It works on several levels: here are three important ones...

1. As described – by stimulating the body's natural pain relieving system – hence release of endorphins. Acupuncture, massage, heat, different types of manipulation and quite a lot of other therapies are thought to work on pain like this too. TENS is good because you can do it yourself at home and do it often.

2. By distracting you from the pain – TENS produces a tingling sensation and when set strongly enough will 'drown-out' the pain. The tingling distracts you from the pain. The problem many find with this is that they feel that getting rid of the pain will mean that the thing that is causing the pain is still there and is not getting fixed – and, it may even be further damaged if it loses the protection of pain. What we now know from research is that many pain problems, especially those from nerves or from joints and muscles – are often way out of proportion to the damage done, and that the pain produced is actually detrimental to recovery. High levels of horrid pain make people miserable, move awkwardly and stiffly, make them tense, stop them resting and sleeping well and so on. High levels of pain like this will actually slow the healing response. Important pain is never completely masked – it will always come through and warn you to be a bit careful (see information leaflet – *'helpful and unhelpful pain'*)

3. Scientists can now scan the brain and actually 'see' the areas that are working when we feel pain or any other sensation. If a subject is given two sensations at the same time – one vibration or TENS (pleasant) and the other painful (e.g. a hot probe) – and the brain scanned, it is found that circuits for pain only operate when the subject is attending to the pain, and that when the subject attends to the vibration or TENS – the pain circuits stop almost completely. This means that when TENS is applied it is good to spend a few minutes every-so-often really concentrating on the tingling sensation. This stops the pain circuit from operating and also stops the pain circuit from becoming established long term [see hand-out 'pain memory'}. TENS therefore helps switch off the pain circuits and prevent the problem lasting a long time or becoming permanent. There is now a great deal of research that shows that good early pain treatment PREVENTS pain becoming established and therefore prevents it becoming a 'chronic pain problem'. The message is 'shut the pain up early' – and use anything that helps or works.

For TENS to work best:

Put the electrodes where they feel they are helping the most. This is often simply over the pain area. I get patients to show me where they would rub or massage the pain – and then place the electrodes around the area indicated. If this does not work well, it's good to start moving the electrodes to different places. This can be just away from the pain, or along the nerve that goes to the area of the pain. It can also be over the area where the pain is actually coming from. Sometimes TENS even works well when the electrodes are placed well away from the area of pain. I will help guide you with best placements.

It is important that you feel comfortable with the sensation and understand and feel happy with how it works. Studies on animals are showing that TENS can 'unwire' pain circuits very well – but only if nerve circuits that come down the spinal cord from the brain are able to operate normally. Nerve circuits that come from the brain *down* to the spinal cord are called 'top-down' circuits. In humans the activity of these 'top-down' circuits is hugely influenced by the way we feel about something and what we may think about it.

For example in pain experiments where subjects have wires attached to their skin from an apparatus that produces electric shocks it is found that when they are told that what they are going to feel will be very mild the subjects are less anxious and report only mild sensations. In other subjects *exactly the same amount of current* produces quite awful pain when the subjects are made anxious by telling them to expect a nasty sensation. How well pain therapies like TENS work for you are strongly influenced by what you think and feel about them. If you are not sure about anything or if it does not make sense – you must tell me so we can discuss it. Remember, our expectations, beliefs and feelings seem to have a strong affect on the top-down circuits which in turn have a powerful effect on the pain-unwiring mechanisms of TENS/other pain treatments.

To start with, the current must feel good to you.

I will have shown a few of the various sensations that you can get from the machine. There are many possible settings, but there are two extremes:

1. Pulse rate setting 70-130 Hz.

This is set with the right hand dial and it means that the machine is sending out between 70 and 130 electrical pulses every second. This is a SMOOTH current setting. It feels smooth – people often like this setting if they feel they want their pain stroked rather than pummelled or massaged deeply. The dial on the left – the 'pulse width' - I set at between 220 and 250 when we did it together. If you find that when you turn the current up (the dial on top of the machine) muscles start twitching under the electrodes and you don't like it much – turn the pulse width dial down to around 60-120 setting. This will stop the twitching but the intensity will drop away too – so turn up the current again using the top dials to the intensity you like. The key thing is that the current feels good to you. If you like it, your pain unwiring circuitry is likely to as well. Remember the importance of the 'top-down' currents and how your thoughts and feelings can influence them.

2. Pulse rate setting between 2 and 10 Hz (right hand dial).

This produces a far more jerky or jabbing current, which to some people feels quite aggressive. If it feels good though, it's fine. Again, muscle twitching can be decreased or eliminated by turning the 'pulse width' dial down to 60-120.

A big question is how long and how often to use the machine?

There is no general or exact prescription but start with these guidelines. Don't have it on if it's annoying you – it must feel comfortable (but see below) and the pain must be improved if at all possible. The idea is that the sensation of the machine successfully competes, even the smallest amount, with the sensation of pain so that it lessens. If it is working – do it! This means that many people use them fairly continuously for a while. However, check your skin is not getting irritated by the electrodes and the current – to keep the skin comfortable it is worth lifting and moving the electrodes from time to time. I usually suggest every hour or so.

Some very recent research is guiding us further with the best use of TENS. I may have advised you to go with this method straight away, but both can be combined.

This regime is simply 15 minutes on nice and smooth – 70-130Hz at a 'comfortably strong' intensity. This gets the 'endorphin' system going to start with.

This is then followed by 15 minutes on 'intense' – with the pulse rate set at 2Hz, the pulse width high at around 250-260 and the intensity up so that the current is 'acceptably uncomfortable'! This stimulation method has been found to actually de-activate the pain system so that it unwires itself. In animals it has been found that doing this regularly has long-term effects on the wiring. The recommendation is that you do this up to 4 times a day – especially if it is working well. It is very important that a) you focus and concentrate on the current (it's hard not to!) and b) you feel positive about the sensation, not anxious about it – remember the 'top-down' currents discussed earlier.

I have had many patients with horrid constant high levels of nerve pain (like sciatica) who have got excellent relief by having the settings very 'aggressive' and at a very high intensity for long periods of the day. This is great because nerve pains are renowned for being very difficult to help – even with very powerful pain killing drugs. What is being found is that the quicker and earlier that the pain can be controlled – the quicker the recovery. If it's working – Do It!! Anything that makes the pain lessen is changing the processing of the pain and helping to stop it become stubbornly wired into the nervous system.

If your pain is coming down well the idea is to get your system to take over and to try and become less dependent on the machine. Often, as you get to know what works for you, – you will find that when you use the TENS you get pain relief more and more quickly and that it lasts for longer and longer afterwards. This means shorter and shorter but more and more efficient use of the machine. Your nervous system actually learns, or becomes 'conditioned' to stop the pain more and more efficiently with the machine. It starts to forget how to turn the pain system on. As 'pain-on' *unwires* so 'pain-off' *wires* in the nervous system.

If you have had a great deal of pain for a long time sometimes it can be difficult to unwire the pain circuit. It is worth reading the 'pain memory' handout [see **]. TENS may still be helpful in reducing the level of pain to more manageable levels so that you can function better. Getting the various settings right may take a while so it is worth being patient and keeping trying rather than finding that it doesn't work and giving up quickly.

Louis Gifford

Falmouth Physiotherapy Clinic

Section GE 4
Read what I've read

GE4.1 Shopping Basket

Jones M., Rivett D. (2004) Clinical Reasoning for Manual Therapists. Elsevier

Gifford L.S. and Butler D.S. (1997) 'The integration of pain sciences into clinical practice'. Hand Therapy 10(2): 86-95.

GE4.2 Biomedical compartment 1

Stam H. (1994) Frozen Shoulder reviewed. Physiotherapy.

GE4.3 Biomedical compartment 2

Red Flags: A Guide to Identifying Serious Pathology of the Spine, 1e (Physiotherapy Pocketbooks) by Sue Greenhalgh MA GD Phys FCSP and James Selfe PhD MA GD Phys FCSP (22 Feb 2006)

Red Flags II: A Guide to Solving Serious Pathology of the Spine, 1e (Physiotherapy Pocketbooks) Sue Greenhalgh MA GD Phys FCSP and James Selfe PhD MA GD Phys FCSP (2009)

Waddell, G. (2004) The Back Pain Revolution. Edinburgh. Churchill Livingstone.

RCGP (2000) Clinical Guidelines for the Management of Acute Low Back Pain. Royal College of General Practitioners, London

GE4.4 Biomedical compartment 3

Jones M., Edwards I. (2002) Conceptual models for implementing biopsychosocial theory in clinical practice. Manual Therapy.

GE4.5 Biomedical compartment 4

Comprehensive essential reading listed at start of chapter

GE4.6 Psychosocial 1

Paul Watson's three chapters in Topical Issues in Pain 2 (two are with Nick Kendall) and the chapter in Topical Issues in Pain 3 – with Chris Main, 'The distressed and angry low back pain patient'.

GE4.9 Psychosocial 5 Pink flags!

Seligman M. (2002) Authentic Happiness. Using the new positive psychology to realize your potential for deep fulfilment. Nicholas Brealey Publishing, London.

GE4.10 Disability compartment

Simmonds M. (1999). Physical function and physical performance in patients with pain: What are the measures and what do they mean? Pain 1999 - an updated review. Refresher course syllabus. M. Max. Seattle, IASP Press: 127-136.

Watson P. J. (1999). Non-physiological determinants of physical performance in musculoskeletal pain. Pain 1999 - an updated review. Refresher course syllabus. M. Max. Seattle, IASP Press: 153-158.

GE 4.11 & 12 Impairments compartment

Bou-Holaigah I., Rowe P.C., Kan J., Calkins H. (1995) The relationship between neurally mediated hypotension and the chronic fatigue syndrome. JAMA. 274:961-7.

Butler S.H., Nyman M., et.al. (2000) Immobility in Volunteers transiently produces signs and symptoms of complex regional pain syndrome. <u>Proceedings of the 9th World Congress on Pain, Progress in Pain Research and Management, Vol 16</u>. Devor M.,C., Rowbotham M.C. and Wiesenfeld-Hallin Z.(eds) Seattle, IASP Press: 657-660.

Calkins H., Rowe P.C. (1998) Relationship Between Chronic Fatigue Syndrome and Neurally Mediated Hypotension. Cardiol Rev. 6:125-134.

Freeman R., Komaroff A.L. (1997) Does the chronic fatigue syndrome involve the autonomic nervous system? Am J Med.102:357-64.

Schondorf R., Freeman R. (1999) The importance of orthostatic intolerance in the chronic fatigue syndrome. Am J Med Sci. 317:117-23.

Stewart J.M. (2000) Autonomic nervous system dysfunction in adolescents with postural orthostatic tachycardia syndrome and chronic fatigue syndrome is characterized by attenuated vagal baroreflex and potentiated sympathetic vasomotion. Pediatr Res.48:218-26.

Topical Issues in Pain 3 chapter 2 page 67

GE.13 General Health

Bortz W. M. (1984). The disuse syndrome. Western Journal of Medicine 141: 691-694.

Buckley J., Holmes J., and Mapp G. (1999). Exercise on prescription. Cardiovascular activity for health.   Butterworth Heinemann.

Case Histories

Sections 1-4

Case Histories 1
ACUTE

Chapter CH 1.1
Scott's acute low back pain – the 'twisted ankle' approach

Scott's a typical Australian, he's over here in Cornwall trying to tell us 'poms' all about his new marketing programme and how his company's going to save the UK economy. He's got a good sense of humour but, like most Australians, is full of bravado overlying a deep sense of fear and insecurity!

Let me start with some natural and fun prejudice and then I'll behave properly! However, there's nothing like setting the scene and catching the attention for the educational 'play' that follows.

If you're Australian and starting to feel offended don't be, because I will be having fun with our 'home-counties' folk (er, remember Vivien in the Volvo back in chapter 1?) the Cornish and all and sundry too.

My lessons from Scott will be as follows:

- understanding the application of the shopping basket to the acute pain sufferer

- seeing how self-help can apply in the acute situation

- there is no need for any modalities or hands-on techniques

- normalising recovery

- understanding the 'twisted ankle' approach to acute low back pain

Scott – the chat

Scott's in the waiting room ten minutes early; I know it because I can hear him from my room where I'm working with another patient. So that's about fifteen paces away through two closed doors. He's asking the receptionist if I'm going to be long because he's in agony. There's the occasional tense 'Oh Jesus' going on and I can hear the receptionist offering him a glass of water.

Fifteen minutes later he's sat sideways on the edge of a chair, he had walked in crab-like, rather heavily flexed and held onto the walls a lot as he came along the corridor.

'I'm from Brisbane Louis. I see you were in Adelaide a while back.'

He's seen my certificates.

'Yes, I spent three years there but escaped because it was hot, flat and there were no bends in the streets!' I quipped.

We both laughed and he settled to tell me his story.

It turned out that he'd never had back pain before but this had been getting worse for the last five or six days. This morning was the worst it had been and he'd manage to get an appointment with me. He was 35 years old, reasonably fit looking and told me he'd been shifting some furniture last week and felt a bit stiff afterwards and the next day. Since then the pain had slowly spread across his back into both buttocks. He described the pain as a really nasty 'deep gnawing ache' but when he moved it was like a 'stabbing knife' that took his breath away.

'Anything going down the legs?'

'No.'

'Pins and needles, funny feelings or loss of feeling anywhere?'

'Can you go to the loo OK, back and front?'

'Fine, but could hardly get off the toilet this morning.'

'Cough or sneezed by any chance?'

'Wouldn't dare, Christ!'

'General health OK? Anything serious wrong? Operations? Things in the past that might be of importance?'

'No fine, but wrote off a car once, just bruised and shaken up for a bit, that was it.'

'That's good and you haven't had any accidents like that or falls out of the ordinary recently?'

'Not at all.'

'Doesn't sound like it but are you on any tablets for anything, or anything to help the pain?'

'Oh, I did have asthma for a bit when I was a kid, had one of those puffers and for this back pain I took one of the wife's paracetomol this morning, complete waste of time.'

'Got that. Have you been sleeping OK?'

'Yeah, no problems but since I did that lift I've been really stiff getting out of bed, hardly get my socks on and this morning I've not been able to get straight.'

'So for the last few days, apart from this morning, you've freed up after getting up by the sound of it?'

'Correct, took about twenty minutes until this happened today.'

'It doesn't sound like you've been to a Dr at all?'

'No, wanted to skip the pills and get it fixed.'

'Good, so have you any thoughts about what you might have done or what has happened?'

'Well, yeah, I thought I'd only strained it like you do and it'd get better in a week or so but this morning's really scared me. I thought about going to the Dr because it feels like it's broken or something's out and I've bust something big time. My neighbour back home in Toowong when I was younger had a back pain for months and could hardly move, yet they kept telling her to get moving but it turned out she has some rare spinal disease. That's kind of in the back of my mind since this morning.'

'Right, got that Scott, you know when you moved the furniture do you feel you used a lot of force or was it awkward in some way? What I'm getting at is from what you did would you have expected to hurt yourself?'

'Oh, right, yeah, she had one end of this wardrobe and we were moving it out the bedroom, round the open door and we had to twist it awkwardly. I was up front holding this thing all twisted and at the same time I'd forgotten to move the bloody great cheese plant and it was in the way, so I'm there kicking this thing in this crabbed up posture for about two minutes. Christ was I cussing.'

'Did you feel something there and then?'

'Nothing more than a feeling that I'd just worked the back really hard, thought nothing of it after ten minutes.'

'So I'm now building a good picture, noted that you're a bit concerned about what's happened this morning. And I'm sitting here thinking what your understanding of physiotherapy for your kind of back pain problem might be?'

'Ah, that you guys use machines and give exercises rather than cracking it off or tying the patient up in knots.'

'No, that's the sort of thing that a Kiwi physio'd do to an Aussie or vice versa! We tend to be more subtle.'

I go on.

'OK Scott, two things from this. First, I'm going to do some key checks for anything serious (and if I'm the slightest concerned I'll get you to go up to see the Dr). Secondly, if everything's okay, which is likely from listening so far, I'm going to see what you can do movement-wise and we'll take it from there... By the way, have you been going into work these last few days?'

'Absolutely, once I'd got over the stiffness I was pretty good, occasionally a bit stiff getting out of the chair but then I'd move around a bit and it would free up and I'd forget about it.'

'Work's good then, you enjoy it?'

'Absolutely best job I've ever had, weird for a small Australian marketing company to have its northern European base all the way down here but everyone's brilliant and we're going places too.'

I nearly said something about cheap rents down here but decided against it. You can only take the piss out of an Aussie in pain for so long...!

'OK, good. So what have we got to get you back to – what do you get up to physically – any interests hobbies, activities, sports?'

'Two major things; I windsurf, I also sail and usually race two nights a week. We do a lot of walking too. I'm also doing some decorating at home right now, that's why I was moving the furniture.'

'Rate yourself fitness wise?'

'Well, pretty good, although I don't get out of breath for long, unless I do a jog or bike ride and that's not very often at the moment.'

Let's take a break and see where this has taken us as far as the 'Shopping Basket' is concerned.

Shopping basket

Biomedical: no obvious red flags, no serious disease, morning stiffness is typical of an acute back pain, no leg pain is a good thing but wary here as this has the sniff of 'disc' and could develop into nerve root pain (very flexed and shifted to the left, can't get upright, can't get socks on etc.)

This is familiar – therefore a 'common presentation'.

Need to check neurology even though no leg pain. It serves as a baseline, it is 'neurologically reassuring' red flag wise and there could be loss of conduction (I have seen plenty of acute back pains with no referral that have loss of reflex or motor weakness appropriate to nerve root injury).

This is an 'acute' injury situation so should respect the tissues – as per a twisted ankle. So think possible inflammation and swelling (can't prove) and early stages of healing but safe to start getting gradually going. Forceful techniques and rigorous movements are unnecessary and virtually contraindicated to me, think, 'I wouldn't do that to an acute twisted ankle' and you've got my point – thanks!

Pain mechanisms – yes, all involved, generally adaptive and classically because of the acute nature of the problem, nociceptive mechanisms are a consideration and tie in with the tissue thoughts. I also have 'potential nerve root' in the back of my mind and therefore thoughts about 'peripheral neurogenic' mechanisms are not unreasonable.

It is early days but Scott's apparent high concern from the morning event is an issue in 'facilitation' of central mechanisms – i.e. encouraging pain rather than inhibiting it. But having said that his reaction hasn't been going on long and should ease up as things progress.

Some key things to consider in the light of what we know about acute injury to tissues and to nerve:

- the tissues may still be in a state of gradually increasing inflammation – this could keep on rising for a few days (refer to chapter 13.2 and note the 'box' that outlines the stages of healing that I have on my white board)

- a nerve component could well be present – he doesn't like bending (nerve pulling) or coming upright (nerve compression)

- the typical early nerve related pain delays its 'build-up' sometimes

The point in time: 'Scott' is at is the beginning of a possibly rising graph (see chapter 13.1 – 'The Toblerone recovery'). This could be the start of a quite natural symptom 'build-up'. It has a clear potential to increase and spread distally into some form of sciatica or nerve root pain. That's a big reason why it is important to:

a) Not do strong techniques and get blamed for it happening when it could be happening anyway.

b) Do a thorough neurological examination and tell your patient what you are finding as you go. You want him to leave the session knowing about his muscle power, sensation and reflex status.

c) Give an adequate explanation that covers the possibility of spreading and increasing symptoms. Yes, I know that is a negative message but wait until you see what I do shortly, thanks. Over the years I have made massive efforts to take the pressure of me and give the patient a realistic view of their situation. In the last twenty years I have had very, very few patients who have come back worse and not understood why they were worse, or who have blamed me for being worse. Like all therapists I have had my fair share of disasters.

Psychosocial: the main issues that crop up from the 'ABCDEFW' so far are:

- 'A' (Attitudes and Beliefs) – some concerns and worries about what is going on but looking to be reassured and with the red-flags so far there's nothing serious to worry about. Reassurance is high on the agenda though.

- 'B' (Behaviours) – it is hardly fair to judge this on just one morning's new experience.

Looking at the last few days since it happened his 'behaviour' has been fine, he's carried on at work and accepted and got on with the stiffness. His food/drink/drug behaviour isn't an issue either. He did make mention of being cured and that physios use machines but also exercise. I feel he is the sort of chap who will be happily guided by my findings and reasoning.

- 'C' (Compensation and Economic) – is not relevant at this early stage and isn't likely to be unless he has to take time off work.

- 'D' (Diagnosis and treatment issues) – nothing of huge importance here, he hasn't seen a Dr but has some concern about missing a serious diagnosis due to his neighbour back home's experience.

- 'E' (Emotions) – he's clearly upset and a bit reactive, at least in the waiting room but with me he's soon settled. His worries about serious pathology have been noted and will need to be checked.

- 'F' (Family) – I haven't delved into this much as it's so early days. Seems to have a happy relationship with his wife.

- 'W' (Work) – all positive news at this stage.

Disability/Functional restrictions: I have a clear idea of the physical activities he does and therefore the level of function to aim for as he recovers – windsurfing, sailing and walking. I will get more details if necessary at an appropriate time. Note for example that windsurfing involves awkward carrying of the board and sail down the beach, sailing is often a lot of flexed sitting and pulling of ropes and winching – quickly, suddenly, hard and often in a flexed posture. Cycling and jogging may be useful to get him going and fitter at some stage.

Impairments: the list will mount with the physical examination. At this stage I could include, loss of flexion, extension, posture, left sided shift, awkward gait etc. There's a good overlap of these with function. I'll revisit after the physical examination.

General Health: seems pretty good, he's used to being physically active and enjoys it so it shouldn't be too hard to get him involved in a self help/exercise/graded exposure type programme.

Pain: pretty obvious, location wise and the clear 'sharp' and 'ache' distinction. Some help here is important and the use of appropriate anti-inflammatories should prove helpful. He has a typical morning stiffness 'inflamed' type presentation. He may feel better with, dare I say it, a lumbar support for a few days! 'You can't do that Louis, they've been shown to promote passivity and illness behaviour and there's no good evidence.' Yeah right! What's the key here? Simple, it's 'If it feels good – do it ' (you'd happily support a sprained ankle and it seems to me that 'taping' is back in, or does that help lymphatic drainage – claims recently withdrawn!)

The physical examination and early management

I nearly always finish the 'history taking/subjective' part of the assessment session with this:

'Right, is there anything else you want to tell me, anything that you feel I might have missed, or that you're still concerned about?'

Believe it or not quite a common one is 'Oh, do you want me to undress?' Probably not what you were expecting but worth a quick mention here. There are a great many patients who hate showing their bodies, who have rather awkwardly placed tattoos or who have their 'inappropriate' underwear on or off! Undressing is to 'Where you feel comfortable.' This usually means it's fine for trouser bottoms off and leave top on. If there's a big deal in the thoracic spine and you want to look get the patient to slip there top half-off so you can see. I would hate to be a young girl in bra and pants standing around while some unknown physio watches closely every movement and every fold of flesh. Be sensitive to this please? How would you feel?

Back to Scott...

He struggles to get his trousers off and by the time he's done so I've seen a heap of awkward movement. The key is that it's not—'not moving'.

'Right Scott I want to have a careful look at your movements and if you don't want to, or are concerned about anything just say so, you just do what you feel you want to and tell me about it. I'll probably get you to try movements in different positions but we'll see how we go. Are you up for that?'

He grimaces a polite 'I'll give it a go but I'm a bit concerned' type of look.

'I'm also going to do some nerve tests and I'll explain them as I go along.'

He nodded.

After watching him struggle to walk again I almost immediately got him to stop and stand. I let him lean forward onto the couch which I'd raised to a comfortable height.

'Ah, that's better' he muttered.

I'm thinking right, 'crutches' and grab a pair that are in the corner of the treatment room. I adjust them and give them to him.

'Try leaning on these and if you feel like it see what they're like walking.'

He stands and looks at me 'Cor that's better, though I'm entering the world of the disabled a bit here Louis!'

He said it with a grin.

'Simple things often help us to keep going, or at least move around with a lot more comfort and you're unlikely to need them for long!'

'You reckon?'

'Well you might get hooked on them, find that everyone helps you and takes pity on you and takes you out for meals and then I'd have to really question the Aussie ethics!'

As we're taking the mickey out of each other he's giving walking up and down a try and finding it a great deal easier. For one thing he looks less shifted and the other he's more evenly weight-bearing and smoother. He's still flexed. I can't emphasise enough what producing a sense of 'security' or 'safety' does to alleviate tension and increase confidence.

'Right, let's try a few standard movements while you're on the crutches, first up show me how upright you can comfortably go?'

He pushes rather tensely on the crutches and comes up to about 10-15 degrees off upright. I pull his shirt up and have a look at his back it's quite kyphotic and he's also dipped his pelvis forward by bending his knees a bit.

'Go back to where's comfortable Scott.'

He relaxes forward and his knees straighten up

'What about going forward, do you want to have a go? Get the crutches at a good angle to support you if you do.'

Forward he goes – it's all hip; his back is unchanging intervertebrally. He goes to the point where his head is parallel to the floor.

We do the same with side flexion to which he dips his knees but rotation does show more freedom towards his left, shifted, side.

My thoughts now...

> In the back of my mind is the red flag, 'persistent severe restriction of lumbar flexion'. I'm looking forward to seeing if any intervertebral movement occurs with a change in posture.
>
> I need to do a good neurological and explain it to him, plus discuss any thoughts that he may be having as a result. I nearly always do my neurological examinations for the lower limb in sitting with couch raised and feet off the floor. I adapt of course if the patient finds this impossible to be comfortable in.

Onwards...

'Right Scotty, the next thing is that I want to look at a few things sitting like this.' I sit up on the couch with my thighs fully supported. 'Do you think you could manage that for about three minutes?'

'Let's give it a go.'

He sits up and finds it best to grasp the edge of the plinth and be slumped in the back and lean forward. He takes some pressure through the arms just like with the crutches. He gets comfortable and I do his calf and quads reflexes which are fine.

'OK, good reflexes equals good nerves, these two reflexes test the two main nerves that supply the legs – to the muscles to make them work and to the skin and all the tissues so you can feel your legs and know where they are.'

He nods.

'The point about this is that when a back is injured it can also compromise the nerves and stop them working properly; if the nerves are all good with these tests it's a big confidence booster for me and of course for you too.'

I then do a quick sensory check with light touch and also all the standard muscle tests sitting – quads, hip flexors, abductors, adductors, hamstrings, foot dorsiflexion, eversion, inversion and toe flexors and extensors. I do calf standing (usually before getting them to sit – and in Scott's case while he's standing with the crutches). All tests are fine and I again reassure him that the nerve tests are all normal.

I then check some components of the 'slump' test to see if there are any neural 'sensitivity' issues. As an aside, don't forget that sometimes when there's a lot of acute pain, a positive neural tension test may relate to 'secondary hyperalgesia' – it may be a false positive. Even so, it could also be an early sign that some neural irritation is involved and therefore add the potential thought that an early 'disc' situation is a possibility. Remember disc material that escapes imbibes fluid and swells, then the immune/inflammatory response may start. The inclusion of a mechanical or chemically mediated irritation/damage to the nerve should always be in the back of the clinician's mind I feel.

Scott's still sitting slumped and I ask him to slowly lower his head. He doesn't really think and drops it down fast and bang!

'Yow! Bloody hell that hurt my back, that was the knife pain alright, shit!'

I explain the simple physical connection between the head and neck and the nerves in the back and that there's a pulling effect – that the pulling is normal but that it's very common for back pain to occur when the whole area is sensitised.

'I'll put that one in my shopping basket – I'm collecting up some of the findings as we go along and putting them there – the point is that I'll keep an eye on that and you can too by testing it from time to time. Right, let's go more slowly this time and see what happens.'

He now tentatively lowers his neck again and it's not half so sharp, in fact as he stays at the point of discomfort he finds it lessens a little and he can go a bit further.

'Next part of this is to see what happens when we move the nerves from the other end.'

I sit next to him and explain the sciatic tract; I then slump like he is and slowly straighten my knee and tell him about hamstring tightening but also that the sciatic nerve is being moved.

'Now let's start with the left.' (I choose the left because of his shift to the left and assume that because of this it's likely to be easier and freer, though it needn't be.)

He slowly extends his left knee and it goes to full extension with a slight pull in the back of the leg.

'Can you normally touch your toes?' I ask.

'Pretty much, easy to my ankles, then an easy bounce and I can put flat hands down.'

That gives me an idea of his normal hamstring/sciatic tract extensibility.

He now does the right knee extension and at about 30 degrees off full extension he goes,

'Louis, that's pulling in my back and increasing the pain a bit.'

'If you're OK, just see what happens when you slowly pull your foot up towards you.' I'm still next to him in the same position as he is and I demonstrate.

'That's increasing it more, how weird is that?'

I've seen enough now and get him to relax back down. I explain the foot's role in moving the nerve and that the response is common.

As an aside here it's of interest to note that one of the few physical 'yellow flags' is SLR being positive for producing back pain. I haven't tested SLR I know but when the slump is positive like this quite often the SLR is too. A big bite of caution, remember Vivien in the Volvo, every test hurt like hell yet a day later it had all settled. The massive spread of sensitivity that is possible in some acute low back pains is astonishing. That this sort of sensitivity has meaningful anatomical, pathological, or injury related consequences has to be interpreted with great caution.

When newly qualified I remember finding acute pain states and marked spread of sensitivity like this very daunting, any inexperienced physiotherapist or any other clinician is quite likely to as well. All I can say is know your Red flags and assess them properly, do a thorough neurological examination, be aware of acute seemingly maladaptive 'secondary hyperalgesia' and use the 'twisted ankle' approach and all will be well.

Be careful not to be seduced into thinking otherwise by persuasive guru type figures, or 'cocky' operators, who claim that they 'cure' in one treatment this type of patient – there is nothing more demoralising than making a patient worse or them not returning for their follow-up appointment. Please don't feel pressurised by the patient who claims his last therapist fixed him, 'I went in bent and came out straight'– most patients forget acute pain very quickly. Patients are often relieved that you aren't going to 'crack' them and openly say so when you state you are not.

I now lower the plinth down and get Scott to wriggle forward so his feet are flat on the floor. He now has to sit with his thighs angled slightly downwards and I ask him what coming upright here feels like. It's easier and as is quite common, he's actually sitting fairly square with little or no lean to the left. I then get him to bend forward keeping his hands on his thighs so he can control the movement and take some tension off his back. What's good is that he can flex right forward, trunk onto thighs.

'I'm pleased to see that.' I say. We also do twisting – not bad and side bending and he goes about 20 degrees each way, mostly by rocking his pelvis and weight transference. Again, there's little sign of intervertebral movement happening.

'I'm wondering if you can get comfortable lying on your back or if not on your side?'

'When I found I could hardly get out of bed this morning, I managed to get to the loo and back to the bed. After that I only managed lying on my back with my knees bent up. My wife Demelza, she's Cornish by the way, she put a pile of pillows under my knees and that helped me relax until I got up to come here.

I thought about using my low 'traction' stool, which is adjustable up and down, but decided to try simple crook lying first. I soon had him comfy on his back, the key being the raised head end of the plinth plus several pillows adjusted until he felt comfortable and relaxed.

In this 'non-weight bearing' situation it was going to interesting to see if any reasonably good movements of the back were going to be possible.

'Same rules Scotty, I suggest some movement and you try it. First up let's try lowering one of your legs, try the left first unless you'd prefer the right.'

I didn't expect much but he was OK so long as he did one at a time, putting one down then adding the other was painful. That was in the shopping basket as a useful 'pink' impairment. He could also do 'grab-a-knee' fine (hip and back flexion) and also do one then add the other and do both together. I was happy that his back was flexing OK now. And I told him too.

I wanted to check any further extension possibilities, so in the crook lying with head end up lying position I asked him to attempt a pelvic rock – the way I did this was to put my hand on his lower anterior rib cage in the midline and ask him to lift my hand upwards. I was surprised to find that he could do this with ease.

Next, because of his shift to the left I wanted to see if there was any side bending, especially to the right. In crook lying it's simply 'hip-hitching' – a movement that I tend to think of as an anatomically speaking 'bottom-up' type movement, the movement starting from the pelvis and going up from L5, rather than standing side-flexion which is more top-down. For many patients it's quite a novel movement. Anyway, in this position of lumbar flexion he could go either way once he'd mastered the awkwardness of it.

Crook rotation was freer to the left than the right but the range wasn't bad.

Pause for thoughts... neurologically OK. I can find some simple 'start-easy-build-slowly' movements to do in all directions, his back isn't locked and I need to tell him that, it just doesn't want to move in weight-bearing at the present time. I think he's going to be able to get about better with the crutches and I'm now wondering if he might relax a bit more if I try him with a comfortable lumbar binder.

I leave him lying where he's comfortable to chat.

'Right Scott how are you doing and what are you thinking!' I smile.

'Well, I'm pleased my nerves are OK and I'm seeing that you've been able to get me comfortable enough to move.'

'That's good. Now, what about those concerns of yours, about something being seriously wrong'

'Well, I'm not sure, you haven't really told me what I've done, you know, I'm wondering if my back is 'out' in some way or maybe I've ripped a disc or a ligament in my back.'

'Right, from listening to you and all your answers to my questions I can tell you that I have no fears of anything seriously wrong with your back. I am particularly reassured by the tests of your nerves which were fine but also that the nature of your presentation is very common. Sprain or overstrain is a good term to use here and from what you describe the injuring movement will have done just that. We know that young spines like yours are incredibly strong and can withstand pretty high loads without serious injury. However, twisting and loading awkwardly are classic positions for the back to overstrain in. That means inflammation and early stages of healing right now – think like a cut finger or a twisted ankle, they're both vulnerable for a few days and like you to go carefully, then things ease up and you get going more and more. We use the term, 'start-easy-build-slowly' – it makes sense with a twisted ankle and it makes sense with an overstrained back. Maybe you can see what start easy movements you can do?'

He promptly went,

'What I've just been doing and maybe those ones sitting weren't too bad either.'

That's right, you can also move better on the crutches and I'm going to lend you those to use if they help.'

'I also want you to see that when you did that 'arch-up' exercise to extend your back and then let it go down again, that was the equivalent of being able to go from fully straight to bend backwards (I'm demonstrating as I talk) to all the way down to touch your toes from the back's point of view. What I'm saying is that if we take the weight off your back it's capable of near enough full movement in these two directions, it's just that for you it doesn't like doing it with the weight on in standing. That tells me that nothing is blocked or stuck in your back it's just being limited by the pain.'

I do this because I'm keen to link the movements and exercises he's doing and will be probably doing at home, to day to day functional movements. Scott nods, he's with me.

'Next thing. You may also notice that for common muscle and ligament injuries in sport, the trainers use taping and tight compression type bandages, or elasticated supports. Many people find that having a bit of pressure round the area makes it feel better and they relax and actually move better as a result. I'd like to see how you feel with a lumbar support if you're up for it?'

'Give anything a go...'

'Right, see if you can get up off the couch is the next challenge?'

Pleasingly it wasn't too difficult and five minutes later I've helped him put a simple wrap-around support on and he's moving around with the crutches thinking about it.

'The rules for it are, use it if it feels good, rip it off if it's annoying. Most people find they can be helpful for a while but often get annoyed by them if they're on too long. There are no 'you must wear it at all time' commandments at all. We like the phrase for this stage of a problem 'If it feels good, do it!'

I said he could borrow it until we met up again in a few days so he could see what it was like given a bit of time.

So he went away from that first visit:

- with crutches and moving better and far less tense

- a binder which he wasn't sure about, but could try

- simple movement exercises in raised trunk crook lying and sitting. He agreed 5-1-15 repetitions 'anytime' having tested the number of reps and found 5-10 quite acceptable.

He was going to try and do them regularly through the day and also anytime he felt uncomfortable to see if they helped to decrease the ache and the stiffness.

• the message for movement was, big, floppy, as easy and relaxed as possible movement, not tense. If things felt tense he was to slow them up and not do them so far into range. If they freed up he would let them extend into range so long as it felt good.

• I was quite happy for him to take time out to rest, so long as it was as comfortable as possible. He said work would be fine with him lying on the office floor and he'd take in a few pillows. I also encouraged him to balance the rest with short walks using the crutches

• I emphasised 'start-easy-build slowly' and don't go mad, like a bull-at-a-gate.

• I showed him the typical recovery graph – the 'Toblerone' recovery, and that easing up and flaring up were possibilities and also typical pain behaviours for recovering back pain.

• I explained to him the typical healing stages showing him especially the early phase where inflammation sometimes builds for two to three days before settling.

(He understood that this could happen but with good pain control and being sensible he could well be fine. I noted that deep tissue injuries, like in the back, were far less predictable in their behaviour than simple cuts to the skin. I could have gone on about sensory maps in the brain being excellent and therefore accurate for skin but not for at all accurate for deeper tissues – but it wasn't necessary.)

• I encouraged him to not panic or tense up if the pain took a turn for the worse, but use the resting position, the belt if it helped plus any form of heat or cold that might help too.

• I explained and advised some NSAID's – to be taken regularly until I saw him again in about three or four days time. I explained that reducing pain actually helped to speed healing, which he found surprising.

• I told him that the current way of looking at back pain was to classify it into three, simple back pain, nerve root pain (I mentioned sciatica) and 'serious' pathology. I said that his was classified as 'simple back pain' and that meant think 'sprain, strain' rather than broken, ripped torn and irreparable. He found that reassuring.

• I mentioned that there was a slight 'sniff' of nerve about it and that I was unable to predict whether a nerve in his back was involved or may become involved. I reassured him that at the present time it looked fine but that if he had any further concerns or worries, to phone and leave a message. I always do this with my patients and I mean it. I tell them that I don't want them sitting at home worried, ring and talk and if I'm concerned, I'll see him again immediately.

• I lent him a copy of 'The Back Book'. Roland, M., G. Waddell, et al. (2002).
  The Back Book, The Stationary Office Ltd. It is also reproduced in full in Waddell G
  (2004) The Back Pain revolution. Churchill Livingstone, Edinburgh – a book everyone
  involved in treating back pain and musculoskeletal pain should have and have studied
  in my opinion.

Follow up and recovery

I saw Scott again four days later. He hadn't phoned and he came into the treatment
rooms carrying the crutches, less tense, still rather stooped but certainly not grabbing
the walls and furniture.

'Not bad for an Aussie from a shack in Toowong!'

'Funny, but like you said it was bad for a couple of days, though I have to say those
ibuprofen helped and I kept the exercises going when it felt good to do. Yesterday
was a definite improvement and today I'm feeling far more positive about it.'

He sat down normally and said,

'You know you said about that nerve possibility, does that include pain going into my
goolies by any chance, Christ they were aching for those two days?'

'I think if you tried to look that up or ask a Dr you wouldn't get much response but
all I can tell you is that pain gets referred, meaning you feel it in places where there's
nothing wrong. The best example is pain down the arm from heart problems, that's
'angina', you've probably heard of that – but pain in the testicles with back pain is
very common in my experience and as you've found as the pain settles it goes away.
All I can advise is best to ignore it and let it go but if it keeps coming back a trip to
the Dr may be worthwhile. The key here is that it's linked to the intensity of the back
pain and it doesn't sound like you've ever had it before?'

'Never.'

'Any more questions or shall we get on and see what you can do.'

We got on and I noticed that he had the lumbar support on.

'How did the support go?'

'Good for an hour or two when it's feeling a little achy, helps me relax, then I take
it off and I find I do a few stretches and the sitting exercises and I'm then good for
quite a while. It's been good to have.'

'Do you want to hang on to it a bit longer?'

He did and he thought that it would help him do more and have better posture for a while round the house as he wanted to get back to the decorating. All good stuff, I've no problems with that, after all many builders, weightlifters, motocross motorcyclists and tradesmen have lumbar supports and find that they help. They don't use them as a display of disability or as some form of message to help, they thoughtlessly stick them on when doing a bit of loading, want to feel secure and comfortable and that's it. I'll discuss the importance of a good 'natural' corset later.

Scott took his trousers off and we got on with looking at movements.

I went through the same routine again, walk, standing movements, checked calf, sat down, checked all power and reflexes plus slump as before.

He could just about get to upright standing, he could bend to two to three inches below his knees, side flexion was finger tips roughly to knee joint line on the left, with 'tightness' and 'pulling' but to the right it was about two thirds the way down the lateral thigh – intervertebral wise it didn't go past the midline. Rotation was far more relaxed but most sore towards the right end range.

All the neuro was still fine. The head component of the slump 'pulled' in the back and the right knee extension was nearly full but he did tend to lean back. Foot dorsiflexion added a pulling like the neck flexion. All signs were either stable or improving. Good and he could see this too.

I reviewed the lying exercises and found that we didn't need to put the plinth end up but required two pillows. He could almost get both legs down straight in this position but could when I raised the plinth end by about six inches.

I kept going with the 'nice' movement approach with a focus on freer intervertebral movements in all directions. Kneeling on all 'fours' proved very helpful. In this position he could do arch well after a bit of training to get his head round it and the more we did 'sag' into extension the smoother that became too. 'Arch and sag' was put on his list. I also looked at 'hip-hitch' in all fours, or what I call 'butt-waggle' with the patients. This was especially painful when hitching the right hip (right side flexion/closing down the right side) however, by fiddling with arch/sag (flexion-extension) we soon found that he could hitch well in a few degrees of flexion/arch! He understood the principle of getting the movement going with little or no pain, with nice easy relaxed movement and the biggest movement that felt safe and was comfortably possible.

Although I didn't do this with Scott I also test pelvic rock/arch-hollow in what I call the crook lying up on elbows position. Try it sometime, some people find this starting position a lot easier to get the pelvic rocking movement from. It's also a good starting position for the bottom-up side to side 'waggle.' Side flexion done in flexion, if you ever care to look at the facet joints, is in a much more loose packed position.

He went away from the second session...

Continue the tablets for a couple more days, plus the warning that
sometimes when you stop tablets you can get a little flare of symptoms as
the body/pain system reacts to stopping the tablets.   I often explain it as a
'mini cold turkey' effect. I also tell the patient that if the pain continues to
be a problem over two to three days to take the tablets again consistently
for a couple more days. The whole idea being that pain flare-ups are
unhelpful (think central cell assembly formation as well as pain halting
functionally recovery too) and that it's best to nip them in the bud, but
also to then try and stop the tablets again a day or two later.

Basically I try to help patients stop the tablets as soon as possible but I
also like good pain control too and I make sure they understand this. I
know my little system hasn't any support whatsoever but I also know
that patients feel much happier to be quickly off tablets and coping on
their own, rather than doing what the Dr says, which is usually take the
tablets regularly for at least two weeks (I'm thinking NSAID's here) and
nothing else. By 'nothing else' here I mean no rehab input and no advice
as to what to do. Most Drs, if they do give advice, it's given in about two
minutes and usually in the form of some basic exercise that the patients try
but can't see the point of, that hurt, that don't make sense etc. I have to
say, that it takes time to get a patient onside, understanding what is going
on and getting them to take responsibility. This is pretty unfair on Drs –
they try to tell the patients they've pulled a muscle and that they should
keep going – we are lucky we have time to deal with this better. There
should be a decent physio in every GP practice sorting out all the MSK
patients?

With the 'new' on 'all fours' exercises plus the old with the instruction to
increase the numbers and range gradually. Again, it was 5-10-15 anytime
through the day, 'little and often' and not necessarily all the exercises at
once. With some patients I would give clearer guidance but Scott grasped
it all well.

With a walking programme suggestion – with or without the crutches.
Having found that Scott could be on his feet around the house and at work
for about five minutes we agreed the initial walks would be around three
to four minutes starting at four times a day. I reminded him of 'start- easy-
build-slowly' and 'succeed-not-fail' – so that he didn't overdo it, at least
initially. He also agreed to come in again in one week and that during the
week he would increase the time of the walks gradually with the goal of
fifteen minutes four times a day.

He also agreed to start doing some sit-stands and step-ups working to
'done something' feeling. We tested this in the treatment and he found he
could do about fifteen reps comfortably for his back and felt he'd done a
bit for his legs. He agreed to the 'any-anytime' and start easy etc. principle.

He also told me that he wanted to try doing a bit of decorating and so we discussed taking time to make sure he worked in comfortable positions and took regular breaks.

Following session...

I saw him once more two weeks later but kept in contact with him.

Scott continued to recover but over the next month had two big flare-ups, one following a longer than usual walk/being on his feet (shopping!) and the other for no particular reason. In both instances he took the tablets again for two to three days, he eased back the exercises to the ones he found easy but kept them going, he used the binder intermittently and paced rest/activity sensibly. Each time took about two days to ease back.

At the one month point...

> He was back sailing, he found the binder helped and for the first few sails he avoided being 'in the thick of the action' on the boat. His main role was spinnaker trimmer – which involves standing pulling a rope and letting it go to adjust the sail, all the while looking up at the leech of the sail. So plenty of balance and an upright almost constant posture while concentrating. Evening racing spinnaker legs last about twenty minutes maximum. Pleasingly for the first time he tried it was light winds and he swapped between standing and sitting while trimming.

> Cardio-vascular wise, he agreed it would be wise to get fit and to this end he found cycling the best. He started tentatively but within a week was happy going out for an hour. I suggested he stopped occasionally and walked for a minute or two, did some 'opposite' stretches (extension, twists and side to side) before continuing on.

> I showed him how to get his lifting confidence back. He used theraband under his feet up to both hands to work his half squat and then up tall with comfortable back straight posture which he quickly got the hang of. We did some lifting practice using the chairs, trolleys and couches in the clinic. He could easily see the value of 'planning' lifting and not jumping right in as he had done.

> He got back to windsurfing round the six week mark The key was to carry the board down the beach separated from the sail rather than suffering the awkwardness of carrying the whole board and rig together! I got him to practice testing and lifting the board before he went out.

Points

1. This is an example of a typical acute back. And because there were relatively few 'yellow flag' issues, for example, the patient was happy to take responsibility for his recovery, he quickly understood what he had to do and was keen to be a part of it, he did well and it was easy for me to steer him to full recovery.

2. Full recovery? Ah, good point, because if you really do follow your acute back patients up you'll be surprised how long their problems dog them for sometimes. I only saw Scott three times to cover the above but I also stayed in contact with him for a year. That was easy because I saw him about every other week at the sailing club after racing and we often had a quick 'on the quay' update and problem solving session. At the end of the season I rang him a couple of times. Patients I'm interested in I put a message to myself to ring in the appointment book – often in six months time. I rang Scott about eleven months after I first saw him and he said, 'It's only in the last month or so that I feel it's finally gone and I'm starting to forget about it. It's been stiff in the morning for a few minutes for all that time, after racing the next day it's often been stiff a bit longer but loosened up with a shower. Now at last I'm free in the mornings. Over the whole period I reckon I've had a flare-up lasting two to three days about once every five or six weeks and once I had that pain back in my bollocks.'

3. What about his future? Good point too and impossible to predict, he might be fine but statistically he's likely to have further episodes. I would bet that one day he'll end up with sciatica and/or that he'll go through a period of regular stuck and shifted phases. On his side is that he's active and fit and upbeat, he enjoys life at work and at play.

Louis and I did discuss his use of tissue based explanations (particularly – 'nerves') and he acknowledged that this is the language that most patients understand. For example, how often does a patient come into the clinic and tell you that they think they have pulled a muscle – even though they've had their problem for many months and there was no injuring incident that they could remember?

Louis educated Scott to self help from the first session – Scott knew to help himself through flare-ups rather than to run to therapists to 'fix' him – Louis added that this is the point we hear from many past patients – they learnt self help from us.

Scott could have got better without any physio or medical input? – many acute back pains do   and it was his first episode? Louis commented that he also likes the reassurance and education side of therapy. As regards the 'follow up' – we've been in the same place for over 26 years and it's easy. And you hear how it really is out there recovery-wise!

Philippa

Chapter CH 1.2
Clara's acute whiplash

Clara's situation

Clara was in tears as she came down the corridor to the treatment room. She had a thick scarf around her neck and she didn't look up when I greeted her.

Ten days ago she'd stopped her car at a roundabout and a young fellow in a van had rammed into her. Her car was shunted about a metre into the roundabout. She said the guy just yelled at her for stopping for no reason.

'I haven't really stopped crying and I'm so angry.'

'Tell me what happened.' I said as we caught the tiniest bit of eye contact for the first time. She was sitting clasping a tissue; she looked drained and quite dishevelled.

'The car was my first new car it was only a month old...'

She related a story of being taken to hospital in an ambulance and when she got there she waited for five hours before being seen.

'As I was sat there this head pain welled up, it spread from my neck over my head and settled across my eyebrows. I felt like the back of my eyes were being stabbed. I told the receptionist what was happening and she almost bellowed at me that someone would be with me as soon as they could. I yelled back at her and all the other patients were on my side. After that the headache got worse and then the neck pain spread down my shoulders and I started getting weird pins and needles feelings in my hands. Oh God it was awful and just like all the other times.'

'The other times,' I enquired.

It turned out that she'd had two accidents in the last five years; one where she'd backed into her street too fast and a passing car had clipped the back of her car, the other was a similar rear-end type collision to the current one about three years ago. Both times she'd ended up in casualty, both times they'd hardly looked at her and both times she'd been off work with headaches and pain in the neck for over three months. Her casualty experience was similar every time; no proper examination in her eyes, no x-ray or scan, just a bit of reflex checking, a few arm movements, a listen to her heart and chest and then sent home with painkillers and a referral to her Doctor.

The Dr was similarly dismissive this time, as the other times and told her to rest and take tablets.

'He's seeing me again next week I think. He doesn't really want to see me I know.'

I could have taken the conversation in any number of directions.

'Let's stick with the current accident for now and I'll come back to those other ones later. What's happening with it now and what's been happening since the accident?'

She told me she'd got a friend to come and pick her up from the hospital; that she lived alone with her four cats and that her work was at 'County Hall' – working as a secretary in local government. She told me that it was all getting worse – she could hardly feel her hands now and the headaches went from her eyes/eyebrow area back to the back of her head. The neck pain felt like a constant vice, she couldn't move it and the pain was also across the base of her neck, upper thorax and out to both shoulders. She also said she was feeling pain in her low back too. I mapped it all out on a body chart and constantly checked with her that I had it all right. She gave them all scores of ten out of ten.

'Since the accident are all these pains always like this – what I mean is do they ever change at all, do they move around, or vary in intensity, or are they just constant ten out of ten?' She didn't really seem to listen to my questions but eventually told me it was constant all the time; that she wasn't sleeping, that it kept her awake and that it made her really upset. She kept coming back to the driver swearing at her and the argument she'd had with the casualty receptionist.

'Earlier you said you were really angry, is that all about the driver and the casualty?'

'Partly, I'm also angry that I've now lost the car; that I'm in pain again; that it's going to be like before and take ages to get better or may not even get better and that I'm going to be stuck at home for the rest of my miserable life with this. I'm so mad about it and that bloke, what a complete bastard, he didn't even say sorry, he yelled at me for stopping when the road was clear. He was nothing but a 'dick', a complete 'dick' and the driver behind him who stopped said he was coming up far too fast.'

She was crying again. I continued.

'It's been about ten days now and from what you said it sounds like it's either staying the same or even getting worse, am I right, or is there a sign that something might be improving a little?'

'It's not getting better at all; I can't feel my hands properly and the pain goes from my eyes to the back of my head...'

Like a great many distressed patients she repeated the negative side of the symptoms and didn't really answer the question. There was no point in chasing it further. Here was a highly distressed, angry 35 year old who it was pointless doing anything 'physical' too until I'd heard her complete story and she felt like I'd listened, heard and understood too. At this point there were plenty of 'yellow-flag' issues but I felt I wanted to just dip into a few more before moving on.

'Were you referred here by the Dr?'

'No, I only saw him once and it was painkillers and rest, the usual. I'm here because the insurance company solicitors told me too, your clinic here is on their list apparently.'

'Have you seen a solicitor then?'

'I spoke to one on the phone and he told me that they would be assessing the car to see if it was a write-off and also that they'd soon be getting me an appointment to see an accident specialist Dr.'

'Did you go through all this for your last two accidents too?'

'Well for the first one it was my fault and I lost my no-claims but I did for the second one, although they didn't send me for physio then.'

'What happened?'

'Well like I said, I was off work for ages. After a couple of months the solicitor sent me to the accident Dr who basically said it would take six months and that I'd be 100% then. He suggested I start walking and get moving; that I take another couple of weeks more off work and then think about going back.'

'What happened?'

'Well, I went back to work about three weeks later like he said. It wasn't better and about once every ten days or so I used to have to take a few days off work to get it to settle. I reckon it was a year before I was OK at work and the headaches went away. I spent a small fortune on the chiropractor lady.'

'Did that help at all?'

'Well it must of done I guess. She was a nice lady. She said the accident had put joints out in my neck, the middle of my back, the lower back and pelvis, so most of the work she did was down there.   It always felt good afterwards but as time went on the sessions were very short.'

'I presume she sorted it all out?'

'Well she never really said, I kept going and at the end of every session she always said there was more to work on and to keep coming. I went weekly for nearly a year.'

'So were you 100% between then and the recent accident, that's about two years isn't it?'

'Well, in the sense that I could work OK, yes I was, but she advised I stop doing my walking for some reason, I think it was to do with putting the pelvis out, though it wasn't really clear. Anyway, I was OK but since then I've been fearful of walking or even being on my feet for more than half an hour.   I find that my back starts to ache and then I'm afraid that the headaches and neck will kick-off. I've learnt that it's best to only be on my feet for thirty minutes maximum. Oh, and she didn't like me going to my 'patchwork club' meetings and so I stopped all that too. Again she said it was poor posture and that it would only aggravate the headaches if I kept doing that.'

'So it sounds like you stopped your hobbies, is there anything else you like to do that you've stopped because of that?'

'Well that's it, my life's my work, the cats and my home at the moment. I've put on weight and I think it's down to me not walking anymore.'

'How much did you used to walk?'

'I'd walk every Sunday with my friend Lynn. We'd walk for about two to three hours usually.'

'That's good and the patchwork, how often did you do that?'

'Oh, every night, while the TV was on, probably two to three hours some nights. The National Trust shop used to hang my quilts and sell them occasionally.'

'What's happening with work or what are you expecting to happen, have you contacted them at all?'

'Well, I can't go back until I'm better; I can't even sit for more than five minutes, most of the day I'm either in bed or on the sofa. The more I keep the neck and back still the calmer it goes. I'm finding I have to keep the curtains drawn to, the light makes it all worse.'

(That's a little evidence that her pain can subside a bit at least)

'Any contact with work at all?'

'I rang them and told them I'd a sick note from the Dr and they've just gone OK. I don't expect to hear from them for another week at least. Last time they just said come back when the Dr says you can and that's what I did.'

I could have asked about coping financially and benefits etc. but chose to leave it until another time. I asked all the red flag questions and there was nothing of any concern except the fact that she'd had an accident. All I knew was that the car had been shunted forward about a meter.

'Clara, tell me, after he hit you did you get out of the car and have a look at the damage?'

She had and she said there was a big dent in the back door and all the rear lights had been smashed.

'I'm only asking because I want to get some idea of the forces involved, I know it's hard to tell but what are your thoughts, did you feel a great deal of force at the time?'

It was a bit of a leading question but she said, as many do, that it happened so quickly she couldn't remember. She did say that she saw him coming and braced herself hard. I also quizzed her about the reason for the ambulance and she said that the policeman asked how she was feeling and she had said that she had a headache and her hands were feeling weird.

'He then got me into the back of the police car and called the ambulance...'

From that I'm none the wiser regarding the big question: 'Is it safe to start loading'. (Philippa has just pointed out that this sounds like I am going to going to start her off lifting weights! 'Loading' is the term I've used throughout to indicate that structurally the tissues are okay). I have to say that it probably is, but how do I know there hasn't been serious injury to the neck? Well, the red flag 'cord' type questions revealed no problems with bladder and bowel or lower limbs. The forces of the accident don't seem to have been huge. My only strategy here is to do a full neurological of lower and upper limbs to try and reassure myself and if that's OK I can at least feel comfortable to start some movements.

I now wondered if she was sleeping OK, my guess would be most probably not because of all the pain and that she was doing so little lying down through the day – what better way of disrupting sleep patterns!

'One question while it pops into my head. How have you been sleeping?'

'Terrible.'

'So not at all then for ten days?'

'Well, I get an hour or two in the day, same at night but then I wake up and get upset, then I get exhausted, then I fall asleep and so it goes on.'

'So you're sleeping all over the house, on the sofa, the bed and so forth.'

'Mostly on the sofa in front of the TV.'

'What sort of position are you in to sleep, have you noticed?'

'I've not thought about it but I often wake up on my stomach and my neck is agony.'

It seemed that she had a very long sofa and she could lie out flat on it. Hearing she could get onto her stomach to sleep meant that she must have been turning her neck a bit, possibly quite a bit. I felt a little more confident that neck and spine movements would be fine to look at.

Let's review the shopping basket so far:

1. **Biomedical:** 'Typical syndrome or common presentation?' Answer, yes, but I have no real idea of the forces suffered, there has been no scan or x-ray to check for fracture or nerve impingement in the neck and beyond hearing that they did 'reflexes' at the hospital I have no idea of her neurological status. A thorough neurological examination is a priority during the physical.

   As far as the general tissues are concerned, the concept of seeing a whiplash as 'multiple sprained ankles' in the neck is reasonable. Here at ten days assumptions about inflammation and immune activity, bleeding into muscles and joints, early stage healing processes going on etc. are quite okay. I need to answer the question 'is it safe to start loading?' and feel confident that it is likely to be. Whiplash presentations are renowned for slow and complicated recoveries mixed up with other 'complications'. The important thing here is that I'm seeing her early on and should be able to steer her back to functional recovery and return to work if I can deal with all the yellow flag issues

   Pain mechanisms – as I hope you are getting used to me now, the answer is 'all'. Because it is early there is likely to be plenty going on in the tissues that surround the 'nociceptive' mechanism; the pattern of pain and the 'numbness' in the hands needs assessing in the light of 'neurogenic' mechanisms, but only if it's going to be productive to early management goals – which it probably isn't! Thinking central maladaptive is well worth it here, remember Clara has had neck injuries before and has suffered neck pain and headaches with them. That previous pain 'cell assemblies' have been 'rekindled' is a very real possibility but there has to be care in interpretation so as not to 'belittle' the current symptom picture too much. Thinking like this is all about producing a picture of 'confidence' to start 'loading' for me and then for me to pass on to the patient.

'Output' mechanisms are to the fore and are best left to the yellow flag and physical examination in order to see the full picture. Think altered movement patterns, pain/illness behaviour, distress (which you can link to stress and autonomic activity but to me that can be left to intellectualising in that practically it's unlikely to be of much help but good to acknowledge)

So, maladaptive elements early on? Answer: YES, very likely and to me obviously!

2. **Psychosocial:** I hope you all agree that there's plenty here, even in this acute scenario. Clara could have acute low back pain and have a similar yellow flag profile. What I'm pointing out is the nonsense that sees 'yellow flags' and 'psychosocial' of only relevance to the chronic situation. The big deal is that recognising them and dealing with them confidently early on can prevent long-term pain and disability and get people back to work and normal activities. Review Steven Linton's work from chapter GE 2.4

   'A' Attitudes and Beliefs: Clara has underlying thoughts that she hasn't been properly examined – no x-ray or scan, for example and little time spent looking at her by casualty or her Dr. Her previous episode and subsequent chiropractic sessions may impact her understanding of the spine's strength and stability and should be kept in mind.

   She seems to have a very passive attitude to managing the problem – spending considerable time lying down and not moving, plus has the expectation that work/activity/physical stress will make it worse.

   She appears to believe that going back to work will only be possible once she is 100% better.

   There are hints of 'catastrophic' thinking about the future – the pain will be prolonged and may never go away.

   'B' Behaviours: she is reporting very high levels of pain and constant pain. There is also a marked spread of pain. She has adopted a very passive/do nothing/rest/avoid coping style that links to a belief that movement and physical stress will make it all worse.

   'C' Compensation issues: she has in the past and is again involved in a medico-legal claim. I haven't yet quizzed her about the financial implications of being off work again but it can easily crop up at a later time.

   'D' Diagnosis and treatment issues: she has had a torrid time with the hospital; she doesn't feel anyone, including her own Dr has been interested or thorough, she's aware of them being dismissive and not taking her seriously and she's got the typical pills and rest take time off work approach. That is understandable, because what I'm about to embark on is time consuming! If only those in charge of her management would go: 'My best advice for you is to seek care and guidance for your recovery from a skilled physiotherapist. Their goals are to help with your pain but most of all to get you going again as soon as possible. If they need any further support from medicine and what Drs have to offer they will get back to me.'

In my career I have only had one GP who was any good at this and we had a brilliant relationship to the huge benefit of patients. I fear though that our profession isn't taking on board the 'rehabilitative' approach being advocated and as a result Drs are referring to whoever is the cheapest. In this part of the UK, this seems to be to the lowest bidding 'Any Qualified Provider'. We are being usurped by therapists claiming cure whilst rehabilitation is reality. Sadly the politics and economics dictate the service.

I am very aware that from her previous 'whiplash' experience Clara has been filled with the usual chiropractic advice and diagnostic flim-flam: joints being out, pelvis, leg length etc. on the one hand and even worse on the other, the advice to stop being active and doing the things that she enjoyed and even worse again – them not reinstating these activities at some point. The yellow flag 'D' category uses terms like, 'Dramatisation of problem by Health Care Professionals leading to dependency on treatment.' She's certainly suffered from 'continued receipt of passive treatment' but also, 'Health professions sanctioning disability, not providing interventions geared towards improvement of function' – this too! Shame on them!

'E' Emotions: this is clearly obvious and a big issue in stalling rehabilitation progress. She is not only highly distressed—she's also openly admitting to feeling angry—with the driver, the hospital, her doctor, the prospect of a lengthy recovery period, her future, lack of adequate support and the pain itself. She certainly seems to have 'fear of pain with increased activity'. She is 'more irritable than usual' and there's also plenty to hint that she's 'feeling under stress and unable to maintain a sense of control' and possibly 'feeling useless and not needed' etc. It's important that the reader takes a look at and continually revises the 'key features of the 'ABCDEFW' (chapters GE 4.6 and 4.7)

'F' Family: 'lack of person to talk to about the problem' is the only issue that is obvious in this category and it is a significant one. As social animals when we are vulnerable, support is a vital part of recovery and possibly a fundamental 'need-state'.

'W' Work: clearly she has been off work for lengthy periods for her previous problems and expects the same to happen this time. So far there seems to be little interest or support from work, or any pressure to return to work. Clara clearly feels incapable of working and when you consider her current behaviour (lying down, curtains drawn, not moving etc.) – she is a million miles away from that possibility.

I hope the reader can see the importance here of 'Top down before bottom up.' I am not going to get anywhere with rehabilitation and recovery goals if we don't move forward together and deal with some of the important 'top' issues. I would also like the reader to see that simply 'explaining pain' at this early stage is probably not going to be the answer either!

On the other hand, recall the 'mother and toddler' scenario that I discussed in chapter GE 3.1 – after the mother has had a good look and reassured herself, there's the 'touchy-feely' treatment bit and then the distraction phase where the young toddler is brought out of their misery by the skills and distractions of play, movement, games, chat or whatever is needed. Could this approach apply here, rather than a complex and difficult excursion into anger, stress, tension, blame, the future and so on? The session could well be more 'top down **during** bottom up...?

3. Disability/functional restrictions. This is straight forward so far: she's stopped everything, and she's also been told to stop walking and quilting by the previous chiropractor. That's over two years of not walking for more than thirty minutes! Hmmm?

4. Impairments. The physical examination is to come but I am expecting to see huge losses of range, unwillingness to move and a great deal of tension and fear with movement. Even though she has 'numb' hands I am not expecting to find any blatant neurological deficit. Static muscle testing is likely to be hard to achieve and the possibility of a very jerky 'cog-wheel' type contraction is high. It is worth doing, to put in the shopping basket compartment as something to keep an eye on. As confident function returns I would expect smoother and more confident muscle contractions to occur.

5. General Health. This cannot be very good. She has done little since the previous accident and she admits to having put weight on.

6. Pain. Better pain control and pain management are surely high on the early agenda. The danger is of dealing solely with the pain and not working in an 'in parallel' manner, particularly alongside reactivation and normal movement. An important issue is to find out how she sees 'physiotherapy', how I might help her and what role she feels she has in her own recovery.

Interview continues...

'Clara, have you ever had physiotherapy before? The reason I'm asking is that I was wondering what you think we do and what you might be expecting from me?'

The answer was a little more elaborate than I was anticipating.

'Well I suppose with the chiro last time I was expecting something to be out and that they'd put it back. I went because all my friends at work kept ringing me saying that I must have put something out and that I should go to one, so that's what I did. This time I thought about going back but really I couldn't afford it again and I was pleased that the solicitors had organised me to see a physio.'

'That's good, so what's your notion of physio say compared to the chiropractor?'

'I don't really know but I guess we're all used to physios being involved with sport, giving exercises, putting ice packs on and doing lots of stretching, things like that.'

'So how do you feel about that sort of approach here?'

I was expecting her to say that doing exercise, or being stretched were the last things she wanted.

'The honest truth is that I'm at my wits end and don't know what to do. I'm so despondent that part of me says nothing's going to help but another part of me says I need some help. I just don't want to go through that whole scenario like last time again. I'm happy to try anything I guess. The big thing right now is that I couldn't cope with it being made any worse than it already is.'

'That's really good I was half expecting you to say 'don't ask me to move' or 'don't even think about touching me!''

For the first time she looked up at me and smiled, it was almost a 'just look after me' smile. But note 'just help me' happens when you are in a mess.

But I didn't want that here, I didn't really want passivity but I could understand it because she was in an emotionally desperate place.

The physical examination

'Clara, the most important thing for me to find out about is what we call your neurological status! That's a big word for saying, I need to know if your nervous system is OK and that is surprisingly easy to check, are you happy if I explain as I go?'

'Yes I am but are you thinking I could have damaged my spine nerves?'

'Well, I'm actually going to check because it's a very important question but I very much doubt you have. I see a great many patients like you and because your spine cord goes down through your neck we always do some important checks to see if it is OK. I'll do the tests and I'll tell you about what I find and what it means. Ask any questions anytime, I mean it.'

So, a bit more was to be done than the 'reflexes' that were tested but not explained in casualty.

See all that follows as part of a good neurological examination and reasoning task:

- getting out of the chair, she did this with tension but easily

- walking, she was very tense and stooped but her balance was fine and she turned both ways in the cubicle fine

- walking on tip toes is more of a co-ordination and balance challenge – which she said hurt, but she could do it, her calf muscles and quads must be fine – she could walk backwards fine given consideration for her 'pain' state

- I got her to stand with one hand on the wall for balance and then go onto one leg then the other and then take her hand away from the wall while on the one leg – this was OK, but typical of someone in high distress and a lot of pain

- she could walk forwards and back three paces with eyes closed (proprioception of lower limb fine- confirmed by this and all the above too)

- sitting on the plinth with legs dangling I did:

  - quads and calf reflexes–brisk and normal
  - clonus–negative
  - slowly built up static contraction – expecting the possibility of 'cog-wheel' but didn't get, all fine and I did all hip, knee and foot muscles that I could possibly do sitting
  - sensation to light touch was fine
  - vibration sense was fine too.

- she was clearly hugely protective and tense about moving her neck, shoulders, arms and the whole upper quadrant on both sides, so for the upper limb neurological I veered towards simple reflexes, sensation especially focused on the hands and a tentative attempt at some static tests

- I continued with her sitting and did the triceps and biceps reflexes which were fine (it's worth practicing doing these reflexes sitting; here, for relaxation I supported her arm on four pillows!)

- she wasn't at all keen for me to touch her over the shoulders or the upper arms, so I got her to test herself, 'Just like I did with your legs, I touched you and you thought about whether or not you could feel it normally – if you can do that gently over your shoulders and your upper arms that'd be great...' She said the sensation was really prickly and sore but was definitely not 'dead' in the way the skin goes at the dentist when you have an injection

  (By the way, this is a good way of getting the patient to give you a more 'gross' picture of any sensory loss – to ask them to recall the numbness from the dentist and see if they have anything like that when you touch them. This filters out all the pedantic 'might be a bit weird or a bit dull' stuff from anything really significant. I'm not saying don't get that stuff but quite usually it is far more a result of processing changes due to pain and disuse than any frank loss due to neuropathy. Don't forget to think in nerve innervation fields as well as dermatomes for sensory loss)

- her hands looked quite normal, she couldn't be precise about the numbness, she said it was vague and felt weird

'How was this numbness compared to the numb feeling you get from the dentist's injection?' I asked. 'It's not like that, it's like my hands don't quite feel like they belong to me, they feel distant.'

I then said I'd do the standard sensation testing:

I simultaneously stroked the skin of both forearms and got her to compare, then slowly worked down onto the back of both hands all the time asking her to compare and give me any comment. She said very little and after I covered her palms she went: 'It feels quite normal there.'

Pin-prick was normally sharp on the base of the finger nails and over the creases of the PIP and DIP joints. However tuning fork vibration testing, she said was dulled over the knuckles compared to the elbow and radial styloid processes.

I could only conclude that some loss of fine sensory acuity had occurred. That went in the impairment shopping basket compartment to be re-evaluated from time to time.

To save space I haven't included all the dialogue but as I went along with all the above tests I gave a simple explanation and reassured her that the tests were good. I summarised at the end and made the following points:

'Right, if the spinal cord is damaged in some way that would have been easy to pick up with all the standing and leg testing, but even though you're struggling to do some of the tests because of the pain you actually passed all the cord tests with flying colours.'

'In your arms the only small thing is the loss of vibration sense and the numby feelings in your hands, but this is quite common after whiplash, just like neck pain and those strange eye to back of head headaches are too. I'm going to keep checking on them and if anything's worrying I'll get you checked further.'

My experience here is that as you get going and move the neck and arms a bit more those feelings improve and the loss of vibration comes back to normal.'

I used the arms going to sleep when the circulation gets cut-off example and pointed out that lack of movement often slows the circulation causing odd feelings. I mentioned sitting on aircraft for long journeys and that in some people their feet became swollen, went numb, got pins and needles and so forth.

I paused. She'd been listening well for those few minutes.

'How are you doing so far? Is what I'm doing making sense?'

I paused again and she gave me eye contact.

'You can say what the hell you like here; I know you're going through 'crap'.'

She burst into tears again and I handed the box of tissues to her and she managed a little laugh through it all.

'I was thinking that you might be getting fed up with me being like this. I was determined to be level headed when I came but I just couldn't help it, I welled up in the waiting room and then the floods came.'

'I don't mind you being like this at all, we see patients who have been through the most awful things, some who you wouldn't expect to break down but do, it's normal – we think it's normal and we encourage our patients to see it as normal too. We wouldn't be human if we didn't get upset when something horrid happens.'

She smiled and settled.

'Do you want to stop at this point? Go home, take a break and come back tomorrow fresh?'

'I think that would be a good idea, I feel exhausted.'

'Good, come back tomorrow and come at the end of my list and I'll have plenty of time with you. If you think of something you want to tell me, if you've any worries about anything ask me and we'll go through it all.' I paused. 'I'll tell you what I'm thinking. Two things, first, the human body has an incredible ability to recover, it wants to recover and it recovers best when the pressure is off. In the late 1800's and early 1900's rich folk who were ill used to get sent to mountain retreats in places like Switzerland, all the pressures of the world were taken away so that their bodies could focus all their resources and energy on recovery and rehabilitation. The focus was on good diet, appropriate rest and good quality exercise in the fresh air, sunshine and beautiful surroundings. The second thing is that I think you have an excellent chance of recovering faster and better than last time, we've just got to work together to help you create the best conditions for that to happen, a key is that we've got to give your bodies recovery systems and your resources a chance to work at their best and right now they're not focused on it because you're so upset. The key to you feeling better about it all is to get a bit of progress and I'm hoping we can make a good start tomorrow, we'll see how we go.

She nodded, snivelling a little less and I got the classic response that sometimes pisses you off but in actual fact is quite normal!

'So you think you can fix me?'

What I've just said to her is typical of the therapist thinking 'This little nugget of information will calm her down and she'll come back tomorrow all chilled and feeling more positive,' but unfortunately it doesn't always work like that and the patient in their desperation and rigid way of thinking loses the flow of your logic and entirely misses what you were getting at. They probably think you were 'rabbiting[1]- on a bit'. Yes, you were and I was too!

So, I respond back.

'There's plenty for us to do, I'm looking forward to seeing you tomorrow.

Make it easy – day 2

The initial pleasantries over, I asked Clara:

'Any more thoughts about anything from yesterday or anything from anywhere?'

'It was all a bit of a haze to be honest with you, I was wound up coming here and meeting you wasn't easy and I'd got wound-up and frightened that I'd just be dismissed and told that I was making a fuss over nothing – I had the most horrendous headache and ended up taking the codeine the Dr had prescribed for me. I was pleased I was in bed when I took it because it knocked me right out. That was about eight pm last night and I didn't wake until about eleven am. I'm a bit clearer headed now than I was yesterday thank goodness.'

I decided to get straight on with what I like to call the 'make it easy' approach when dealing with limited and tense movement. It would be good if the reader could go back and take a peek at figure GE 2.7 – Main, Spanswick and Watson's disability model ('MSW model' from now on). The important thing is that pain leads to 'guarded movement and muscle spasm' and vice versa. I prefer the term 'guarded movement' or simply, 'increased tone or tension' rather than 'spasm' during movement because it's a much better reflection of the usual state of affairs with the patient. Any patient who moves slowly and cautiously you could categorise here as having 'increased tone' –there's a constant state of readiness in the 'stop' muscles.

The big thing here is to think at multiple levels, for example, you can think 'nociception' driving pain mechanisms into the cord and reflex tonal increases to protect the structures that have been damaged, are inflamed and are healing. But you can also think that tension is in large part driven by 'top-down' processes related to fear or pain and unwillingness to move or unwillingness to enter the world where

---

1 - *'Rabbiting on' means non-stop talk – it comes from Cockney rhyming slang 'Rabbit and Pork' = talk, hence rabbiting is talking!*

more 'hurt' is a possibility. Recall too that high levels of distress correlate with high levels of pain behaviour. Not moving the neck, head or arms are therefore a form of pain behaviour, they 'show the outside world' that this person has a problem – just like the scarf she rather obviously has round her neck. The 'props of illness' and expressions of a vulnerability state are in evidence. So it would be good to also take a peek at the Vulnerable Organism figure – GE 2.3 for example but also the fear-avoidance model too, figures GE 2.5 and 2.6. They all fit here.

I got Clara to stand; no undressing required here, she's uncomfortable enough with her clothes on, let alone standing in her underwear in front of me. I didn't ask about her headaches, her neck pain or her hands – why up-regulate even further an already up-regulated pain system? My intention was to observe some basic movements and some functional activities, also to see if any opportunity to improve them arose. It may be that I would have to leave it alone.

Think like you would a day one hip replacement patient who you're about to stand and walk for the first time. You don't ask about pain, you just get on and see what they can do. And day one hip replacement has a mass of nociception going on – thanks to the leg being half cut off, chunks of bone removed and new bits of metal being glued and screwed. Go back to the section 2 case history if you like – 'Mary, Sue then me'.

We stood facing and I said, 'I'll do a movement and then you show me what you're happy to do. Before I do, the rules are do what you feel you want to, it's up to you.'

I then put my head down flexing my neck and she managed to lower her chin about an inch. I looked up – her head jerked about half an inch and she screwed her face up. I then turned very slowly about half way left and right. Again, her attempts at mirroring my movement were very jerky; her eyes and forehead showed plenty of tension, she barely moved the neck, the shoulders simultaneously followed to compensate. I slowly shrugged both then one shoulder then the other –same again from Clara, tight and tense. Two ways to go now: first could be, come back to the neck and shoulder movements; second would be to have a look at more functional things like sit to stand, walking or step-ups. I opted for the neck and shoulder again.

I got out what I call my 'shoulder pulley' – it's a simple pulley with two handles tied to the ends of a rope that passes through the pulley. It's the good old fashioned 'frozen shoulder' exerciser with a neat modern addition to make it easy to take home and set up. The pulley has a 'door-jamming' rubber attached to it so you can fix it in a closed door and use it from any height you like. I jammed it in the door at about her head height, held the handles and then stepped back until the tension had been taken up and the relaxed arms were being held in about 20-30 degrees into flexion; I then started pulling the handles, one reciprocating the other, one down aiding the other up.

Clara had a go and although tense managed to pull the arm up into about 90 degrees of flexion.

'That's good – you're looking a bit more relaxed.'

'Am I? Oh, I've never done this sort of thing before, it feels a bit weird.'

I stood next to her mimicking her movements and timbre

'Slooow and heavvvvvvy... as you go... light and easy...' At the same time I slumped and went floppy in the shoulders and head... repeating the words in time with the movement. (If you're aware of it I'm thinking 'mirror neurones' –t he motor neurones and pathways that fire in the brain when you're watching someone and thinking about it, or trying to learn what they are doing. Remember, movement inhibits pain and novel and thoughtless functional movement does especially well). (Figure 5.2 from the chapter on central mechanisms showing the 'inhibiting' branch from descending motor fibres to the dorsal horn may be a reminder!)

After about ten improving slow, but reasonably relaxed repetitions we stopped and I opened the door and shifted the pulley about a foot higher.

'Do you want to have another go?'

I caught her eyes and she could see I was pleased.

'Don't forget, you can say what you like here.'

She didn't say anything she slowly went about trying again though it wasn't so good.

'Try walking on the spot before you start.' I suggested.

After about four or five steps – again, I'm mimicking her timing and pace – I now start moving my arms and beckon her to join it. Soon we're repeating together: 1-2-3-4 up... 1-2-3-4 down as we count the walks on the spot and time the up and down. That produces a better result.

We're keeping going...

'I'm really happy with the way you are moving now.' I say.

Then at last, she says something (note I'm not prompting her by going how's that, are you alright, do what you can, if you don't like it you can stop...? Just try shutting up and letting the brain do its movement thing, try not to interfere with a bit of normal processing and screw it up by bringing thoughts about 'what I might be feeling' into the equation. Therapist shut-up, gob closed, watch and reinforce a little, let the patient find out and work out for themselves what it's like!)

She says:

'This is nuts compared to the chiropractor sessions, in fact it's nuts compared to anything.'

I smile and she lets out an interesting kind of sigh which is more 'let-go' than 'tense-up' in my reading of it!

'Let's try something different, let those go and come and stand again.'

(Tip: don't be tempted to re-test those 'standard test' movements, they will just reinforce tension. Just don't! Forget them – they're not for normal life.)

She stands facing me and I move to just less than an arms width apart.

'I'm the thing in the mirror you try and copy.'

She's getting to know that when I do something in front or to the side she has to have a go at mirroring what I do.

I take my left hand and move it across in front of me to touch her left elbow. I keep my head up looking at her with a slight encouraging smile. She repeats back to me, we swap arms, we go higher up, touching mid upper arm and after a few more repetitions, up to each others' opposite shoulders. I then step back a pace so the reach is a bit further.

This is going well, reaching across brings the shoulder girdle and whole trunk into rotation, the head staying still means that the neck is rotating under the still skull, but it doesn't feel like it. It tricks the processing with some patients and with Clara it was working well. Her neck was rotating with ease probably into about half to two thirds range.

We were now patting each others' flat hands in front of us – two together, left to left and right to right, repeat, just as if we were in the playground at infant school.

I told you this was like mothers and toddlers!

Although we are saying little we're getting on with it and getting on with each other too. Clara is in her own little world and I'm sure will astonish me with some comment at some point. My aim is to get her to the stage of having a little homework and making some choices over what she wants to do.

The next couple of things are my favourites for this sort of tense immovable type neck. The first is called 'hunting and stalking'– a term and way of doing it for the blokes and for the ladies it's 'window shopping!' Sorry, but you'll see why and maybe excuse me.

'I'm going to demonstrate what I call 'window shopping' and if you don't get on with that we'll try 'hunting and stalking.' I'm smiling; she's smiling and shaking her head! You'd be very tempted to ask her what she was thinking right now, but I daren't! What's the point.   I'll discuss things at the end very soon. I wanted to keep the novelty of 'what's he going to do with me next' thing rolling. I hope the reader can see that this stuff can easily be toned down to be not so 'mad' for the more serious patient.

I started: 'You know when sometimes you're walking down the street and something in a shop window catches your eye... you carry on walking but all the while your gaze and attention stay on the object in the window. It may only happen for a few moments, but we all do this all the time; I walk along the cliff path here and gaze out to the ships in the bay. I keep walking but my attention remains on the boat or the view, whatever.'

She nods.

'Imagine my windows here are like a shop window, we can see just outside a myrtle tree and I think it has quite interesting bark on it.'

I'm now wandering up and down the room with my gaze fixed on the myrtle tree outside. As I walk and turn to go up and down in the room my head remains locked in to the direction of the tree while my body underneath does it's thing. There's considerable neck movement to accommodate what is going on, but it's all from the trunk upwards rather than from the head downwards. Think about the standard way we examine a neck; it's head turning on a fixed trunk, when probably our most frequent neck movements are done the other way, fixed head and moving trunk and thoughtlessly! For day to day head turning on fixed trunk think sitting down and someone comes in the room behind you, or all the right and left checking you have to do when you're driving.

When I was teaching the Graded Exposure course I used to get the participants to be involved here. You try it if you like?

Stay sitting and just slowly turn your head left then back then right and just take in what you feel. I get a clear upper cervical awareness and then soon quite a bit of neck muscle tight-awareness at towards the end of range jointy feelings throughout. I then got the audience to stand, and keeping their heads still, to rotate their trunks with floppy arms – the sort of exercise we give patients and the ones that some golfers like to do on the first tee. But note what you feel doing this – for most it's thoracic, lumbar tight waist feelings, hips, awareness of knees and legs being twisted and so forth. Most folk are totally unaware of what their neck is doing – yet, if you're twisting well it's going near full range. The great thing about this simple exercise is that all the sensations from the body tend to 'modulate out – or 'gate-out' those from the neck. When I realised this long ago, I then thought about common daily movements in comparison to 'standard examination' type movements and found I could virtually change the lot. I suggest you do too it can be hugely helpful with the type of situation I'm describing here with Clara. Just take a standard movement and see if you can do it in another way so the 'processing' of it is completely changed. This is exactly what happened when I found I could flex my painful shoulder by bending forward and dangling my arm (see chapter GE 1.1).

With 'hunting and stalking' you pretend to be an African bushman with a spear. You're in the high grass stalking an antelope and you're crouching, your eyes and attention are transfixed as you slowly move to a good position to throw the spear... your head stays still your body moves in all directions.

Back to Clara...

'All you have to do is lock into something with your eyes and start moving around. On the end-wall over here is my chart of Falmouth harbour; just here on the left is where the Pandora Inn is, I expect you know it, you can see it's right on Restronguet creek just here.'

She's looking at the Pandora Inn spot on the chart now.

'So what you can try is keeping your gaze on the pub spot and from where you are simply walk towards it but come in a bit of a zig-zag.'

Just then she rolled her eyes up spontaneously to show that I was nuts. Yes, but when you roll your eyes up at someone your head goes up spontaneously and that's what happened. I said nothing, just carried on encouraging her to see how she got on.

The width of the treatment room was enough for about eight paces or so and she started her zig-zag. Sometimes it works and sometimes it doesn't – but the key is never to say anything about keeping the head still while the trunk moves around underneath. When I ask the class of physio participants to stand and keep their heads still and twist their trunk – a surprisingly large number of them just cannot do it! But if I say do 'The Twist' everybody – they can all do it fine.

It's tricking processing, tricking pain and it can be very good sometimes!

Clara zig-zagged well and as she turned I got her to concentrate on some words on my whiteboard at the other end of the room. I encouraged her to try increasing the zig-zag excursion and again she coped fine. We 'started easy' and 'built slowly'. I hope you can see why I call it 'make it easy' – I could also add 'make it thoughtless'.

She tried looking at the myrtle tree for a few laps and was notably tense as she went passed it, she had to turn her trunk, but that was fine, this was a good start. I was also interested in seeing if I could get any spontaneous extension and 'hunting and stalking' sometimes helps here. With 'hunting and stalking' there's a bit of bent knees slightly bent forward posture – a keep-low-keep-your-head-down posture with slow soft and deliberate steps; all the while keeping the gaze fixed on something in the distance, which brings the head up nicely into some extension. It's like riding a bike with forward or drop-handlebars. Just as I was about to start, something made me want to try a different way, she had a slight look of tiredness or maybe slight confusion.

'Let's sit for a minute. Are you OK, or am I totally bonkers?' I felt it was time to ask before doing anything more.

'You're getting me to move that's for sure and you're bonkers!'

'Spot on! The next thing is agreeing some practice for home to back this up.' I said.

'You can do some of the things we've been doing here at home. I'll show you in a minute and I'll write some things down. I could do just a couple more things and you can choose them as well, if you want?'

She nodded and agreed to see what more there might be, which was a little surprising but very encouraging.

'OK, the big thing I want you to take away from this session is the need to be really floppy and relaxed with movement; to me, watching you move you seem to be very good at it, you've actually been a nice surprise, I've got a lot further than I thought I would.'

She nodded (a spontaneous neck nod, great!). I was sitting facing her.

'More of the 'see me in the mirror' and 'have a go at what I do stuff' now.. '

I sat a little more upright in better posture and she followed.

'Watch what I do first; then try it.'

I then slumped down and went forward to rest my elbows on my thighs just above my knees; I was looking at the floor and then slowly lifted my head to look at her.

'Try it'

Down she went and up came her head a little way. I could see her eyes screw up as she stopped. It was when her upper cervical region started to extend.

'Try again but slump forward to about half way, think floppy everywhere...'

This time she went forward with less tension across her shoulders, at half way she stopped and lifted her head much better. It was slow and smooth. I encouraged her to keep in a comfortable range and keep it slow and smooth and she went from floppy flexion to about mid extension.

Again, in the Graded Exposure class I got the participants to sit bolt upright and focus on their necks while extending to end range. 'Note what you feel and remember it,' I'd say.

Then I'd get them to do what Clara tried – extending from a forward lean position, 'Note what you feel and compare,' was the directive. Most found the lean forward extension far nicer than the upright for obvious reasons. A key point to make though is that there's always some wise-ass in the audience who prefers it the other way, the way you'd least expect! This also happens with patients and the rule is (thinking 'fire-apart depart' and relaxed floppy movement/low tension) use the starting position and movement that the patient prefers, the one that gets the biggest, easiest, most relaxed and best quality; teach the patient that they can try and they can swap if it changes. The patients learn the basic technique, they learn that they can adjust it, do less, go slower, be more relaxed, go faster even – if it all results in *easy movement and mastery*!

Clara came back up.

'I think you're clever' she said.

I shrugged and look slightly quizzically at her.

'I mean I've just realised I'm moving my neck quite well and by really letting go it feels weirdly nice. I don't think I've actually let it go like this since the last accident if I'm honest.'

There was a pause and she sighed.

'My worry is that OK I'm moving it but what's going to happen later. I kind of know it's going to get awful anytime soon and I'm dreading it.'

'I appreciate that completely but one question, what are your thoughts about moving it even though you fear it might be more painful later?'

'It's like I said to you yesterday, I trust you to help me – I have to.'

'Good, so we maybe need to think about a strategy for dealing with it worsening later. Is it worth making a list? Let's get something down on paper to think about.'

We sit together and I ask her for ideas.

'Well, I could knock myself out with the codeine again.'

'Yup! Anything else you can connect with feeling better?'

'Resting and closing all the curtains...' She looks despondent but I nod in agreement.

She's stuck and there's an awkward resigned sort of pause.

'I'm going to see if I can help by looking at in another way.'

I take another piece of paper and write the words, 'Everyday headache' in the middle and circle it,

'I want to make a list of things that make, or bring on a headache, not the one you've had since the accident but a normal one that we all get from time to time.'

I'm doing a 'star chart' and she starts with a few examples from her own experience...

'Tiredness'

'Stress, when I get wound-up'

'When I don't sleep'

'After a lot of TV, sort of doing nothing for hours sometimes'

'When I get my periods'

'Eat too much and always if I drink spirits, like Vodka'

'When I've got flu'

'Sometimes when I go without food, like missing lunch'

'Driving and concentrating for a long time, like computers'

'After a scary movie'

'I used to get them before an exam.'

They all go down on the chart with arrows to the triggers she comes up with.

'That's good, right we're now going to look at more or less the opposite... '

I take another piece of paper and write in the middle, 'When I feel clear headed and at my best'.

'That's easy, when I'm...

'Relaxed'

'Happy'

'With friends'

'After walks on the weekends, well when I used to do them...'

'When I'm sleeping well'

'When things are going well, no hassles, works good, the pressures just right...'

'When I eat a drink sensibly'

'It's basically when I'm fit, well and relaxed.'

Good, one more piece of paper and this time it's 'What might make a headache better.'

'Good night's rest'

'Drinking water'

'Relaxing!'

She's smiling now and I know she can see what I'm getting at.

'Go on,' I urge her.

'Right, er, aspirin and codeine!'

'Maybe even exercise and fresh air?'

'Relaxation, get rid of any stress if you can.'

'Avoid over-eating and maybe alcohol, eat and drink good stuff...'

I'm nodding, she can see where I was coming from and she also generated many of the answers herself.

'Right two things – when you came yesterday you told me you were tense and wound-up, you obviously were and that later, after seeing me, it was really bad and you had to take the tablets.'

'That's right.'

'So comparing how you felt yesterday to today in terms of those things, what's the situation now?'

'Right, today I came in feeling far less tense. I'd had a good night's sleep and I guess I knew you and I felt comfortable, like I knew you were OK and I knew you weren't going to be horrid or anything! The neck pain was really bothering me, it was horridly stiff and my arms felt like lead and my hands were numb.'

She stopped and looked up in surprise.

'They feel normal now.'

It was almost like she hadn't noticed, except for her statement earlier than her neck felt relaxed and it was weird, but now she thought about her hands and arms she suddenly realised they were feeling normal. It had dawned on her at last that it was the movement, the relaxed easy movement that had helped.'

 'Right, you've just found out what my second thing was – yes, movement if it's done nicely seems to help, it does right now and you're going to find out later what happens, you may even think about using some movement if it tightens up again and gets stiff, or even if the headache comes again.'

She agrees and also points out that if it comes to the worst she can always take the tablets.

'Now, of all the movements we've done, do you want to try them all or do you want to pick out a few to do at home. I can lend you the pulley.'

'I'd like to try them all then I can see for myself.'

'OK, that's great, I've got one more thing to suggest and I want your opinion on it and that's how do you feel about starting doing some easy walking again?'

'I'd love to walk again but I'm fearful from what the chiropractor said before.'

'Well, I think you're quite OK to be getting slowly fit again, especially if we start off really easy and slowly build up. I think eventually your back will feel much better for it. More of that next time.'

So here's a brief review of her homework (all jotted on a piece of paper for her reference):

- make it easy principle – start-easy build-slowly, nice, easy, relaxed, floppy movement...

- 'succeed not fail' – if you go nuts and do too much and then suffer, you'll be upset and won't feel like doing it again – start easy!

- pulley exercises – find the height that's nice, you found ten or so fairly easy, keep that your maximum for the first day or two, then you can slowly start building

- see if you can do it 4-5 times a day to start, if they help you relax when uncomfortable, fine, do them, try and see – our goal is little and often

- you can do the touch hands thing I did with you against a wall, stepping back makes it a bit harder

- 'window shopping' – the zig-zag and hunter-stalking

- sitting slump and head up and down, slow smooth and floppy is key

- walking programme (this is what she agreed to start with – 5 to 10 minutes twice a day) pace that's easy and comfortable – goal is 15 minutes twice a day in one week

- regular move and rest rather than prolonged one position

- don't worry if the neck goes stiff, that's normal

- if it flares up, tablets are fine for now, but get comfy in bed not awkward on the sofa

- do anything that helps you relax rather than get wound-up

- come back in a week but phone anytime if concerned.

A comment about 'Physiotools' or other standard software exercise print outs. We don't work in the NHS and therefore don't have to have standard print outs. We find this quite liberating! Our patients' exercises and instructions are drawn and written, with the patient often doing them and adding bits – they are unique to each patient. We have seen many patients, who have seen other physios and the patient says 'We just got handed a sheet of exercises' and in their eyes they are meaningless...!

Early activation was key to get Clara to process her problem differently and quickly. Also, her high pain levels were helped by tablets and Clara was starting to get some control. I felt that discussion of other modalities such as heat, relaxation techniques etc. would have been too much to take in after only two sessions.

Unfortunately Louis did not write anymore about Clara. Hopefully the reader can take a lot of information from the first two sessions and apply the shopping basket approach through future management?

1211

Chapter CH 1.3
Chris: 'tricking pain' or maybe 'pick-pocketing' pain in a twelve year old!

Managing patients with pain is sometimes a rather unnerving balance between hard medicine and the need of some 'evidence base' derived attitudes – what I sometimes think of as the 'automaton' approach – and the complexity of the human with the pain and their often incredible pain behaviour. This is what makes something relatively straightforward quite mystical and confusing. The 'automaton' approach is obviously robotic: 'You-have-simple-back-pain-here-is-a-pill-and-a-booklet-that-explains-it-all-and-my-pathetic-handout-that's-been-sanctioned-by-the-health-authority-and-is-supported-by-the-latest-research... etc.' (Read in a monotone voice!)

One rather crude key is to 'see-through' the sometimes amazing pain related 'antics' that pain brings on and simply get a good answer to the question: 'Is it safe to start 'loading' and get going?' and if it is, to get on with doing just that, often using 'antics' of your own. That's what this next case history is all about – it's about humour, tricking, teasing, playing, having fun, cajoling, communicating and being human with another human. Before starting I am reminded of my father treating me once when I was a youngster; I had the most terrible chest infection, I can recall that awful time when you struggle for every breath. I was highly distressed. The 'right' thing to do might have been to call the Dr. It was the sort of situation that ends up being taken to hospital, given various bronchodilators and put on a nebulizer. What did my Dad do? He tickled the living daylights out of me; I laughed and coughed and coughed and laughed and he didn't let up until I was exhausted – exhausted and clear! He knew that I had to get my lungs clear and he also knew that the easiest way to get that was to make me breathe one hell of a lot more and deeper than I was willing to or could in my distress. That was a never to be forgotten moment!

The following is about a young lad called Chris, who could easily have developed into a disastrous 'complex regional pain' state, or long term problem. Well it could look like that. On the other hand in the hands of experience where logic, listening and watching tells the clinician that the tissues are safe to start loading, it makes for a different sort of challenge. This I hope is an example of the 'art', 'humour', 'cajoling' and 'distracting' that is sometimes required in clinical practice. It's an example of the skills no triple A stars at A level or distinction and degree level can give the budding young physiotherapist. I think it's an example of what Daniel Goleman[1] calls 'emotional intelligence' – the skilled knowing interaction of two human beings. Some of us are good at it and it's natural to us, others can learn to be better and some I'm afraid will never get it. My mother always used to say that it was sad how the physiotherapy profession was demanding higher and higher grades and academic qualifications to be able to train. She believed, as I do that the price was the loss of those who were less academic but far better at being human humans – those naturally skilled in communication, in making people feel at ease and in getting along with people. The term people-people sums it up or 'people-skills' – but it is also 'emotional intelligence' too.

The goal is, as it always should be – the ultimate return to function, via good old fashioned rehabilitation using every trick in the book.

---

1 - Goleman, D (1996) Emotional Intelligence. London, Bloomsbury

I think I learnt, or absorbed most of what follows from what I call 'older generation' physios like my Mum and Dad. They had little fear of structure, they were not constrained by any dogmatic 'manual therapy' system or treatment 'approach' and they almost majestically – but in some eyes naively, looked at the patient and went 'Come on, you should be able to move, let's see what you can do.'

I have to say that often on my courses, a great many more 'mature' physio's used to sidle up to me and say, 'Do you know Louis, I'm so relieved to hear what you're saying. For years I've felt so hopeless in the presence of these young 'Maitland' and what-not physios with all their complicated and fancy techniques. I've just stayed in the background and just got the patient going like you've been saying. They all think I'm useless. So thanks, you've made me feel so much better, what a breath of fresh-air!'

Chris.

(Occasional extra 'thoughts' of mine are in italic so as not to spoil the flow)

In comes Chris, a 'young' looking 13 year old, two crutches, right foot dangling in mid air – plus Dad and his girl friend, Dawn. We do the pleasantries.

'What's happened then?'

Chris sits and looks sheepish. Dawn looks on with a nervy nod of encouragement to me. I try to let the air settle with a smile.

Dad answers...

'...and he's just got into the rugby team at school,'

... were almost Dad's first words and he had a deeply serious look – like his son was either a huge problem or was a pain in the ass to his new relationship! I hadn't quite worked the relationships out at that point? Dawn at least had a nervous smile. Chris looked a bit scared.

Dad sighed 'Friday at school, he fell down the stairs and landed on the side of his right knee, he immediately couldn't take weight on it. I got a call at work to come in to school and we took him straight to the local hospital. We then had to go to the main hospital for an x-ray. No fractures, no swelling, no bruising but loads of pain – he hasn't been able to take weight on it or move it for what, six days now. They gave him the crutches at the hospital.'

(So no reason why the leg shouldn't move or weight-bear – in fact it should and could safely, if the pain would let it)

'No movement at all?' I question.

'No, he can't bend it or straighten it and he won't even touch it to the ground like they told him to at the hospital.'

'Where's it hurt then?'

Chris now pipes up and my attention moves to him, eyebrows raised, I'm now interested.

'Over here' – he indicates the lateral side of his right knee, 'and it's weird down here', he points to his ankle and the lateral side of his lower leg.

'Weird?'

'Yes, it's like thick pins and needles feeling but it hurts and it spreads from my ankle bone up to my knee.'

'What's the knee pain feel like then?'

'It's stabbing, it really hurts.'

'All the time?'

'Oh no, only when I move it or try to put it on the ground.'

'Got you, so, are you sleeping OK?'

'Not really, it wakes me every time I move.'

'Right, so just to check – are you aware of it at all when you're not moving it?'

'No, it's fine then.'

We carry on; he's never had a knee problem before; he's normally fit and active, cycles and doesn't like school! He's not on any tablets but he's seen his Dr, after the x-ray at the hospital, who told him to take anti-inflammatories and see how it goes for a week but to move it if he could. This was in contrast to the hospital who had, surprisingly for round here, told him to see a physio as soon as possible. No one had given any kind of diagnosis, except bruised knee.

So here we all are, slightly tense atmosphere, a slight feeling of no hope perhaps and me looking at this young lad who's not really athletic but is, to Dad's relief, starting to get into something physical and get off the Play Station fixation/screen addiction thing.

I keep looking pleasant and positive.

'I'd like to watch you walking again with the crutches Chris,' I say.

He wiggles about, manipulates the crutches and goes up and down the room happily enough.

'Can you even touch the ground with your tip toes?' I ask.

'It hurts too much...'

'Show me what you can do.'

He walks again without touching the floor...

'Right, up on the couch, legs dangling and let's have a look.'

Up he got, sitting there with the bad leg stuck out at 45 degrees to horizontal, all tense all present and all presenting!

(The knee has no bruising or swelling and looks quite normal – the only thing is that it has a very slight skin blotchy look that comes with lack of use. Think of 'just-out-of-plaster' type skin but not anything like as bad.)

'Show me what movement you can do.'

He moved it about 20 degrees into flexion and then back to the 45 degree position. He winced and tensed a lot.

'Can I touch it?'

'Not there, there, or there.' He pointed to the lateral knee, the knee-cap, the lateral lower leg.   I put my hands around his posterior mid-calf area.

'How am I doing Chris? I'll move around and you tell me.'

I move my hands up his leg and he immediately pushes me away.

'What was that? I say with concern.

'It's too painful.'

'Give me a number from one to 10 for how painful it is?

I'm only gently moving across the skin with the lightest of touches.

'7 out of 10.'

'That's a fair bit!' I'm smiling at him careful to not be disparaging.

I turn to the adults.

'Well, this is 'supersensitive!'

I turn back to Chris...

'In physio and pain science we've got a couple of big weird words for this, 'allodynia and hyperalgesia.'

I'm quietly rubbing his leg a bit more and he's concentrating on me. I keep rubbing.

I turn to Dawn and Dad, taking Chris' attention with me...

'Have you ever met anyone who's had Shingles?'

Dawn has and she nods but she's laughing, Chris picks it up.

(She can see my hands have moved up around his knee a bit more and that he's not noticed and isn't pushing me away or wincing)

'What's so funny?' Chris frowns.

(I can now see he's not very warm towards Dawn)

I answer as Dawn tries to resume a serious face, Dad sits looking puzzled for some reason.

I turn to Chris, 'I think she's happy with the way this is all going and that we're having a bit of fun –even though it's painful, or maybe she's remembered something about shingles, we'll probably find out in a minute,' I quiz.

I thought I'd bring him in on what was happening.

'Hey, the trickery of distraction Chris – go on keep talking, we're getting to know your knee a bit now.' I'm now rubbing away and all around and I'm also rubbing both knees at the same time.

He then pushes my hand away... *(Oops, maybe shouldn't have done that, stop here. I've lost this for now, quick, do something else...)*

'Let your leg dangle now, really let it go and relax.'

I'm holding his foot and gently wafting it 20 or so degrees from dangle position into flexion and then back into a bit of extension – he's letting go and then resisting, letting go, then resisting.

'Deep breath in, hold your breath, blow me away, no spitting.'

We're now blowing at each other as hard as we can. He's relaxed and laughing. Dawn is smiling. Dad's still looking confused and concerned. I'm wafting the knee at least double the amount.

I keep moving his knee, then a few jokes:

> My daughter asked me for a pet spider for her birthday, so I went to our local pet shop and they were £70! Blow this, I thought, I can get one cheaper off the web.

> I was at a cash machine yesterday when a little old lady asked if I could

check her balance, so I pushed her over.

I was driving this morning when I saw a parked AA van.
The driver was crying uncontrollably and looked very miserable. I thought to myself, that guy's heading for a breakdown.

Chris, me and Dawn are laughing away, Dad's still dead-pan.

All the while I continue to 'pick-pocket' his leg (move it without him noticing!)

Dawn is muttering 'amazing' and smiling carefully now.

(I now have this little fear that they're embarrassed and thinking it's all in his head, Dad might even be getting annoyed. I need to give the pain some credibility.)

We're still laughing and holding our breaths and I'm wafting the leg about 40 to 50 degrees quite well and I've got the other leg going in rhythm with it... kick-kick-kick. I stop.

'Time to do some testing now Chris, I want you to tell me whether you can feel me normally when I touch you lightly.'

I gently brush my hand up and down the lateral and medial sides of his good left leg. (It's nearly always best to do good leg first when there's hypersensitivity – so they know what's coming)

'Is that OK?

'Yes, tickles a bit.'

'Compare that to this.'

I then go over to the bad right leg – up and down on the medial side of the lower leg (that's an area of no pain report).

'How's that?'

'OK'

'This?' I go up and down on the lateral side – up and down where he reported it as hypersensitive about five minutes ago.

'I can feel that, but not here' – he indicates a patch over the mid lateral peroneal area about jam-jar lid size.

I look round at Dad and Dawn with my 'sensible' mode switched on.

'There's maybe a 'nervy' element to this, which would make it make sense – you know I mentioned Shingles just now, it's when a nerve gets a virus in it causes blistering in the area of skin that the nerve goes to?'

Dawn nods and says that her Mum had it round her waist and frowns with the recollection of the problems it caused.

'Well, I don't know if your Mum had awful pain with it – as a great many do, but what all those who get it say is that even the slightest touch can be incredibly painful – even just blowing on the skin can be painful – it can be agony. The amazing thing about it is that the horrid soreness and sensitivity carry on after the blisters clear up. The skin looks normal but it hurts like hell! That's what pain scientists call allodynia – remember the word I used ten minutes ago?'

They nod, I look at Chris and he looks puzzled…

'Test now Chris' – what was the other word I used just now, eh?'

'Thought you were listening! Pressure's on, have to hurry you.'

He hasn't a clue.

'Right 10 to me, minus 10 to you – it's H-Y-P-E-R-A-L-G-E-S-I-A – how do you say that for 10 points.'

He repeats and doesn't do too badly!

'Well done, yes, hyperalgesia – it means supersensitive and often occurs when a nerve is upset – you're problem has a touch of it. What was the other word we said for it just now – for 10 points?

'Allodinnereria or something?'

Ok, 5 points – you're minus 5 score now, but still 15 points behind me though, you better concentrate!' I go on.

(All the while I'm still moving both his legs and changing my handling all the time)

'So when a nerve is upset it can give you patches of skin that you can't feel but also some patches that are super-fantastically sensitive – think our words hyperalgesia/ allodynia. So you've got two nervy things now eh? I do the thumbs up, a bit of a wink and an eyebrow up smile. I want him (and the adults) to know I'm getting a handle on things – I'm confident so far and that they're all a part of the reasoning process.

(You may be thinking this flow of labelling towards 'nerve' is a bit drastic, agree, but let's see where it goes, it doesn't have to at all)

'Let's check out a bit more – I've got to do some more nerve testing and also check the knee joint out if we can – to make sure nothing bad is wrong there'… I pause.

'You could have banged the nerve round here when you fell (point at the head of fibula where the peroneal nerve winds round) just like when you bang your funny bone at your elbow and it hurts and fizzes down your forearm into your little fingers – you must've done that?'

He nods with a yuk type frown acknowledging that he knows.

(I want them all to have a good logical view of cause, effect/diagnosis and then a pathway out of it. The notion of useless/maladaptive pain and get it moving is the key.)

'Hey, let's go on now and check the nerve with some fun stuff.'

I pull out the tuning fork.

'Middle C!'

Bing! I bang the fork on my knee and it buzzes a way. I put it on his left (good) knee cap.

'Buzzing? Yep?'

'Yep'

I repeat on his left malleoli, left big toe MP joint and his forehead!

He's laughing.

'Got the idea of what it feels like!'

He smiles with enthusiasm and wants me to do more! I start on his right knee cap, he frowns…

'Hardly anything'

I repeat on the malleoli and the big toe MP joint.

'Maybe just a bit…'

'Legs gone a bit dumb Chris!'

Dad's still looking concerned but Dawn is looking fascinated.

(I'm not worrying at all here, a leg that hasn't moved for nearly a week, that's been constantly held in an awkward position, is bound to show odd/abnormal responses, plus…

I'm thinking more and more there's a bit of 'fib' and over-egging it, as I'm sure you might be. On the other hand there could be plenty of top-down related aspects like fear and altered sensory processing plus the mix of the on-going attention and concern from Dad and Dawn. Now, like many therapists and Drs do I could have had this sudden urge to try and 'prove' the kids was a fake. For example, I could try the good old hard jab in the 'so called numb area' with the pin-prick and make him jump – (kids of his age and sensitivity can't usually over-ride a nasty pin prick and remain not-bothered). But this type of approach doesn't help one bit. **What you think about the situation is irrelevant.** *What is relevant is finding and giving the lad and his processing system a chance to normalise and get going again. Staying in his current state of disability, if it goes on much longer could have nasty long term consequences. I'm thinking CRPS here. My job right now is to do some good basic testing as far as I can, then reassure and then get the lad a lot further on if at all possible. Weight-bearing and normalising is essential.)*

I get the reflex hammer out and bang his good knee – huge kick-up and a big laugh by Chris and Dawn – Dad's dead pan still (wow!). I do it again for another laugh.

Then I do his good ankle – all very good.

Over to the 'bad' one now – big jerk there, great and no 'ow' as I smack the previously super-sensitive patella tendon area.

'Hey, let's do it again!'

Bang-bang – jerk, jerk, we're all laughing, even Dad's got a glimpse of a smile. I do the calf – all good too.

I lower my voice to a touch more serious and turn to the adults. 'Right, I do all these tests to find out about the problem and first up to reassure myself that nothing serious is wrong, or that there is something of concern and that I need to refer the patient back to the Dr to find out more and maybe have some tests.'

'OK, so these reflexes being good are very reassuring.

(The clinician reader may disagree with my logic here – but in the bigger 'pain' clinical picture good reflexes are very frequently a useful tool to pass on some positivity – a 'pink' flag if you like. In these circumstances it was a useful 'ah, at last, something that works really well' moment. And somebody has checked!)

'I'm going to do a few gentle tests to your knee now Chris.'

He's still sitting with his legs dangling (not sticking out at 45 degrees anymore – or not quite!). I've got the plinth well up and I'm on my low stool – my heads at about his sitting waist height. I place the heel of his good left foot on the stool between my legs so it can take the weight and he can let-go. (If you don't like a kids foot between your legs stick a pillow there first!). I gently grasp the upper end of his good side tibia.

'Floppy, floppy, floppy... I'm going to pull and push it a bit to show you what a cruciate ligament test feels like – heard of those?'

'No.'

Dawn and Dad have, they're nodding.

'Test! Two words for super-sensitivity from earlier, one is allodynia the other is...?'

'Hyperaleesha or something.'

'OK, not bad, 5 points, you're now on zero. What did I call these ligaments just then... come on brains...'

He's laughing and I'm doing the test, pulling and pushing the tibia gently and building it as he relaxes...'

'Crush-e-ate was it?

Hey, another 5 points – but it's 'crew' as in ship's crew, 'she' – like Dawn over there and 'ate' like you just had a piece of toast. 'Cruciate!' I won't tell you how to spell it unless you're really keen and want 10 points.'

He does, I spell it, he gets it right and he reckons he's now winning.

'Cruciate! It's the one that footballers tear when they fall and badly twist their knee – they usually injure other ligaments too and there's a whole pile of swelling. So here's another positive – your knee's not swollen so it's unlikely you've torn anything, but we're still going to check it out.'

I start gently pulling on his left tibia again, forward and there's a nice glide.

'I need to get it to knock a bit' I wink at him, 'Feel this...'

I give it a quick little jerk and there's a nice anterior cruciate 'knock' as the ligament tightens up.

'Great!'

I then give it a quick jerk backwards and the posterior cruciate gives a nice knock too.

'Great!'

'Feel the knock?'

He laughs at the weird sensation and that he did indeed.

I give him a naughty smile because I know he knows I'm going to do the same to the right knee! I put my hands around his knee – he's trusting me more and lets me do it without batting an eye.

'Right, gently forward and back – bear with me Chris – I promise I won't rip your leg off!'

I slowly build his confidence and end up giving it a nice little jerk in both directions – they're identical to the left leg.

'Feel the same as the other one to you?'

'Yes,' he agrees.

Sure? You don't have to agree with me – last chance. I'll do it again –sure?

'Sure!'

(I hope you can see that all this handling is as much treatment and desensitising and me taking things further and further – as actual investigation I know the cruciates should be fine, but wise action is always to check, you never know what may happen after a session like this)

I then show them all a model of a knee and point out the cruciates in a way that makes sense of the simple tests.

'Right, things are looking up, now for the summary and the plan. It looks to me as if you've fallen and banged a nerve on the side of your knee – a bit like banging the funny bone in your elbow.   So no wonder you've got pins and needle feelings and it's got a numb patch – we've all done it and one time or other. But the nerve isn't badly damaged because you've still got good reflexes. Next thing – your knee isn't badly damaged, there's no swelling and all the tests I've done are good. So here's the big question. Why does it hurt so much and why can't you move it or put any weight on it?'

I go on...

'Remember the shingles we talked about – huge amount of horrid sensitivity and pain yet no evidence of anything bad going on in the skin where it hurts; so nerves can have minor bangs and knocks in some people and cause heaps of pain and all this super-sensitivity to touch and move – yet in others there's a quick bit of pins and needles and it's all forgotten.'

'Key thing is that the best way to go now is to get you going and you won't hurt it or damage it I promise. We'll go as slow as we need to.'

The adults are nodding away now.

(The clinician may be wondering how I can make such assumptions about a nerve having not tested muscles yet. The picture here is of a young lad, with loads of pain, unable to weight-bear, unable to move it, who would hardly touch it himself – to get anything valuable out of classic static muscle testing is very unlikely – but getting the muscles contracting may well be one route into getting the problem working, moving and processing properly again. If it was peroneal nerve then if it was severe you'd expect difficulty with foot and toe dorsiflexion etc. Chris was holding his foot up fine. Further testing could be done later but if I can get good function, power loss will reveal itself. Whatever, the key thing is action!

How to look at this? To me – it would be easy to look at him and say he's amplifying things, he's wimping it big time, he's trying to get out of things he doesn't like, he's got footballer-like-agony-fall-over-and-die-after-tripping-over-a-puff-of-air-contagious-syndrome. There's a pile of things going on around the family (maybe banishing from the room would have sorted it all out, but I doubt it) – that stuff is maybe all fine, even entertaining when you're in the mood to think like this, but very dangerous if that's the only way you think. (Yup, I do think this stuff, it's OK – I like to amuse myself with what I see as being 'instinctive' intolerant thinking! (There's a research project for someone!) Dangerous thinking? Yes, if that's all you've got, because it doesn't help you to help anybody in any way at all. The colour of your mind and your attitude to the patient just cannot produce any useful interaction and if anything, the patient is highly likely to get worse – both in their pain level and in their pain behaviour. It's my belief that this attitude could be a significant factor in maintaining the level of disability (foot off the floor and in the air) and it soon becoming a very difficult to deal with CRPS 1 problem.

Best think neurophysiologically a little perhaps? It might be a more productive way of looking at things.

*I'm thinking – here's a nervous system that has had some kind of shock – pain somehow has been created – perhaps he did pull, knock, or whack his peroneal nerve? Perhaps he didn't? Whatever, the top-down response to the shock of the fall has sensitised the system somehow. The key is that **what's in front of me is what I've got to deal with** and I've got to get this nice, but slightly fragile looking kid going again, get his mind off the pain and relieve a lot of the tension that surrounds him and get him going – at the same time keeping a careful eye out for something physical/anatomical/biomechanical/medical that may emerge as we go along.*

*Clearly, his nervous system is on high alert, movement and physical stress around the knee area is high on its **inhibition agenda** and pain response and sensitivity is high on the **facilitation agenda**. High attention is too. Everything needs modulating down and off – and using normal inputs via physical movement may be the best way to do this – combined with the on-going chitter-chatter distracting orchestra I'm conducting.*

The approach and the style is a mixture of acting, art, confidence, trickery, distraction, humour, cajoling, explanation, chat, rests, changes, novelty, being human, getting on the right wavelength, keeping trust and so forth. Plus some very basic physiotherapy skills and some that are the product of a bit of ingenuity. Nice! Fun? Yup! In the textbooks? Never!)

My one slight concern is that this pain could be very reactive – especially if I 'lose' his trust and our relationship goes a bit ... or it's more reactive at some 'tissue' level than I'd thought... The big thing is that even if it is, I know I won't have done anything that can possibly injure it.

Here we go...

'Right Chris' – let's start by seeing what'll move'

He's still sitting with 'the' right leg held out semi-dangling. I'm pumping the couch up as high as it will go... pump... pump... up he goes... he's smiling...

'How high will it go?'

'Prepare to be squashed on the ceiling'... I'm giving a little laugh... Then he's up as high it'll go... (my plinth will go up pretty high)

I sit on my stool in front and well below him now and start moving his lower leg forward and back very gently, he quickly spasms and the movement is resisted... he wants to push me away again...

'See if you can let go if I go very slowly... I promise you it won't do you any harm...'

At the same time I very slowly move him into flexion ... I'm going back under the table about 10 then 20 degrees and then the spasm is hitting quite hard. I'm not talking or asking about pain (just reinforces the pain facilitation circuitry from top-down). But, while he's saying it's painful, he resists me with strong contraction which in turn puts a great deal of pressure/stretch/force through the very structures that hurt – which in turn should make it hurt a lot more!

Different tack now...

'I want you to keep it still now when I try to move you.' The leg is dangling fairly relaxed – good!

'Feel the resistance as I build it up and match me; don't try to beat me, match me... concentrate...'

I slowly increase the pressure pushing back into flexion. I'm growling at the floor to keep him amused...

'You've got it, good, now feel for the change in direction of pressure and match me, you mustn't let the leg move at all, keep it still.... me against you...'

He's getting it well, strong contractions now and I'm pushing hard on the lateral side of his foot... then sliding round to pull on his heel... back to the lateral side... back to the front... then round medially... my hands start to move up his leg to give the pressure. I'm turning into a bit of a witch, growling and grunting and getting him to work harder... I'm now pushing hard around his knee area to get him to resist – the area, you remember that I was barely able to touch earlier.

I've got him giggling now and he's having to use his arms to keep his balance and hold onto the couch... I'm now mirroring what I do with his right on his good left leg – so we're doing both together...

'Concentrate on the left leg now, here we go push, push! PUSH! I'm shouting as I change the directions – I get sharper with the onset of the pressure (on both legs) – he's working quite hard and his balance is getting seriously challenged as I change directions and the zones of pressure... I'm making lots of noise as I apply the quickly changing pressure... he's starting to grunt and laugh too...

'If you fall off the couch it's your fault not mine... 'I'm pushing this way, that way, all ways! 'Hold, resist! Resist! Hold! Hold! ... It goes on.

I suddenly stop and as the commotion effect is slowly dying away I'm straightening his knee out to about minus 30 degrees... then flexing it way under the bed... He's hardly noticing and looks over at Dad and Dawn; it's almost as if there's a moment of calm as 'the eye of the therapy storm' passes over us and the adrenaline and endorphin rush it caused floods the scene – numbing any sensation! (or something like that – I am joking!)

'Come on Chris, on your back now' – I throw a couple of pillows up to the end of the couch. I'm still holding his ankle as he lies down onto his back from the high sitting position, but I keep holding his leg and don't let it go with him – he's lying on his back now with his leg out in abduction and lower leg still dangling down off the couch in flexion... there's a calm moment. Chris's head is back on the pillows and he's staring at the ceiling looking a bit stunned... and then I slowly lift his leg and put it on the side of the couch – it's relaxed in full extension – hmmm, good! I turn to Dad and Dawn and raise my eyebrows and smile. They look a bit gob-smacked.

'I think we are getting somewhere at last.' I smile.

I now bend his leg calmly and fully, there's no resistance at all, it's as if the shock of all that work   has taken every last ounce of resistance out of him precipitating a pleasant and overwhelming passivity! Remember he's done virtually nothing 'exciting' or sudden for around six days – that's a very long time for a 12 year-old. I have to keep him going. I need to work on the weight-bearing quickly before any inhibitory 'recovery' occurs – I need to make this relevant to walking if I can.

I hold him by both ankles and I come round to the foot end of the treatment couch slowly pulling him down the bed by his feet. He's laughing... I'm now pushing him up the couch and the pillows drop to the floor, he's laughing even more as I'm pulling and pushing him, the pressure's going well down through his legs as I push, then pull and traction the legs – there's plenty of force and I'm brimming with confidence now – all of I've got to do is transfer this to standing and walking – but he's enjoying it so much that I have to keep going! I continue to pull and push him and 'the folks' are laughing now too!

Dawn laughs and says 'Mind your pants!'

'Right, come on Chris we've got to put all this good work into practice – your knees are taking plenty of weight through them with me yanking you around, up you come...'

He's up sitting looking a little disconcerted at the thought of having to walk but I don't really give him a chance, couch goes down, down, down (my couches are hydraulic foot operated and go up and down at a fairly quick pace) and stops with a bump as it bottoms out. He's giggling again and I'm smiling.

Without time to think about it I've got him standing up, but the cautious standing and walking inhibitory patterns are coming back and his knee isn't taking too much weight.

I'm standing next to him now and holding him round the waist close to me, swaying side to side and pushing him onto his right side, chatting away...

'How's your confidence about getting better? Scale of one to 10, 10 is 100% confidence of getting back to normal, back to rugby and running around without thinking about your leg?'

'About seven,' he says a bit sheepishly.

'Seven! Is that all, what about the other 30%?' I'm humorously sarcastic now but I'm pushing him along. We're starting to walk and he's hobbling. I open the treatment room door and we're off down the corridor.

'Second door on the left into the gym, let's go...'

We're in and I'm helping him up onto the cross-trainer – he's a bit small for it and he's starting to go backwards with the foot-pads!

'What are you doing dude! Grab the handles, pump the arms and help the legs. He's struggling to get the hang of it but it's distracting him and he's trying to get the machine turning by pushing weight down through his right leg – he's getting going a bit and I'm helping him by pumping the arms of the machine.

'Lean left, right, left, right, push down, down, down... go, go, go... you're doing it...'

I'm encouraging him... he's struggling with the size of the machine but he's going for it... We're doing it for about 2 or 3 minutes and I want to get him off and walking again.

'Off you come now Chris, let's get out of here and get going.'

We're now going back down the corridor and I'm not touching him and he's walking but hobbling a bit.

Back in the treatment room and I've had enough and have got to get on with my next patient.

'Here he is guys' and Dad and Dawn applaud and make encouraging noises.

'Right, he needs to get going now, forget the crutches and get moving again. I want Chris to make the decisions.' I look at Chris and wait for a nod... 'And I don't want anyone having to nag. You're getting going and you're going to be fine, but I need to see you again in about four or five days time to see how you're going and to re-check the knee.' I look at Chris, 'Is that OK with you?'

'Yes!'

'100%?'

'Yes'

'Yes!' we high 5 and as they go out.

'Remember any problems or worries phone me – if you get the answer machine, leave a message and I'll call you back – I mean it! I don't want anyone sitting at home worrying, OK!'

Follow up

The appointment is 8.15 Monday morning of half term. Dawn's brought him over and they're sitting in the waiting room, no crutches. Chris is smiling.

'I'm getting a new camcorder.'

'What's all that about? What is someone miserable like you going to do with a camcorder?'

'Film my Grand Theft Auto!' He smiles.

'Eh? What to show your friends?'

'Yeah!'

He looks so animated... and I'm thinking how bloody sad is that?

I aim some good natured sarcasm at him...

'So Chris's a Game-boy addict then eh? Goggle chops?'

Dawns nodding, like this is THE biggest problem with the kid.

'Come on let's have you down to my torture chamber and see what's happening...

He's walking normally and I'm behind him, Dawn's behind me.

'Looking good, how many out of 10 now?'

'10!'

'Good lad – you should have had a bit of faith eh?'

He's now in the treatment room and up on the couch.

'Get off! Walk! Up and down the corridor – off you go.'

He's looking normal.

'Run! Go on... run!'

He's running up and down and I'm now chasing him.

'Turn back...' He's now chasing me...

'Turn and we're going back the other way... turning more and more, faster and faster...

'Jump, jump! JUMP!'

We're back in the treatment room and I've got him hopping on both legs, then on one then doing burpees and he's doing it, but he's hopelessly unfit looking!

'You're rubbish' I'm going...

'How old are you? – 9 was it?'

'12!' he shouts...

'Oh and I'm 58 and I can do a better burpee than you! Hey you're so not-fit dude!'

Dawns nodding and going...

'His Dad just can't get him to do anything... Dad goes to the gym three times a week and tries to get him to go but he's gaming-gaming-gaming all the time – can't get him to exercise enough, he's really worried about him.'

I'm smiling now at Chris.

'You are bad! Addicted to thumb exercises and succumbing to goggle-out-dull-kid-boggled-up-grumpy-dumpy-yawn-all-day-no-need-for-legs-disease eh?'

He's laughing but I am thinking this is a bit sad, but like his Dad said last time, he's 'just' got into the rugby side – like it was a big relief that at last he was doing something physical.

'Come on, I want you to really get into being more physical   get back to rugby training and get down that gym with your Dad... How about you make an activity diary and phone me in two weeks and tell me day by day what you've been doing? Let me be your 'activity' monitor? The deal's this: at least ten minutes activity every day but I want you to really do twenty to thirty minutes minimum – and I think even that's pretty pathetic!' I'm smiling and winking – but he knows I mean it.

'Come on mate!'

'Right, I've got to make a few checks on your knee – up on the couch, on your back!'

I'm hoping the reader is thinking, like me, that these tests – given that he's not complained of any problems since seeing him five days ago and all he's just been doing with me – are unlikely to be abnormal in anyway. Still, it's a good thing to do, overall for me and also for the lad and his family to know that there's nothing detectably wrong. I test the collateral ligaments and the cruciates, I have a good feel of full flexion and extension with a bit of rotation added in both directions to put a reasonable bit of torsion on the joint and see how it responds. He doesn't bat an eyelid and I'm happy.

Did he phone me, did he heck, but I phoned him recently, two years on and he's now 14; he got through most of the game-boy phase, or less obsessively and has been really enjoying squash and badminton. Luckily he lives on the edge of town and all his mates have bikes, so he's often out with them.

Case Histories 2

SUB ACUTE

Chapter CH 2.1
Dylan - Part 1

'One morning I shot an elephant in my pyjamas. How he got in my pyjamas I'll never know.'

Groucho Marx

'Politics is the art of looking for trouble, finding it everywhere, diagnosing it incorrectly and applying the wrong remedies.'

Groucho Marx

Hopefully, this case history is dominated by a physical findings dominated 'shopping basket', meaning there's a strong focus on the 'impairment' compartment. When I interviewed patients 'live' in front of groups on the Dynamic Nervous System courses I used to say to the audience 'Try and follow where my brain's going and see if you can anticipate my next question or line of enquiry. I'll pause occasionally and ask you what you might want to ask – but the patient is not allowed to answer the question, we discuss the question first and if it's relevant we may even answer it without asking the patient! The key thing that I want to know is WHY you are asking the question you want to ask and why ask it now?' It may be possible for you to follow this along and think where your own reasoning is going and what you'd like to know next and why.

Dylan is 15 years old and a keen cricketer and rugby player for his school. He says he's a fast bowler and likes going to the gym to work out.

He reported having a left sided 'groin strain' that came on about two months ago. There was no specific incident but he said that the pain had come on after playing cricket.

'What, immediately after?'

'No that evening.'

'So you can't recall any incident during the game?'

'No.'

'The pain's in the left groin you said?'

'Yes, deep in here.' He points more to his upper inner thigh rather than right in the groin. I'm thinking, maybe it's in the adductor tendon area, or musculotendinous junction rather than on the bony insertion.

'Have you had a good feel around – is it tender there?'

'I have but I can't find anything.'

'Ok, I'll check it out later. I'm thinking fast bowling you come down hard on your left leg at the point of bowling if you're right handed?'

'Yes.'

'So what does it feel like?'

'It's an aching feeling, almost a throbbing ache when I get it.'

'So it's not there all the time?'

'No, only after exercising, particularly running or even jogging for about five minutes.

Oh, and I recently had a bit of a kick around with a football with some mates and it was really sore and stiff. I could hardly move it or walk for about an hour.'

'What straight away after?'

'No, after I got home and had sat down, that was about two hours after the kick around.'

'OK that night and the next morning and day?'

'It remained a bit sore that evening and was stiff and sore the next morning but once I was moving it slowly freed up.'

'What about the day after that?'

'Back to as it is now.'

'... and how long was the kick-around for?'

'Probably an hour or so.'

(So this 'after-use-stop-get-up-feel-sore-and-stiff-and-into-the-next-day' response shows that it's a little reactive and fits into a moderately typical 'inflammatory' type response – although even this could be a 'pain memory' type mechanism. I now have 'hip' in my mind slightly but adductor muscle and groin are too. I still want to clarify something that I'm a bit puzzled about.)

'You said just now that you feel it after jogging for about five minutes? Do you mean the ache and throbbing come on there and then, or afterwards?'

'There and then.'

'So if we went for a jog right now it would come on?'

'Yes.'

'Have you tried carrying on to see what happens – meaning can you run it off or does it just get worse and worse?'

I haven't tried, well except when I ran around a lot with my mates and it was then very stiff afterwards.'

'Yes, but did you feel it while you were running around then?'

'No, actually I didn't.' He looked puzzled because he was seeing what I was getting at.

I just raised my eyebrows… 'Don't worry Dylan, most pain problems don't quite fit with what you'd expect... you're not mad! And I'm not thinking you're mad, but pain can be a bit!'

He looked pleased to hear that.

(I hope you're all thinking that one explanation for this 'loss' of pain while playing soccer relates to simple inhibition/gating – for example the endorphin pain-off system being promoted by the enjoyment, the focus of attention. If you've ever been running you'll know how your brain gets bored and tends to wander – one minute being out in the environment to look at the view or the passers-by, or cars... the next wandering around your body listening to bits and pieces, to feelings in your legs, to your breathing, to any little ache or pain... then into your head to try and sort something out that's bothering you. Now, playing soccer, there's no chance of that freedom of the mind to go wandering off. Running = somatising[1] IN... Soccer = somatising OUT!)

'It sounds like you've stopped all exercise?'

'I've stopped and rested, because when I had it before I rested it for two weeks and it went and was fine. The problem this time is that it's gone on for two months now.'

'When did you have it before?'

'About a year ago.'

'... and any incident back then?'

'No, same again – a bit of a mystery why and then it was after rugby not cricket.'

'Had you been doing much cricket at the time, I'm thinking net practice, indoors etc.?'

'I'm in the school gym nets every spare moment I can be. I've got a good mate who's as keen as I am and he's a batsman.'

(So, plenty of repetitive forces through the left hip then and as he's 15 he still has epiphyses – I'm particularly thinking aggravated epiphysis perhaps or at worst slipped capital femoral epiphysis which can occur in adolescents)

'Ok, and you haven't done any games at school recently – it's rugby this term isn't it?'

'That's right – I've not done anything.'

'Gym at all?'

'No.'

He looked a bit sheepish.

'No, why not?' I half seriously joked.

---

1 - Somatising – meaning focusing on the body and what's being felt there.

He shrugged and smiled.

'So you've been two months waiting for it to recover and it's not improved at all?'

'No, but I went to the Dr with my Dad to have him check it out.'

'What did the Dr make of it?'

'He thought it might be a hernia and I had to go for a scan – but there was nothing wrong – so he said see a physio.'

'How long did all that take?'

'About four weeks until he suggested physio…'

(As an aside here – astonishing! This sort of thing happens every week at work – the Dr not really listening and examining properly and also taking ages to get to the point of some 'action' – with the usual wait-and-it'll-recover approach. If the Dr had simply got the kid to show him exactly where the pain was – in the very upper medial thigh, not the groin or anywhere near the inguinal area – surely the time and expense of referring and waiting for a hernia scan could have been avoided and active rehab got on with weeks ago?)

'Oh, I forgot to mention, I can cycle OK, but I tried swimming and it hurts when I do breast stroke.'

'Right, is this an instant pain while you're doing the stroke, or an 'after-pain' like you got after playing soccer?'

'Instant – when I bring my legs together – I feel it.'

'Is it the same every time or does it ease up the more you do?'

'Well, I've only been once and as soon as I felt it I did a few more strokes and it was the same, the rest of the time I was in I stuck to crawl and it was fine then.'

'Could you just clarify what that pain felt like?'

'It was a sharp twinge deep in the spot here.'

'Do you get that at any other time?'

'I've had it once or twice with awkward movements; once I think I was getting out of the car from the middle of the back seat and I extended the leg to get over a pile of bags and shopping, I felt it then very briefly.'

'Right so we've achy pain after walking and soccer and an occasional sharp pain with some movements. I think it's time to have a look and find out what's going on, but before we do I'm just wondering what's going through your head about this thing?

What do you think is going on?'

'Well, I just thought I'd over-strained the groin again like I must of before and that rest would get it better and I'd be off back to normal again – but it hasn't. Then when the Dr went on about a hernia I was a little puzzled and then a bit concerned about maybe having to have an operation or something. While it was a relief that the scan was OK I'm still left wondering what's going on and why it's not got better.'

'Are you confident that it'll get better?' I slipped this in: knowing that patient confidence about recovery is a powerful outcome predictor.

'Well I was when I first got it but I'm starting to get anxious about it being a long term problem now.' There was a pause then...

'I really love my rugby. But I understand some things take time to heal.' He looked down and his voice lowered.

'Well, it's had plenty of rest, it might be more appropriate to get it going now in a gradual way. You're right, being young you should recover well and yes it may need a little more time. Because there's not been a specific incident it's unlikely to be badly torn but the continued and regular pounding it gets may be a factor, especially on your growing bones.'

His faced brightened a bit.

'Before we start, have you ever had anything else like this in any other areas of your body – aches and pains that have come on without any apparent injury for example.'

'Well I had back pain last Easter'

'That's about four to five months ago' I say out loud... 'Tell me about it?'

'I just woke up with it one morning, it was really stiff and sore in the base of my back – it went on for a couple of weeks then went.'

'So you couldn't put it down to anything by the sound of it?'

'Well nothing obvious but I had been doing a lot of rugby training at the time... '

'Any more or different from usual do you think?'

He frowned a bit and looked up,

'Not really.'

(I don't question further, rugby is the ultimate 'feel nothing at the time most of the time' game and the body gets wrenched and strained into all sorts of positions. For Dylan, he could well have overstrained it without noticing it.)

'OK, I might have a quick look at your back shortly as well and just to check once more – you've never had back pain before this, or anything else you can remember when you were younger...?'

'No I haven't.'

'And the back's absolutely fine now?'

'Yes!'

'No problems as far as you know when you were very young, no spells in hospital for anything 'hippy'?'

'No!'

'All the family's hips and backs OK, Mum, Dad, brothers, sisters?'

'They're all really fit like me, or like I was anyway.'

(I'm thinking any juvenile, congenital or familial hip related problems – Perthes disease, hip dysplasia or slipped femoral epiphysis – that could have left him with a vulnerable hip for example.)

I then did all the standard, general health questions and asked about medication etc. All fine, he's a fit young lad who's neglected his fitness for last couple of months.

(Thinking about his problem at this point – there's a degree of 'post-activity' reactivity which needs acknowledging and lightly monitoring if I get him to start getting going again. It also looks as if there's a mechanically patterned and mechanically sensitive element to it – so I'm expecting to find a direct relationship between physical stress in the area of the pain and an instant pain response at some point when doing the examination.

I'm also thinking that this isn't typical of a groin strain and that with no obvious injuring incident that over-use may be an aspect of it.)

'Right, good, let's carry on and get going with having a look at it... '

He takes his things off and we get going. I start with a bit of simple 'routine' before expecting to go more specific.

'Let's have a look at you walking up and down...'

He strolls about normally...

'Tip-toe walk now...'

Fine.

'Bent-knee-low-down-walk – just like Groucho Marx!' I quip. He looks at me puzzled... then I show him...

'Sorry Dylan, American 1950's and 60's comics, who did zany things, ignore me. All fine so far?

'No problems.' He's still looking at me like I'm a weirdo! I'm just smiling.

He does the low walk fine.

'Don't worry about me but a little madness helps when you're working with pain all day long for years and years... It's a wonder I'm not madder isn't it...?'

'Right, try this...'

I face him, then standing on one leg – I flex the other knee to chest, as high as I can and keep repeating it. He mimics me but in a rather half hearted way.

'That's looking a bit pathetic! Get the knee up any higher?'

(He looks surprised and a bit unsure and I'm thinking he's been very protective of this and is a little fearful of pushing it... I'm still working my leg up and down trying to keep him in rhythm and mimicking my range of movement... He gets going a bit....

So if you're thinking that I might stir him up – I'm not too bothered, as I know that after running around and kicking a football with his mates is far more 'physical' stress than any examination movements that I'm likely to do and that even if it does get stirred up it should settle quickly. He'll be able to cope with that if I communicate well)

'All OK? Manage that? Right, try this now... '

I start doing active abduction and as before I have to get him going to push it a bit as we repeat the movement together I get more and more vigorous and he follows – he's fine and no discomfort so far. I then start doing large hip extension movements – 'big curtseys' as I call them. My leg's extending back and forward keeping the back foot on the ground and the trunk nicely upright and I swap from right to left all the time. He's getting the idea and we're both warming up a bit now.

'So far so good then?' I do my usual, eyebrows-up expression communicating a bit of positivity and ready-to-move-on. He nods.

'Let's have a look at this now.' I'm doing the splits to a point where I can comfortably feel an adductor stretch then lunging to left and right to add a bit more.

'Dylan, I'm doing the splits to the point where I start to feel a *normal* stretch on the upper inner thigh muscles and now I'm slowly and comfortably lunging to the left and right to feel what it's like with a little more stretch and compare one side to the other. You have a try and tell me what happens?'

He's doing it – I'm waiting for a response.

'Both feel the same' he's saying, a bit puzzled.

(Note, this could have been positive if I'd gone straight to it from 'cold' – I could have 'warmed' him up by doing the other movements. Not to worry but the thing about this is it's quite 'Pink' for the adductors' stretch capability and sensitivity)]

'Right, stay there (he's lunged to his right) and what I want you to do now is try to press your left foot into the floor and build up the pressure – the idea is to work your adductor muscle in a stretched position to see if it complains – got the idea?' He repeats it on his right leg to compare.

'No pain; both feel the same!' He's looking a tad incredulous.

'Great! Don't worry Dylan, nothing ever fits the textbooks as it should! And you know what the less we find the better!'

I now get him to twizzle round from the splits position to stretch into right hip extension.

'Stretch it, then tighten into it and press your right toes into the floor with the muscle like before, remember what that was like – then twizzle 180 degrees round the other way and compare the good right to the left. He's got the idea now and a few moments teaching him to mimic me slowly makes for faster responses as we go on; he's now in a full left leg extension position with the left leg back pushing down against the resistance of the floor as strongly as he can – it's outer range hip flexor testing. Testing resistance repeatedly and through range is on my list.

'Well?'

'Nothing!'

'Ok, let's try jogging on the spot now.' I'm jogging away and he's catching on and quickly doing it with me.

'All OK?' He nods now with an accepting shrug. I start hopping on one leg and he follows. He's looking happy so I assume all's OK. I then hop higher and dip a bit lower on the one leg. He stops.

'The ache is just starting to come on, just like if I jogged for five minutes.'

I've now got the adduction swimming movement in my head and am thinking forget the static muscle tests and do some through range resistance.

'Are you OK to carry on, the pain coming on is useful now and will help me to analyse it but you may be a little sore afterwards, as you were from the football. Are you OK to carry on?'

He was fine; the pain was a mere 1-2, 'Just noticeable' he said.

I did a quick check of his back posture and standard back movements which looked fine. *(Try NOT to find anything is key! BUT be open to revisiting if it may help).* I then got him to sit with legs dangling on the couch and typically for a large, strong-legged youngster his legs were well out in abduction. I gave static resistance to hip adduction and abduction and both were positive for the groin pain, just like the breast-stroke swimming plus more – it hurt in both directions! I then repeated, this time with resistance through range from as much abduction as he could get sitting to knees together and then from knees together out into full sitting abduction. I started with resisting adduction.

As he built resistance I got him to push against me and bring his legs together rather than to build statically and not move. If it's any help, for static contractions I use the command 'build as I build, and 'match me don't break me' as I increase the resistance. I also tell the patient that if they don't like the feeling of strain and want to stop to just ease up.

The pain was worse in resisted outer range adduction and by about half way in it went off and was nil by the time his knees touched. I repeated doing abduction – from knees touching out towards his active abduction limit. Again, the groin pain came on at about half way out and increased to the end of range! So testing abductors created adductor area pain and testing adductors produced it too. To me this sort of 'impossible' test result is more the rule than the exception (especially in shoulder testing!). It makes a bit of a mockery of the 'Cyriax' protocol that uses selective and localised forces to isolate to a specific musculotendinous unit and expect pain to fit with where the forces are directed.

(If only the clinicians who swear by this precise diagnostic stuff would see that the brain has a very poor representation of deep structures – it's impossible to be precise for 'inside' stuff for most of us– (though there's always some hippy exception). Think skin injury if you want precision, or a wound in one of your orifices – don't dentists have it so easy? You almost want to shout at the tissue – 'Hey you, get yourself a homunculus will you, yes you!' Maybe just think of this type of response as a mere 'misread' and don't get worked up about it—just pop it in the 'Impairment' compartment of the shopping basket— it's a finding to note, maybe to address and maybe to monitor! Intellectualising it to a structure is generally not necessary unless you've got a syringe with a needle or a scalpel in your hand.)

At this point in time I'm starting to find a bit of an appropriate pain response, albeit a bit scrappy but it's helpful, it's even helping to 'make features fit' a little – to use a good old Geoff Maitland phrase. Yes, it could be 'joint' I hear you thinking and that is a consideration on the reasoning list as we've already discussed. What's interesting and very positive is how confidently and how hard Dylan could work the active standing hip in extension (working all the hip muscles for sure but bias towards hip flexors and adductors) and in abduction (bias to the adductor muscles) – with not even a whiff of the pain. Once again, this type of discrepancy in response to physical testing is commonplace and there's more to come.

Before getting Dylan to lie down, to take the examination further, I decided to quickly review active hip adduction and active, resisted and passive, lateral and medial rotation in this very convenient sitting legs dangling position. Active leg crossing is a good way of quick testing active and functional adduction and it allows the patient to give their evaluation. Dylan found it far easier putting his right leg over left than left over right – in fact he could only just manage it! Just like an OA hip! When I see this in OA hips I then get them to do this: for a left leg, in this sitting position, bring your left leg up to put your left foot on your right knee or just above it and then lower the left knee towards the floor. It tests lateral rotation and abduction simultaneously and is commonly very difficult with stiff hips – some can't even get their foot onto the knee! Dylan got his foot up alright but as soon as he lowered the left knee it gave him a really sharp jab in the adductor pain area. Ah! Interesting! His right leg was fine and he could lower the knee to nearly the horizontal, as most flexible hips do.

All this goes in the 'Impairment' compartment. 'To be worked on/monitored!'

Next, the 'in-sitting legs dangling position' – do/test: hip rotations. I got him to do it actively – foot out for medial rotation and then the usually much more awkward to do foot across for lateral. Dylan's medial rotation on his left was sharp at about 20 degrees whereas the right had about 45 degrees of movement (good range!). Lateral rotation was unremarkable. I now did the medial rotation movement passively and got a full 45 degrees but with the pain only at the end of range. Lateral rotation again was fine. Static testing by pressing the outside of the foot for medial rotators produced his pain, as was lateral rotation resisting on the inside of the foot, but far less so. You'd expect this to be the other way round... another 'well that doesn't quite fit with anatomy' finding – medial rotators are mostly the gluteus muscles on the outside of the hip! Don't panic; just chuck it in the Impairment compartment! If you are panicking you've got far too much 'what's the cause of this' thinking going on in your head.

Now if you've been concentrating you might be thinking hang on – lateral rotation is fine here but he could hardly do that left foot up on right knee then let left knee lower out into abduction just now – the movement contains a great deal of lateral rotation of course. Try it! So what did I do? I repeated the passive and active tests with his trunk flexed over his thighs – active and passive were both painful. So, that's in the Impairment compartment too! Why did I do it like that? Because the leg up foot on knee movement is near enough full hip flexion. Tip: remember to look at movements in the standard way but also look at reversing them... Like lumbar flexion, standard examination is trunk forward and down; reverse it – pelvic thrust! So to remember the Tip – think '**bottom up AS WELL AS top down** for all movements. (Remember my shoulder pain that got me thinking? There you go!) It would be quite fun to try doing your next examination with a patient using the very opposite movement sequence from standard... try say, a neck for starters! (see chapter CH 1.2)

I thought for a minute that it would be worthwhile getting him to show me his bowling style to see what effect that might have had on the pain and to see what he actually did. But the old 'manual therapist' in me wanted to feel his hip and do the standard lying supine and prone tests. Since his standing hip movements were so good I was interested to check the hip rotations in the full supine position and also check ab and adduction here too. As you might expect it confirmed that they were okay – no wonder he was comfortable standing and walking and doing all those standing active tests we did.

I now got him to lie prone to check further – doing prone hip extension and abduction; and using the 90 degree flexed knee as a lever did medial and lateral rotation in this 'hip neutral/nearer extension' type position. There were no problems, however back over in supine lying, left hip flexion plus adduction easily reproduced the pain and was significantly limited compared to the right. Hip abduction at 90 degrees flexion was tight and reproduced the pain easily, reflecting the active foot-on-knee-and-then-drop-the-knee test done sitting. Adding rotation to this abducted position further provoked the pain quite markedly. Finding pain with physical testing by fiddling with combinations of movement was something I got very good at thanks to working with Geoff for those couple of years. In some problem presentations it can be very useful, especially those associated with high end sports performance. Dylan though was quite straight forward to me, but I've seen many like him who've had 'courses' of physiotherapy or 'other' treatment – where the whole focus was on treating the site of pain and the 'diagnosis' (adductor tear/strain). Sometimes the urge to give a diagnosis completely traps the therapist into localising the treatment and missing the bigger picture. OK, hang in there...

I palpated the painful area he indicated and with really deep pressure produced some sharp discomfort. Dylan looked pleased and said the usual... 'That's the first time anyone's been able to find anything there.'

I go: 'Hang on a minute, I'll repeat that and I want you to remember how hard I was pushing, the type of pain and the intensity because I'm then going to go to your right muscle and do the same thing for you to compare it to... '

After repeating the pressure with his guidance he said, rather forlornly...

'It feels exactly the same as the left.'

Now, if you get good at finding the pain for the patient with your thumbs and you want to take the easy option 'That's the spot, that's the problem, I can feel a knot, that's where we treat' – then DON'T! Go and do what I just did – palpate the other side and do it in such a way that asks for exact comparison. If you want to be honest and not make so much money but see the bigger picture DO go and do what I just did!

'What did the physio find dear?'

'Oh a knot in my crotch Mum.'

'Bowline? Reef? Sheepshank? or was it something fancy like a Carrick bend?'

(Sorry for the joke! Check out the Ashley Book of Knots for Sailors!)

The knot in the muscle, the ability to find something in the right spot, a 'Pot of gold' rather cynically pops into my head right now. Since becoming more and more sceptical I have made great efforts to show patients that although the tenderness found is where their pain is, it doesn't take a minute to find it exactly the same and sometimes even worse – on the other side! I always allow the patient to make a comparison and to think about whether the difference is due to my firmness varying or not. The main point is it's yet another finding for the shopping basket to hold onto if there is a difference.

I didn't palpate his back; I didn't want to find anything there if I could help it. Well I'd found enough and there was plenty to get on with, if I really got stuck and felt I had to I could always revisit.

Time to take a break.

Chapter CH 2.2:
Dylan - Part 2

Shopping Basket analysis!

Let me now make a list of things to work on from a shopping basket perspective and also discuss how I tackled it all.

1. Biomedical

    a. Safe to start loading, yes.

    b. What's going on then? He's got limited hip movements and various positive muscle and joint signs. Let's be honest, I don't really know what's going on but I know there's plenty to get on with. I've got to get him super confident in his left adductor region again and fearless of continuing his sport at the level he's doing it and more. He's young and should recover with a good graded rehab approach was a constant background thought. If he fails to improve it may be worth an x-ray or scans. It could be over-use and at his age growth plate epiphyses can be vulnerable. This may be a factor especially with high impact sports like rugby and that fast bowling action repeated so frequently.

    To put serious 'hip' in perspective of someone at this age – in my whole career of seeing this sort of problem I can remember only one youngster with groin pain and a slightly odd presentation who turned out to have a distinct pathological cause. It had been missed by his GP. After an x-ray it turned out he had a benign tumour in the head of his femur! The consultant wasn't keen to operate but said he'd keep an eye on it. Ten years later he came to see me with a neck problem and told me that the hip had been problematic on and off for about two years, he kept up all the exercises and shifted from road running to cycling which helped. He also said he'd completely forgotten about the problem until the neck started and he thought of me! No the pain didn't return at that moment and he had gone back to running.

    c. Now some important 'pain mechanism' points! The statement above that there are 'joint' and 'muscle' signs – in terms of pain, it could be that some, or all of the positive tests are a reflection of 'secondary hyperalgesia' or, if it's easier to follow, see it as referred sensitivity into the 'positively' tested muscles. There may be nothing wrong with them. So, if you had to pin me down to where in this lad's body I would take my mini-submarine to have a look: from what I've found I would say that the hip was vaguely at the centre of the problem (primary hyperalgesia therefore 'true positive') and it's clearly stiff and pain is produced at end range of some tests. I would also say that the pain was wholly a referral pain – rather like those occasional hips you see where all the pain is in the thigh and knee and the patient can't believe it's their hip that is the cause.

    So if we're talking primary and secondary hyperalgesia and referred pain there must be 'central' mechanisms to consider. The notion of adaptive v maladaptive is important here – and I would argue that the processing system is doing its best to tell him the tissues aren't quite right. The problem is that to Dylan, they're not giving him a 'move me' message and he's just assumed he has to rest and take it easy. Output mechanisms – well yes! You can work those out and don't forget to think about what he's thinking!

The big point I want to make is that just because there's a clear on-off pain with testing – don't immediately assume that the tissue tested is at fault/injured/pathological.

   d. I need to discuss the findings with him and make them make sense, even give him a simple diagnosis 'If you saw a Dr this is what they would diagnose,' but with me my physio diagnosis is the list of all the hip and muscle tests that are stiff, or hurt and that are waiting to be improved. They're all in our 'Shopping basket'.

2.   **Psychosocial**

   a. Some obvious trepidation to start with during the physical – so being protective and avoidant/resting behaviour – because it worked before. Now seeking advice on this, so not a problem. Certainly not a 'passive coper'.

   b. Bound to be pissed-off/concerned/frustrated to some extent because he's not doing the sport he loves. Getting him going and fitter immediately should make him feel better. A bit of success should produce a bit of 'Belief and Optimism' – remember BO!

   c. Return to full confidence is vital to keep in mind here. It means that he needs to gradually put the hip/groin 'to the test' with ever increasing intensity.

   d. Although I haven't discussed it, Dylan is like most athletes – keen to do all he can to help himself.

3.   **Function/activity restrictions**

   a. Not only has he stopped playing the games he enjoys, he's also stopped going to the gym and keeping fit which he's quite capable of doing.

   b. Jogging, running... to be tackled immediately!

4. Impairments

    a. There are plenty of seemingly relevant physical findings, some relate to joint, some to muscle/tendon and some to a bit of both and some show pain on-off consistency i.e. have mechanically patterned responses.

    b. There's the loss of range and modest stiffness/pain towards adduction and with the hip rotations – most particularly in the hip flexed position; there's the resistance through range response to abduction and adduction in sitting and most of all the static resistance to medial and lateral rotation done sitting.

    c. Some of the responses may well reflect tissue changes; others may be secondary hyperalgesia – tissues normal but sensitive to mechanical forces – stretch, loading, touch etc.

    d. Graded recovery of hip fitness looks vital. In its current state it is best described as vulnerable.

5. General Health

    a. He cannot be as fit as he normally would be and has neglected keeping fit.

    b. Getting going with general fitness immediately is a priority and should make him feel better in himself.

6. Pain

    a. At this stage the best approach is to restore the impairments in parallel with general fitness and observe the pain. He has plenty to work on. His route to recovery can be plotted and explained by a modification and massive simplification of figure 17.3.

Thoughts: if you reflect on the findings and the sorts of things that provoke the pain, there are usually some features that don't fit in most patients' presentations. For example, for Dylan, how would fast bowling have brought all this on? Fast bowling isn't in flexion adduction or sitting positions! Well, watch a right handed fast bowler in slow motion on YouTube and after he lets the ball go his trunk flexes down and to the left over the straight left leg. In fact there's a massive jarring of force going up through the whole leg into the pelvis as it flexes and rides over the hip joint. So it's a hard jarring already in some flexion, then flex and side flex and rotate to the left until the trunk is almost below the horizontal, the left hip goes into flexion-adduction and there's bound to be some internal hip rotation to... then the right leg comes through and the bowler starts to come up again. Dylan's action was just this when I looked at it the following treatment – plus he turned his left foot in as he planted it – medially rotating the hip then doing all the above on it. Pop that in the shopping basket!

One other aspect of this is that loss of adduction is common in osteoarthritic hips and easily reveals itself if you get the patient to do what I call my 'hip-drop' test. It's very similar to the Trendelenburg test which tests for weak hip abductors but with a different interpretation and different instructions to the patient.

For the Trendelenburg test you simply get the patient to stand on one leg and if they can keep the pelvis level they're fine. If they've got weak abductors on the standing leg – the opposite 'hip' to the stance leg drops down and the patient struggles to stop it! Sometimes it is very subtle. Anyway, think weak muscle due to hip disease (but is very common post hip surgery) and also due to neuropathy – these muscles are supplied by L4, 5 and S1 – but mostly think L5 clinically. So they're very likely to be weak in common lumbar nerve root presentations but largely get ignored, not tested and not worked in standard 'sciatic' treatments and rehabilitation.

Quick test: 'Where do you go to test L5 myotome?' and the usual poor answer, 'Somewhere in the foot Louis, is it evertors or invertors, or maybe the big toe extension, oh and foot dorsiflexion?' Exactly, you fiddle round in the foot and forget that it's the hamstringsa nd all three of the glutei but mainly the two abductor muscles – medius and minimus. L5 is a part of all foot movements.

The nerve that supplies the hip abductors is the 'superior gluteal nerve' and leaves the lumbo-sacral plexus at a spot just above the piriformis – a spot that's often sore and very tender in a great many patients! I wonder how many hard and deep thumbs and points of elbows have caused a bit of a neuropathy here! Those mythical money making muscle knots again? 'Look Deirdre, you've got piriformis syndrome, but in reality (and in this historic maritime town of ours) what you've really got are two half hitches and a bowline in your buttock! I'm going to work them loose and then we'll be able to untie them for you!'

In the 'hip drop' test I get the patient to stand on one leg on a book usually about one to two inches thick to start with. Then, keeping the stance leg knee dead straight, I ask the patient to see if they can lower the free foot to the floor and touch it – but with the heel so as to not cheat by extending the foot. This effectively tests the weight-bearing hips' ability to adduct. It is very commonly stiff and painful in arthritic hips but also in conditions where pain is on the lateral side of the hip. This is because the test works and stretches these tissues too. One classic diagnosis is 'trochanteric bursitis', a diagnosis which to my mind really means pain in the lateral hip area of unknown cause. Invariably with this 'diagnosis' the tendons of the gluteus muscles are tender and in particular where they attach to the greater trochanter and distally. What's good about the test is that the book/little platform can be raised and lowered to find the patient's limit but also to find an easy pain free range to start working from. Always check the good side first, which is what I did with Dylan.

He was able to do a good hip drop from about a two inches high book on the right but on the left was only about half that and it hurt.

Early management

If it was old manual therapist me I would probably have got stuck into mobilising and trying to free his hip – into flexion adduction and maybe rotation in flexion and then re-tested some of the sitting findings. But my priority at the end of the treatment and with only about five minutes left was to get him to get going. Besides, since biasing to keeping my hands-off patients in the sub-acute and beyond situations far more, I've been pleased to find that simply getting patients like Dylan going and more confident leads to many of the 'positive tests' sorting themselves out to quite an astonishing degree sometimes.

Dylan enjoyed the gym and was pleased to hear I wanted him to start getting fit and that next time I'd get more focused with his 'stiff' hip problem. He could clearly see what I had in the 'Shopping Basket' and we discussed it all. 'Shopping basket' was a term that I'd introduced to him when I found the first 'positive' pain producing sign – the sitting ab and adduction tests. It went something like this:

'Everything I find that might be relevant to your problem I put in what I call my 'shopping basket' those two tests are in!' I said and then went on... 'It usually gets slowly filled with things to do, to work on, to desensitise or get fitter and freer in some way. I'll make a mental note of them all and you can too, come the end we'll see what we've got.'

Back to the present now: 'I think it would be worth you coming back in three or four days time so we can really get going, my allotted time with you is running out now so how about the following between then and now'

This is the essence of what we discussed:

a) 'Get going again at the gym; the rule here is 'start easy' and then 'build slowly.' The worst thing is to overdo it, make it all worse and then be put-off going again. I'd much rather you did 50% less of what you think you can do for the first few sessions and then gradually start building from there. If you're embarrassed to be in the gym with your mates being wimpy then go when it's quiet and they're not there.'

b) 'Next rule: when we use movement to help recovery and where there is pain we have two ways of tackling it. The first is by what's called desensitising – that means bringing on the pain and repeating it until the pain eventually goes – you get slowly get used to it, rather like those who swim in the sea all the year round. The problem with this approach is that it can make the pain worse and worse rather than better. The trick is in choosing the right time to do it and that is rarely straight away – so we are very likely to come back to it later on.' The second way of tackling it is via what we call the 'fire apart-depart' approach *(use figure 14.2 from chapter 14   it's a good hand-out)*. Normally when you do a movement or activity and it hurts, the circuit in your nervous system for the pain wires itself up with the circuit that produces the movement. This rule is called 'circuits that wire together fire together'. It's rather like every time you hear a certain piece of music it brings a specific and sometimes strong memory flooding into your head.'

If you do the movements that hurt in a slightly different way it's possible to do them with no hurt, for example, not doing them quite so hard, so far into range, or with so much force. This is 'fire-apart-depart' and this is how we're going to start all the exercises with you – so that they don't hurt, but are working the area we want to get freer, less sensitive and fit again. I'd like you to take this simple rule to the gym – use any machine, do any exercise but when the exercise involves the left leg, do it in a comfortable way with no pain. It means you might have to play around with the exercise, the amount of weight, how far you go through range and so forth. I'd much rather you did lots of mini circuits of the leg machines than did lots on just one of them. We know for example that five minutes jogging brings it on, we also now know that it comes on after doing several minutes of stretching then hopping on one leg here with me and so on.

Dylan understood and was pleased.

'Should I swim?'

'Crawl, yes and cycle, yes and rower... same rules for all... get the cardiovascular system going is what we want but keep the rule going – keep comfortable. You should find more out about it too.

'What about actual jogging but just doing a minute or so?'

'Great! – make a start on the treadmill and give the cross-trainer a try as well. Try starting with about two minutes. If you do several circuits of all the exercises you can repeat the two minutes a few times. I'd be interested to hear what happens.

Second visit – 4 days later:

Dylan walked in and sat down.

'How've you got on, did you manage the gym at all?'

'All fine, I've been twice and out on the bike twice as well, I didn't get to the pool for a swim. I've got going and feel a lot better in myself, I've kept it all short of any pain so I've no idea what it's like except I've been crossing my legs to test it and it actually feels a bit easier. I also did five repetitions of the two minutes on the cross-trainer during the hour and a half I was there yesterday.'

'Great, if we add all the two minutes up that's ten minutes running in total and no pain.'

This is typical of these sorts of pains that take time to come on doing an activity (or inactivity) – if you stop before they come on, then do something else for a while or rest, you often find you can go on again for roughly the same amount of time without pain.[1] I hope you can use the same principles for those who cannot sit – in

---

1 - *see chapter 14.2 'Pete' — a calf strain where this 'principle' of run with no pain under the normal pain onset time, then walk for a while, then run on again, was very successful.*

a 'reverse' kind of way. Tip: if you do this – the patient must have a timer that pings when time's up!

I then repeated all the shopping basket 'Impairment' tests I'd noted and found them to be more or less the same responses as before. Interestingly, a slight shift further into range of the pain responses and having to push a bit harder to get the pain response – especially with static medial and lateral rotation sitting, which was encouraging but nothing spectacular.

I decided it was important to 'set the scene' for his problem as I saw it and also think about and discuss some kind of recovery time and recovery pathway. In this instance it's easier said than done and 'response to input/treatment' over a few weeks may be the only way to have any idea. I have to say that some form of young persons' 'hip' issue (dysplasia, epiphyses etc.) was in the back of my mind. On the other hand getting him a good deal fitter in the hip and the whole lower quadrant would be essential for the kinds of high impact sports he was keen on and if there was a significant problem progress would be hampered at some point. Dylan was definitely one to follow up and keep in touch with.

I also decided I wanted to get him exercising, instead of me 'doing a technique' on him and then reassessing some of the salient 'Impairments' – just like Maitland, do-test-prove-repeat, but here with the patient doing the work and therefore able to take it home with him.

'Right Dylan, I think you've got a fairly clear picture from last time of what we found.'

He nodded.

'Here are my thoughts as it stands now. First, great that you've got back to the gym, if you're going to carry on doing rugby and fast-bowling without setting yourself up for more problems it's essential you're fit and a lot fitter than now. We also know that fit people heal a great deal faster than the unfit and that exercises creates chemicals like endorphins that control pain and too much inflammation – they help get the healing environment just right. So, good start.'

'Your findings indicate several things': this is a summary of what I discussed/told him

   a) 'Your left hip is a bit stiff and painful, the key movements are; when you cross your legs; when you bring your foot onto your right knee and drop the left knee; when you do that hip drop on the book; when you're lying and you let your leg go out sideways and when I take your knee across your body towards your shoulder.'

   b) 'You've got some muscles which produce pain when we get them to contract – like those tests I do to you when you're sitting. Remember, muscles are made of tendon and muscle and that tendons are very tough – that's good but they heal quite slowly which we need to be aware of.'

   c) 'You're young – which is an advantage because the young heal very well and usually quickly. However, it's gone on a bit long with you, so it's a little hard to predict how long it's going to take. It's going to be far easier to have a better idea when we get you going and see how you respond to getting the hip freer and the hip muscles stronger. We're going to get going with that right now.'

d) 'The big thing may be that there's been a bit of hip stiffness and weakness for a while and that's made it vulnerable to becoming painful again.'

e) 'We'll still call it a 'groin' strain but as you can see there's a bit more to it than just the adductor muscles.'

We then went to work. I wanted to get his hip muscles working against some resistance without pain. I used blue Theraband elastic tied low down to the leg of the treatment couch and looping around his lower tibia/foot. He did standing ab and adduction – from outer to inner range with no pain – he could do hip flexion and extension through range a large range too... it all went on the 'to-do' list in the context of 'start getting the hip muscles fitter'. I also got him to try abduction in side lying. Side lying doing hip abduction is a quite useful test position because you can do the leg lifts in a huge arc from approx 90 degrees of flexion way into extension – let the knee bend if it wants to because of tight hamstrings. Dylan found that doing abduction in flexion through a horizontal arc of about 45 degrees brought on the pain... from there to neutral was fine. So his exercise was abduction in pretty much neutral to get the leg going. He understood the principle and could find the position fine.

If you've ever had problems with patients twisting their trunk to do this it really shows that their leg wants the help of the hip flexors. Now, I'm not a great one to want to really 'isolate' things as you've probably gathered, but I'm quite capable of being very precise and isolationist if I need to be. Anyway, that aside, if you want to make sure you work the hip abductors and keep the tendency to cheat and use the hip flexors by twisting – have the patient lie on their side with a wall behind them and make sure the trunk is pressed against the wall at all times. Further, if you want to stop the leg drifting forward – get them to keep the heel on the wall as they go up and down.

Clearly, if abduction in side lying is too difficult or painful – I'm thinking of my old hip OA and my post hip replacement patients – obviously the easiest starting position is standing. Remember, that for every movement that the body has you should have in your head a 'hierarchy' of difficulty and that means making the most of as many different starting positions for that movement as you can. Be inventive so that you can always find a position that the patient can do the movement from with ease. 'Make it easy' is an important part of the start of any graded programme as I've already discussed.

Back to Dylan: I then repositioned the elastic and got him to do through range resisted ab and adduction and both rotations in sitting legs dangling position – elastic round foot, but for ab and adduction it can go round the knee somewhere or stay round the foot,. We soon found that he could do full range pain free adduction and abduction by getting him to lean back slightly. If he brought his trunk forwards it was far worse. This simple change obviously shifts the pelvis a little and changes the dynamics of the hip movement. Try it, see what it feels like! He could actually work the elastic quite strongly by leaning back on his hands to support and relax the trunk. It was exactly the same for the resisted rotations. They were all on the 'to-do' list.

What's good about this sort of starting position fiddling is that it often reveals a potential pathway for exploring 'desensitising' when the time is right. Thus, 'fire-apart-depart' here is doing it while leaning back. Exploring desensitising nudges into the pain by bringing the trunk forward... further and further. So, it usually start -off right on the edge of the discomfort and as confidence and vigour builds the patient goes further forward into gradually more pain. That's nicely graded. You could try 'flooding' by going for it right into the thick of the pain, so for Dylan's hip that means do it in lots of flexion. To me flooding is exactly what the McKenzie approach does, fine if it works, but its friggin' fireworks when it doesn't and for me it's usually 'fireworks' and a very disgruntled patient. Why doesn't it work for me anymore? Answer, because I don't believe it's a good idea to do it like that, the patient picks up on my uncertain bravado and hey, they get worse. Proves it's all to do with processing and gating to me, read the McKenzie debate:

http://giffordsachesandpains.com/download-material/the-full-mckenzie-debate/

Right lets now end the session and finish the story of Dylan.

At the end of this second session this is what he had on his sheet. It was actually my stick men for the quick visual reminder plus appropriate words, like 'fire-apart-depart', 'start easy, build slowly', 'nice, smooth easy relaxed', 'work to done something feeling'... 'Succeed-not-fail' etc.

Fire-apart-depart:

- **Standing:** elastic for hip abduction, adduction, flexion and extension

- **Side lying:** hip abduction trunk against wall

- **Sitting leaning back:** abduction, adduction and rotations

Try 3-4 times a day; start easy with 20-30 repetitions. If OK start building reps and times you do it per day. Try to build it up and get to that, 'done something feeling' to start with.

- carry on in the gym and build as you feel

- treadmill – up it 30 seconds every time you go... goal 4.5 minutes by next time – a week... or as you see fit... try adding the cross-trainer too, but start round the 3 minute mark and build from there

- Ring me if any queries or concerns.

Note in the whole session I didn't address anything to improve the range of movement. Why? Because this stage was 'fire-apart-depart' and in order to start stretching he would be going into pain. Save that for next time, or if 'touchy' and poor progress – perhaps even longer.

Don't panic, I do teach the patient stretches into pain at the same time in this sort of thing, but here I didn't and I've given you the reason why!

Third visit – one week later

Like most sportsmen and women Dylan got going and couldn't help but put it a little to the test as he'd found it all going easily and to plan. He'd even started using the hip ab and adductor machines at the gym, leaning back was a little difficult because of the fixed back-rest but now he said he didn't need to because there was no pain doing it. Great, what about the running/jogging and the cross-trainer? He was up to ten minutes three times on the circuits on both machines. Great, what about the elastic exercises? He'd ripped the blue elastic and was now using an inner tube. Great, what about crossing his legs and had he tried the foot up drop the knee in sitting or the stand on the book and drop the leg down. Crossing his legs was easier but he hadn't tried the others.

I then had a look at him and the hip-drop was nearly the same on both legs – that went on the 'to-do' list occasionally. I showed him how he could do it without being on a book i.e. 'Latin-American style hips darling' – the cha-cha walk! (I omitted the 'darling'!)

Sitting foot up and drop the knee was half way there, sitting in full trunk flexion there was still pain at end of range etc. They all went on the list of things to do. He left with some simple stretches to extend the range and the 'desensitise' approach – push into pain and repeat, gets easier and freer or simply stretch sensation on and sensation off with no lingering discomfort for more than ten minutes. I like patients to do stretching a few times a day and not get obsessed by them... so three times a day and spend about five minutes doing them as well as doing them as part of his normal stretching warm-up routine in the gym.

We discussed bowling action and his 'turned-in' foot position and we practiced slow-mo with foot turned about 45 degrees to start with, then brought it in to neutral or just out so he got the feel of it. Now, while he wasn't bowling, was the best time for him to start to try and imprint a subtly different bowling action, but as we all know changing a well ingrained motor habit isn't very easy – witness the agonies top golfers can go through when making drastic 'swing changes'. Here's what helped. This was about three or four months after he first came to me – he was back into rugby and luckily it was winter so the only cricket was practice, mainly with his mate, in the school sports-hall practice nets. What we did was make a card-board cut-out of a giant footprint—it was about four feet long—and got him to place it, tilted up at a slight angle about four feet to the left of the bowling wicket. In this way the foot was firmly in his line of sight on the run up! He told me it made the whole thing easy. Amazing, I guess we could have made it gradually smaller and smaller until it wasn't necessary... in a graded exposure/learning/neuroscience way of thinking, but he found that when he got on the pitch he was doing it without thinking about it and ceremoniously burned the foot. One problem with stuff like this is that it is a reminder that there's a problem, so sometimes it can work against you.

So to backtrack a little:

- he increased his running in a similar way to 'Runner Pete' in chapter 14.2

- he also started varying the pace, change of direction and built up to sprints and acceleration practice as he would in normal rugby practice but just more gradually

- he kept with the stretches by simply adding them to his normal routine

- about one week after this third appointment we dumped all the hip elastic exercises

- this was the last session I had with him, from here on we had two telephone conversations, I phoned him.

  (If you do it the other way, silly though it may sound, some patients start getting you in mind and start to dwell on the problem! So, mostly I tell the patient that I'll call them sometime to see how they're going, but they're free to call me anytime)

- after the phone conversations he reckoned it had taken about three months to get to 'forgotten about it' stage, but about three weeks or so after first consult to feel pretty much 100%.

LOUIS GIFFORD ACHES AND PAINS

CHRONIC

Chapter CH 3.1
The Ghost of Mr Grubb – 'Grouty'

You may remember Mr Grubb from chapter GE 3.2, the chapter on 'pain behaviour' and you may also recall 'Vivien in the Volvo' from chapter 1.

Mr Grubb was the patient at Geoff Maitland's practice, who was a chronic pain sufferer and had marked maladaptive pain behaviour – recall that he took nearly ten minutes to get to the cubicle and get comfortable, his body chart was nearly completely covered with shading, indicating some symptom or other. I called him an example of *'the hardest patients on the planet'*. His movements were incredibly tense and jerky, he held himself all the time, he wore a lumbar binder on the outside of his shirt, he used elbow crutches to walk and he'd had the problem years and years. He'd seen everyone and he didn't really listen. These patients appear to be disasters but when the pain is coldly ignored, there's no sign of serious pathology – they've had all the scans and x-rays and all the treatments you've ever heard of and some you've never heard of and quite often, they're still expecting someone to be able to find out what's wrong and provide the 'cure'.

The Mr and Mrs Grubb's of the world are very hard to deal with using standard practice and most are realistically only likely to benefit from CBT/pain management approach in specialised units. Even then the results may not be that marvelous.

Now, unlike Mr Grubb, Vivien in the Volvo's pain had started hours before I saw him, yet he was similarly physically 'locked-up' and could hardly move, he grabbed onto the furniture, he was bent double, grunted and groaned, he held his breath, held his back, swore and cursed – in an almost identical way to Mr Grubb!

 So a simple observation is that a great many maladaptive on-going pain states may be a reflection of an early stage of healing and recovery that they've become stuck in! To a distant observer, without any knowledge of the background, Mr Grubb and Vivien are almost identically afflicted.

The key from this thought is that it makes one possible avenue of treatment a bit more obvious – to shift, or transition to the next phase, then the next and so forth. This way of thinking sometimes makes it an easy way of explaining things and the reason for the approach you're going to offer.

The ghost of Mr Grubb is Mr Grout, and this is no longer Geoff Maitland's practice all those years ago but here in my practice about eight years ago with me a good deal wiser. 'Grouty' sits facing me, he's overweight and sweating, he holds his breath, speaks and holds his breath, the one crutch he uses falls on the floor and he struggles and squirms to pick it up. To witness it is movement palaver and the inner thoughts are that there's never a dull moment and never anything straight-forward with pain problems – ever! He rocks slightly in the chair and repeatedly tries to take the weight off his back by pushing through his arms. He ends up leaning away from me and putting the pillow I offer between his legs. If only I could get this on film?

I will summarise the early details of his problem:

    1. Twenty year history of back pain, became constant ten years ago and was

forced to retire. Now on income support and has a disability allowance He's 45 years old, married and living with his wife, who works as a classroom assistant in a local school. He has a son and a daughter in their late teens who are both at school. His mother-in-law lives at home with them and he immediately expresses his dislike for her.

2. He has no hobbies now but used to walk the dog for an hour every day and used to read a lot. He stopped that in the last four to five years. He used to work as a driver for a local fruit and veg. supplier and socialised at least once a week with a few of his work mates. He no longer sees them.

3. He's had three operations on his back to remove discs from nerves. They all made him worse. He now has pain from upper thoracic level to his feet. It's worse in his back and buttocks. He can't feel his feet very well. He takes eight codeine a day and occasional oromorph. Has tried amytriptyline and gabapentin. He rarely sleeps in the bed and spends most nights (and a good deal of his days) in his 'recliner'.

4. He doesn't go out of the house now and finds being on his feet ten minutes about the maximum. He usually uses one crutch. He can sit in his recliner for several hours before wanting to get out – which is usually very difficult. He gets out of breath very easily and is thinking of getting the social services to put a stair lift in for him.

5. He has had physio, OT, pain clinic (TENS and acupuncture and given gabapentin), osteopathy, chiropractic, acupuncture, the 'healing of the stars' lady and tried homeopathy remedies. Nothing helps and exercise makes it far worse.

6. He says, 'I've been told my back has got osteoarthritis and that I've got to live with it.'

7. ... and so on...

When I got to this stage I thought about running through all the ABCDEFW questions, or getting him to fill in the Linton and Halden Yellow flag questionnaire... maybe getting him to do the DRAM (Zung and MSPQ questionnaires)... even the Tampa scale of Kinesiophobia[1] – all useful starting scores and great to assess any areas where I could help or that others may be required. But I didn't because I was thinking, on the one hand, 'what on earth is he expecting from me I wonder?' and on the other, 'the only way I'm going to get anywhere is if I can get him actively engaged in recovery. That could be a big ask!'

'Grouty (he'd asked me to call him that) I'm sitting here wondering what you're expecting from me and also, why you've come – seeing how you've been so unsuccessful with physio and other treatments in the past. Has someone sent you

---

1 - See http://www.tac.vic.gov.au/files-to-move/media/upload/tampa_scale_kinesiophobia.pdf

or have you decided to come yourself?'

'A week ago I got up and the wife had gone out with her mother so the house was empty, it was nice. I got up as I usually do and had a shower and looked at myself in the mirror, it wasn't pretty and, well, it upset me. I thought about all the treatments and surgeries I've had and how they all seemed to just push me further and further down the slope to, well, to nothing, just more pain and a kind of sub-existence. So in desperation I went to the Dr and told him how I felt. This time I got a new bloke who was even worse than the others. He wasn't even interested in me and said, 'What do you expect me to be able to do for you?' So I said, 'I'm desperate, surely there must be something,' and he just said 'You've had them all Mr Grout, there's nothing left that medicine can do, that's it, you need to learn to live with it, you need to lose some weight and do some exercise, get fit and help yourself.' If I'd been more agile I'd of punched him, as it was I told him to 'get fucked' and left as fast as I could muttering that I was going to report him.

Anyway, I've been mad ever since and I've been giving it some thought and wanted to give treatment one more go and your name cropped up – apparently my brother-in-law came to see you with his bad back last year and he's been brilliant ever since.'

'So here we are, I'm a physiotherapist – what are you thinking in terms of me helping you?'

'I know you can't fix arthritis of the spine but there might be something you can do to help.'

'OK, but what's your experience of physio in the past – I know it didn't help but what happened?'

'In the last twenty years I've been referred to physio probably at least ten times and it's nearly always walking in the bars and a 'back' exercise print-off, you know ten three times a day, oh and I had a course of eight hydrotherapies once – which was quite nice at the time. There was once when a fellow tried to crack my back off but I just tensed up too much – no one's ever managed it, most of those other therapists do really gentle stuff that's like, well I could do it at home with a feather duster probably and anyway I was always a lot worse whatever they did. There was one fellow who persisted with trying to re-align me which I fell for.'

There was a pause and he took a deep breath.

'I'm so desperate, I just want someone to try and help me.'

He struggled to speak and I said.

'I know you do and I'm going to tell you a story in a minute of someone just like you and what happened to them. I'd then like you to consider the story in your own time and come back and tell me what you think.'

Before I tell you the story, it seems that over the years some of the Drs and therapists have suggested you do exercises and get active – have you given that a try, and what happened there?'

'Look I'd love to get active and lose weight but as soon as I do anything it makes it worse, besides I get nagged at home about doing too much.'

'In what way?'

'Well everyone tells me not to all the time and the kids tell me think what I'm doing is pathetic I think they laugh at me if I'm honest. I don't blame them, I'm just a nuisance, I don't interact, I don't help even if I want to they stop me. They don't understand. No one understands. Even the bloody job centre doesn't. I mean how can anyone work with pain from back arthritis and three failed operations?'

It seemed there were plenty of barriers to him helping himself – the 'F' for family being one and the blue and black flags were others.

The reason I decided to tell him a patient story was because I wanted him to hear a possible pathway that could improve things and one which was the only realistic way forward. It was to show him that he had an opportunity to improve matters if he wanted to take it. By using another patient example and asking him for his opinion I wouldn't be telling him like the Dr's have, I'd just be showing him an option to go down.

The example was of a patient, just like him, who made slow but massive changes to his life and improved well over quite a long period.   The patient made a lot of changes himself, learnt the skills of graded exposure, learned to direct his own programme and gradually learned how to cope far better and get fitter.

The key thing about these sorts of patients is that a 'patient orientated approach' is essential. This is one where the clinician acts as a facilitator, listens more than talks, gives guidance, acts as an educator, but massively tries to avoid using what's called 'advice-giving,' 'telling' and 'lecturing' like the recent Dr did. Where the only helpful way forward with a problem is with an approach that requires the patient having to change their behaviour and make a big conscious effort – just being 'told' to do it hardly ever works. Take dieting and giving up smoking! Even the words 'you will die and become very ill soon if you don't diet/give up smoking' – doesn't bring about the desired effect for a great many. We are all good at making an effort for a day or two, but to keep something going for a long time isn't at all easy. In order to succeed some of the important ingredients with chronic pain are:

- the patient has to understand and see the importance of the process that will help them (graded exposure/rehabilitation) and what they're going to have to do

- they have to see that its value

- they have to want to do it and have to find the right time to do it

- there needs to be a plan of action prepared and ready to put in place

- the patient needs support and guidance – someone close to 'hold their hand' while they get going and to teach them what to do – that's the therapists role but those at home are massively important too

- any barriers to the process need to be addressed and dealt with if at all possible

I would recommend that all students of physiotherapy should study and be examined on 'health behaviour change.' The best practical book that I've ever come across on this topic is by Stephen Rollnick and his two colleagues, Pip Mason and Chris Butler – 'Health Behaviour Change': A Guide for Practitioners. Churchill Livingstone, Edinburgh. I have a 2002 edition.

With Grouty I used and built up the graph shown in figure GE 2.4 in chapter GE2.2 – but hugely modified it to fit with Ray's story I was about to tell. Ray was purposely very similar to Grouty – and this is a summary of what I told him...

... 'Ray' had a long history, could hardly move, had sharp pain and huge tension with pain, there'd been lots of unsuccessful interventions and lots of therapy with limited success and lots of mind- bending drugs. Ray was similar in age to Grouty and had been involved in an accident at work (welder at the docks) that had fractured his pelvis. I saw him ten years after the accident and he'd been off work and in a great deal of pain the whole time.

I showed and explained to Grouty Ray's story by building the graph which I drew freehand and wrote on. Here are some of things I wrote:

- no instant cure arrow, not possible – I told Grouty that Ray was shocked at this...

- bottom left corner is start... fitness on the vertical axis, time on the horizontal

- slow start – I drew a very gradual series of long slowly rising steps – so there were obvious periods when nothing moved on, I drew dips, to show backward progress at times...

- I wrote near the beginning 'relaxed/low tension movement practice' and said he had to relearn to stand, to walk and to move around with normal tension and movement patterns

- further to the right I wrote small gains in confidence... and also, 'starting to accept' slow progress is OK...

- a third step at about six weeks – start walking programme one to two mins, two to three times per day

- noticed sleeping a bit less in day

- fourth step – now has exercise programme – stretches and some light resistance, start very easy build slowly...

- walking ten minutes with no sticks... at six months.

And so on. Nothing negative, everything realistic, set-backs, pain up and down, frustration normalised etc.

(Note I picked a particularly slow progress patient on purpose – I wanted Grouty to get the reality of recovery and that if he did start a programme and was quicker to progress, it would be more pleasing)

By the time I'd finished the story I'd drawn three graphs gradually getting steeper and steeper – that covered about eighteen months.

There were words like:

- pain far less of a problem, back in control
- far more confident physically and socially...
- better atmosphere at home
- smooth and relaxed movement
- swimming twice a week, walking with wife for up to two hours
- thinking of building up to jog/running despite being told never to by two consultants
- lost three stone
- came off all the drugs (the hardest thing of all)
- started teacher-training course – something he'd always wanted to do.

I then said…

'Grouty, that was over five years ago, Ray is now a full time technology teacher up at the local school, you wouldn't know he had a problem.

I gave Grouty the graphs and all the notes I'd written. I told him to share it with his wife and to come back and tell me what he thought about it and what she had too. He could come back anytime, with, or without his wife – that was up to him.

I also said that the key thing about Ray's journey was that I helped him a great deal in the slow frustrating early stages and I also helped make sure he wasn't downed too far by failing, getting mad and giving up. I also told him that Ray was around and he'd more than likely to be happy to chat about his experiences.

I asked him if he wanted to ask anything or make any comments.

'Looks like there's nothing you can do,' he said pointing to the 'instant cure not possible line.'

I pointed at the other line and said, 'That line is something to think about.'

Grouty left with a sigh, he didn't look that happy. He flinched and groaned and grappled with his stick down the corridor, just like when he came in. I thought I was unlikely to see him again. Maybe I should have done a bit of movement with him, shown him that he could change with a bit of guidance? However, that desire to make an instant change is a 'show-off' throwback from old manual therapy days and inappropriate here and what if I failed anyway.

Note that what I'm doing here with Grouty is sometimes called '**setting the agenda**.' We both need our expectations of therapy to match, which is why I asked him about his expectations of physiotherapy and it's also why I've needed to explain, via Ray's narrative, what I can offer him as well as what I am not prepared to offer him.

So Grouty had gone and before the next patient I jotted his name and the date in a little book I have called 'patients'. It mostly contains the names of patients who have interesting case histories. At the back there's a list of those I want to contact and follow-up which I often do, may be a year or more after last seeing them. It's the only way I can really find out what happened. Grouty's went in the back.

So here's one follow-up conversation from long ago... (c 1990)

'Hi, Louis here, the physio – you came to me a year ago with your back pain, I was wondering what happened and how you're getting on?'

'Oh, yeah, I remember, yeah, you stretched my leg a load, it helped a bit, but amazing – two weeks after seeing you I went to see that healing lady over on the north coast (of Cornwall) – cured! Walked in doubled up, walked out straight, only £5.00! ... felt this weird warmth in the back and was out in five minutes...'

'You mean 'The Healer of the Stars' lady who drives round in a Rolls, who inherited the healing gift from her mother, is that one?' I ask.

'Yeah, that's the one you should refer patients to her...'

'OK, glad you're better.' I put the phone down gently.

'Fuck!'

Ah, I thought I'd sorted that guy... Those early follow-ups and those sort of responses were among many of the reasons why I became so sceptical about what I was doing and what everyone else was doing too. Walking in doubled up and coming out straight in five minutes just wasn't biologically possible to my way of thinking back then... understanding processing change a few years later made a bit more sense of it. The other thing is that many of us can be a trifle generous with the truth from time to time, humans are well known for 'colouring-in' and adding a tad of 'make-up' to embellish life experiences from time to time. Having been to an ex-patient's Christmas party many years ago and introduced... 'Hey everyone, this is Louis – the back man – I walked in doubled up and walked out a spring-chicken, 100% ever since.' The reality was four treatments over about a two months – he had been doubled up for about six months so we did well…

(I wonder what Vivien in the Volvo remembers. Or, Wersey in the pub!)

The interesting thing about healers and the like is that for every apparent evangelical miracle there's a pile of highly dissatisfied, disgruntled, ripped-off and disillusioned refuse that's never heard about or reported. James Randi has followed up a great many of the so called 'healed' and found that the whole thing is a scam and a set-up[1].

Anyway…

Grouty came back three months later. I hadn't phoned him but it was the same pain behaviour performance as before. He eventually sat down with the tension, grunts, groans and stick flying.

'The mother-in-law died about a month after I saw you.'

'Oh, I'm sorry to hear that.'

'Yes, the Dr's and nurses who came were very good with her in actual fact, even the Dr who ignored me. She had a massive bleed in her brain and we looked after her at home, she only lived two weeks.'

He went on…

'Anyway, sad though it was for my wife and the family it's changed the atmosphere at home, my wife's in a sense freer, she spent a lot of time with her mother who was pretty demanding and really never did much to help herself. Typical. Anyway, you don't want to hear all that, but in the last couple of weeks I've been thinking about that patient of yours, that Ray who retrained and became a teacher after years of back pain like mine. My wife is still sceptical but I realise that it's worth a go so long as it's not sheets of bloody exercises that make me worse... and I need to ask you some questions.'

He'd written them down.

'Off you go.'

'Right first one, did Ray have arthritis in his spine like mine? The thing is that if he just had pain and no arthritis, he's bound to do better.'

'The answer to that is yes he did, he had what's called 'spondylosis' of his whole lumbar spine and the base of his neck but worse at his lower back levels.'

'That's the exact diagnosis they use with me.'

---

1 - *Type 'James Randi healing' into Youtube search and be amazed and disgusted at what you see revealed. Or get hold of Randi J (2011) The Faith Healers. James Randi Educational Foundation for more details. I think it's essential reading.*

I then showed him some x-rays I have of the backs of active people – Wallace (see figure xx) being one of them. I also showed him the very useful lumbar scans of identical twins[1] – one of them was a very active farmer, the other was a desk bound journalist and they were 50 years old at the time of the scans. Both show evidence of obvious degeneration, disc bulging and spondylosis. You cannot tell which belongs to which, yet physically they experienced very different loads and forces over a great many years.

Grouty was fascinated.

'My next question on the list is – surely being more active is going to make all the arthritis, the wear and tear a lot worse?... but I'm now also wanting to ask – why do I hurt so much then?

'I'll answer the last question first.'

I use the XXX on the computer explanation (see chapter GE 5). But note I missed out the bit at the end that says that says that 'your pain can recover just like your mother-in-law's neuralgia pain did.' The last thing you want to create with this sort of patient is any certain notion that the approach will lead to the pain going – but see my answer to his question about the pain going below...

This is the essence of my answer about wear and tear and activity...

'The answer to whether arthritis, or wear and tear is made worse with being more active needs to be divided into two. The first is about the actual joints themselves and the second is about the pain.'

1. 'There's no evidence that wear and tear is made worse by normal activities, in fact there is increasing evidence that loading is essential for the health of the spine and back regardless of wear and tear. A simple way of thinking about it is the stronger the muscles are, the stronger the protection to the joints, bones and discs of the back. There is evidence that very high levels of on-going strenuous physical activity increase the risk of back injury which is why there are maximum lift recommendations for industry for example[2]. The big deal for you is that a basic principle of nature is that the more the tissues of the body are used the stronger they get – regardless of wear and tear. The key to getting fitter is gradual over time, not sudden, whatever the state of the tissue, and that's exactly what Ray did.'

   I show him my picture of the feet of the *'lady who walks the cliffs.'*

---

1 - *You can find these on page 94 of the 2nd Edition of 'The Back Pain Revolution' by Gordon Waddell. Churchill Livingstone, Edinburgh.*
2 - *See the 'Return to Work' section of Gifford L S (2013) Topical Issues in Pain 5, CNS Press, Falmouth*

2. 'Now the pain aspect of arthritis – does it get worse the more active you are? The answer is on the one hand—yes, if you are sensitised as I've just explained with the keyboard and the computer—but on the other, the answer is no – if you gradually build up and get going, then you can get used to it, like Ray did and you find you can gradually do more and more. The pain overall has a mind of its own to some extent – as I showed you on Ray's graph he occasionally had set-backs where the pain got worse but we worked out how to deal with them and he got better and better at it.

You see that picture of *'the lady who walks the cliffs'* – I had a patient about two years ago with feet just like hers, riddled with arthritic changes and she was also racked with pain in them, she'd spent a fortune on treatments, on shoes, on supports for her feet and nothing had helped. She had loved walking and she was quite distraught that her feet were going to spoil the one thing she wanted to do in her retirement – walk. When I saw her she was barely able to walk 100 metres and not only that, if she did it would leave them sore for hours and sometimes days. I got her onto 'Ray's' graph and she slowly but surely built her walking up. It hurt a lot to start with but she set her levels so she could cope and gradually she built it up and up. She can now walk happily for two hours and doesn't worry about her feet anymore. With the right pace to build up, patience and a bit of determination most people find that they eventually get better and better. I could put you in touch with her to chat about it anytime you want.'

Grouty then looked up and said, 'Will the pain go then?'

'I'm not going to promise you anything about the pain – look, you've had surgery and a whole raft of therapies most of which were unhelpful and those that were helpful only improved things for a little while but were of no overall benefit. With standard treatment, even with some of the best known pain killing drugs, your pain is hard to help. What I can tell you is that most patients who succeed like the feet lady or Ray – they'll tell you that the pain is far less of a problem. Some patients report that the pain as good as goes, others that it doesn't go but seems to become far less threatening. Some say it gets to being like that ringing in the ears problem – 'tinnitus' – it's there all the time, but because you just get on and don't think about it you don't notice it. When you go and look for it, it's still there, singing away… and pain can be exactly the same.

There was a silence, Grouty rocked back and forth and massaged his back. I was thinking to myself that getting these sorts of questions from this sort of patient was quite a breakthrough! They often glaze over with any form of explanation, don't even ask questions and make statements like 'I am in pain you know.'

(In my experience, when patients start asking questions like Grouty is here – I'm more likely to be able to help, usually they don't and here there is far more complexity surrounding the problem. Having a nearby CBT based pain management unit to refer to is probably the best option)

'Have you thought what you want to do, or thought about what Ray did and how he got there?'

'I've been thinking about it every day since I saw you. In fact I tried to get going a bit on my own after my mother-in-law died. I did it by walking for a few minutes every day but I just got worse and got despondent, so with that I actually found Ray's story hard to believe really. The only reason I'm back is because you said he'd speak to me, so I felt he must be real and that speaking might be worthwhile.'

'That's really good that you tried, tell me more about what happened.'

(Note how important this question is – for years I'd have taken the patients statement as a big 'no-no' and a reason to avoid walking, but when you question further about what happened, it's often worthwhile... possibilities are raised.)

'Well the first day I took the stick and walked up the road for two minutes then back again. I was in absolute agony and had to rest for a couple of hours. I did it again in the afternoon and it was the same.'

'The next day I almost didn't get out of bed but I made myself. I had a hot shower, felt a bit better and did the same walk again and again in the afternoon, that evening it was all worse again.'

'So how was it during and immediately after the walks day two compared to the first?'

'Well, I have to admit that it wasn't so bad but the evening it went mad again.'

'So, have you ever noticed this sort of sudden increase in pain on days where you do very little walking?'

'Well, yes, it's like this all the time, I can go quite well for a while then it's really bad.'

'When I first saw Ray, he had the same problem and I showed him the 'Toblerone' pain graph.'

(I then explained the 'Toblerone' graph, not 'Toblerone recovery' to Grouty – see chapter 13.1 and especially figure 13.8 and modify the chat to showing how normal on-going pain behaves)

'Grouty, the big point I'm trying to show you is that it could have been the walking that made your pain worse, or it might have just been going to do that anyway – because your sort of pain, Ray's pain and all the other's like you – have pain that wanders about for seemingly no reason it 'Toblerones' unfortunately.'

'Anyway, I think you've done really well but I'm going to make some suggestions that might help a bit. You can think about them and try them if you want.'

'Go on then.'

'When this happened to Ray, he got mad like you did and we then used the 50% rule. The 50% rule is simply this – for walking, you work out the amount you can walk every day and manage no matter whether you're on a bad day or good day – it's always best to think about what you can manage on a bad day.'

I pause and wait for an answer...

'Well that two minutes up and two minutes I could manage but after four days it just got too much, so how about three minutes?'

'OK, three minutes, now we apply the 50% rule and that means halve it – so the starting walk time for you is round about one and half minutes.'

Grouty rolls his eyes and goes...

'Well, that's pathetic.'

'Well, the 50% rule has been worked out by clinicians who work with your sort of problem day in day out with a great many patients over many years and they find if they don't set it that low the patient fails, gets a flare-up and gets fed up and gives up... '

'Just like I did when I tried!'

I smile and I can see he understands.

'So I try again but do less.'

He then frowned and said, 'Why don't all the Drs and physios and all those other practitioners do this stuff if so many 'clinicians' have been doing it for years and worked it all out like you said just now... '

'That's a very good point and I wish they did know about it and practice it but they mostly feel their treatments are better.'

'You know Louis, I went to this fellow who told me a joint was out of alignment in my back, I might have told you about him last time, this was about six or seven years ago and I went to him for over half a year. I was frightened not to go I think and you know the treatment I had lasted barely five minutes. In the end it made me angry, with him and also with me for being so stupid. I now think those people are taking the micky and rip people like me off... '

'Well you may be right, all I can say now is to give this a try and see how you go, a little success and reaching a goal is a great thing, it's encouraging and hopefully will spur you on to do more. Have you any thoughts about a 'goal' in relation to walking?'

(Dwelling on the past and getting mad with what happened usually isn't helpful. Though getting something off your chest can be... Therapists also believe that they

fix people – I used to until I listened and followed them up!)

'The corner shop is about a five minute walk away, that'd be ten minutes in all.'

'Good one, when you go home I'd like you to think about other similar activity goals – things you'd like to do again but ones that are small and realistic. For this corner shop walk it would be good to come up with a deadline for when you want to achieve it by, what do you think?'

'Well it depends on how I get on I guess, how about two weeks?'

'Well that's fine but in my head I'm going to apply the reverse 50% rule which is to double it. That's four weeks! You don't have to take any notice of what I say, but we have a couple of little sayings here, one is 'Start easy build slowly' and the other which follows 'Succeed not fail' this is especially important when patients are really sensitive and reactive and have been for a very long time... '

The next thing to work out is what's called 'incrementing' – it simply means the amount by which something you're trying to get better at is increased and how often. For example, Ray started his walking programme and increased it by thirty seconds every three days to start with, after two weeks he increased it to every two days and so on.'

We discussed the incrementing and came up with: staying with a minute and a half for the first week to get going, then incrementing by thirty seconds every two days for the second and third weeks, and in the fourth week increasing by thirty seconds daily. In that way he'd end up with roughly ten minutes of walking. We also agreed that it could be adjusted.

I then spent a few minutes writing down what we agreed – with the walking baseline, the deadline for the walking to the corner shop and a table for the increments[1] and that he's going to think about some other goals. I write the two 'sayings' above at the top.

'Now, how about we look at some of your movements?'

You may be wondering where the physical examination's gone, well it hasn't gone anywhere, I haven't done one and I'm not going to go anywhere near a formal examination as it's totally inappropriate. Step in to the Biomedical shopping basket compartment for a moment – think, serious pathology, red flags, diagnosis, tissues safe to load, stage of healing, pain mechanisms... , now step right out again and don't start thinking 'Rottweilers'. There's nothing of value except as an intellectual exercise. Now step into the Impairment compartment – think what you might find – yes, loads, don't even go there, step right out again. Now step

---

1 - See chapter 13 part 3, page 285 in Main CJ, Spanswick CC 2000 Pain Management an Interdisciplinary Approach. Churchill Livingstone, Edinburgh. The chapter on 'Physical activities programme content' is by Paul Watson and is essential reading for goal-setting and incrementing. There are plenty of case studies and clinical examples.

into the General Health compartment – don't even step in! Pain? Yep, everywhere; which leaves – psychosocial – assume it's brimming and note that you're gathering material to put in there all the time and lastly the FUNCTION COMPARTMENT – it's huge, and that's the best place for a rehabilitationist to start (see figure GE 2.15) and we already have with the walking, but remember the key thing about the chronic pain related disability model (chapter GE 2.6) is that the first thing after the pain is 'guarded movement and muscle spasm. That is a good place to start with Grouty.

Grouty struggled out of the chair to stand and I indicated to come over and sit next to me on the treatment couch.

'Grouty, with have another saying here and it's **'Smooth relaxed, floppy easy movement'** and I'm going to start looking at that with you now – remember I put that on the graph with Ray?'

He did, I raised the treatment couch so that it was slightly higher than the chair he'd just been sitting on. I then put a chair in front of him so he could hold onto the backrest if he wanted to. I went round to face him and put one foot on the chair to stabilise it – 'Grouty, we're going to have a look at getting up from sitting. Ready when you are.'

Up he came with an awkward sway a grunt and a screwed up face. He pulled hard on the chair and lent on it when he was up.

(It may be worth reviewing the patient 'Jude' in chapter 17.1 because the approach here with Grouty was very similar – taking a movement that was extremely tense and breaking it down until a movement that wasn't tense was produced. I like to think it's what a good neuro physiotherapist would do and one day what a good pain therapist would do too!)

With Grouty I was going to be slightly different to how I was with Jude – there I instructed her, here, I want Grouty to find out for himself. 'Telling' and then trying and 'not getting it' can be very disheartening for some and anyway, 'telling' or being 'told what to do' is exactly what Grouty was fed up with. He needed a 'try it and see' approach.

'Was the height too hard?'

'A little I think.' He puffed and grimaced. I raised the couch about four or five inches.

'What do you think?'

'I'll give it a go.'

'Good.' I offered encouragement.

He sat, one arm grabbing the chair and the other searching for the surface of the couch so he could lower himself slowly. After a moment's pause he got up again, the height increase had made it easier.

'Good, that was smoother, less tension and you didn't do that breath holding either.'

After a few repetitions he was getting the hang of it and I encouraged him. He agreed to practice occasionally at home, not thinking lots of repetitions to 'get fit' but thinking practice to get smooth and relaxed. He reckoned that the arm of his armchair would be about a similar height. I showed him that he could use pillows to make it higher or more comfortable.

We then spent a little time walking and ended up with him holding the backs of two chairs that faced away from each other. We ended up just doing simple weight forward and back, swapping between right leg in front and left.

'This reminds me of the parallel bars at the physio!'

'So you've done this sort of thing before then?'

'No, not at all, they just got me to walk up and down and as I did they kept saying, head up look forward and relax your shoulders. They nagged me to get even steps I seemed to remember. They plonked a chair at either end and left me to it quite often.'

'Oh, right. Can you see why we're concentrating on just forward and back right now?'

'Well, yes, I've not realised for example, that I was holding my breath so much… '

He again agreed to 'practice' at home whenever he wanted to.

(It's best to think 'little and often' when learning something, and to use the word 'practice' is much better than seeing it as an 'exercise.' I try to get patients to see that they can do this sort of stuff anytime round the house – and to take a few minutes to work out a few practice 'stations' – like in the kitchen, even the bathroom and so on. 'Practice' is far less of a chore than 'exercises' – especially when the patient can see the relevance of them)]

I then got his piece of paper and wrote 'practice' – sit to stand from chair and weight forward and back holding on… ANYTIME! I also wrote key=nice, easy, relaxed, floppy movement.

I then spent a few minutes discussing 'progression' with him and he soon gave me 'going lower' for the sit to stand, and 'stepping right through' and 'less weight through the arms,' for the forward and back movement.

We stopped there and agreed to meet in a week. Out he went hobbling, grunting and gasping with his stick.

This 'exaggerated' movement pattern – this 'illness behaviour' is often far more than just an ingrained 'pattern of movement.' As Waddell noted[1] (see chapter GE 3.2) 'illness behaviour' or the 'behavioural signs and symptoms' strongly correlate with high levels of emotional arousal, distress and issues like 'disease conviction.' Unfortunately providing positive information has little effect on this type of patient and their movement patterns. We'd love to think that they would suddenly get the message that their body was safe but just hurting and then spring to their feet and run out of the clinic, but they don't. Dealing with their distress and emotional issues may help but, as Paul Watson has said, 'Physical activity is perhaps the most powerful component in pain management programmes. Increasing fitness is important not only in reversing the disuse syndrome, but in giving a powerful signal to patients that they are beginning to regain a degree of control over their mucsculoskeletal system. It is therefore extremely important from both the physical and the psychological point of view.[2]'

The following week Grouty settles in the chair in his usual way and we get to review his progress and it's what I usually expect with the 'novelty' of the first week and when I perceive that the patient is 'getting the idea'. He's managed the daily walking, he's keen to show me his 'practice' movements and he's got two goals. The first is to be able to walk into the treatment room here without his stick, the other is to be able to go straight up and down the stairs rather than going sideways as he has been for the last six or seven years.

It feels like we are on our way, following Ray along the slowly inclining curve. Grouty demonstrates good smooth sit to stand and forward and back weight transference; the walking is manageable and he's started to notice the Toblerone pain behaviour for what it is rather than always linking it to some activity related issue.

I was keen to make sure he had a 'flare-up' plan in place for the inevitable pain exacerbation— which could de-rail the progress and dampen his enthusiasm. I also thought it worthwhile mooting the idea of seeing a relaxation therapist (remember 'Blame' who helped Kate in chapter 17.8?).

The basics of flare-up management suggested by Chris Spanswick[3] are:

- don't panic: this will settle and get better

- use physical and mental relaxation skills

- try stretching exercises or any of your exercises that feel good

- may need to rest but two days in bed maximum

---

1 - *See Waddell G 2004 The Back Pain Revolution. Churchill Livingstone, Edinburgh, p 193*

2 - *Watson P 2000. Part 3 Physical Activities Programme Content. In: Main CJ, Spanswick CC 2000 Pain Management an Interdisciplinary Approach. Churchill Livingstone, Edinburgh, p285*

3 - *Main CJ, Spanswick CC 2000. Pain Management. An Interdisciplinary Approach. Churchill Livingstone, Edinburgh p 278.*

- try to avoid the sense of failure or giving-up and just see the flare-up as a set-back or a 'pause' in the progress

- try to keep active and pottering if at all possible

- cut back on exercise programme

- as settles try to get slowly back to the exercises and activities

- use painkillers that you find helpful

- use heat/cold, TENS etc.

- it's really good to manage yourself through a flare-up – rather than returning to the Dr or a therapist.

Louis didn't finish writing Grouty's story and I don't know what happened. How long did he see him for, or the outcome? And more interestingly what happened on the way. But knowing Louis I think he would have helped Grouty to make some changes. I hope that the 'Ray' story and his success became the 'Grouty' story and a similar positive result!

The pain timeline with typical injury (information for patients)

1. FREEZE PHASE = STOP, DON'T MOVE, TENSE:

- instant pain with any injury or potential injury

- instant concern, directs attention

- try to help self or request help

- Normally lasts a few seconds or minutes to a maximum of a day or so. (Classic example, low back pain when it suddenly comes like a 'knife in your back' and you freeze in a bent position and drop to the floor...)

2. TENSE AND WARY PHASE = REST MOSTLY, BUT MOVE A VERY LITTLE FOR ESSENTIALS:

- acute injury pain (tissues 'weaker', inflamed and early repair...)

- lasts hours, to a few days, to go on longer is unusual but does happen.

- usually two types of pain:

> a. Ache, throb 'look after me' pain and ...

> b. Sharp, nasty with gentle movement.

(Example, low back pain still hobbling round holding onto things, getting sudden sharp pains, can't get straight, restless... like 1. above but not quite so bad...

3. RESTLESS, GET MOVING, START TRYING IT OUT, DO MORE AND MORE PHASE:

Early to middle recovery phase pain that has 4 components. I call this as the 'restless' phase of recovery:

a. Achy, stiffy **'move me'** pain... had enough being still... get up...

b. Achy, stiffy, throbby **'that's enough movement for now'** pain... have a rest...

c. Sharp pain at end range movements **'careful with me but try me a bit and see if I give a bit... '** 'Mechanically patterned' pain that improves at the time of repeated movement and with regular repetition gradually allows more movement. Stiffens up afterwards but gradually over time improvements are made.

d. Sharp or intense pain **'that's-enough-of-doing-that-now-you-idiot'** type pain. Mechanically patterned pain that is very sharp and builds with repeated movement. Usually with sudden high forces and indicates that repeating at lower forces and in a less abrupt way would be better.

4. END PHASE HEALING: The relatively pain-silent phase.

- loss of constant awareness pain – now's the time to start testing it out a bit and then get really going... but occasionally if you do overdo it I'll make it ache so you're 'careful before doing it again'... type pain. Eventually this reaction disappears and all that's left is end range sensitivity which can also lessen if trained into and 'desensitised'.

- because of scar some residual sensitivity may always remain

- the more appropriate the training at the appropriate time the better the end result.

'OLD BUT NEARLY READY'

Case History 4.1

Derek: 'tension and grunting' – undoing a bad habit!

La-la-la-laLa-la-la-la
Nowadays we often gaze
On women over fifty
Without the slightest trace
Of wrinkles on their face
Doctors go and take their dough
To make them young and nifty
But Doctors I defy
To tell me just why
No matter how young a prune may be
It's always full of wrinkles
We may get them on our face
Prunes get 'em every place
Prohibition worries us
But prunes don't sit and brood
For no matter how young a prune may be
It's always getting stewed

Song of the Prune (Extract 1)
(Crumit / DeCosta)
Frank Crumit - c. 1928

Listen on youtube:
https://www.youtube.com/watch?v=TgVlRvl2DI0

if you have to, but don't! This presentation is so common and thinking like that will not help at all, you'll just get angry with the patient and alienate yourself from him, resulting in a totally unproductive consultation. The patient in front of you – from their chemistry right through to their personality and their behaviour is your challenge, try and enjoy it. Oh, and if you can't – you'd better forget working with pain patients, especially those with chronic on-going pain because they're nearly all like this. These folk represent one of the biggest challenges in medicine, they can be some of the hardest patients and they can easily be made more pain disabled by the attitude and words of those who are supposed to be trying to help. But I didn't think Derek was in the 'no hope' category just because of this 'discrepancy'. I certainly wasn't writing him off.

So how should we explain what this 'movement/pain-behaviour' discrepancy is all about? For me, it's all about gating – gating of pain from reaching consciousness and context! Hence, undressing is pretty much a well entrained programme that needs little concentration, like riding a bike or driving a car it can go on while the brain is pre-occupied with something else. Here with Derek, our talking and chatting went on, I think the topic was still on the useless Dr consults and the lack of any interest or investigations – about which he was quite animated. As the brain is only good at focusing on one thing at a time, the fairly emotionally charged conversation had priority and the pain was kept reasonably well out, or at least the crappy, grunty, tense, sharp, jerky movement accompaniment was (gates closed). Now, when I he had his clothes off and he was standing in his underwear – which is quite a novel and perhaps almost a slightly vulnerable making situation and I was asking him to try different movements, the attention was full-on at the site of the movement; the pain-gate's associated with the movement and the area were all wide open. Combine vulnerability/novelty feelings with the focus of attention on the problem and it's hardly surprising that his 'pain-gate' was now wide open. With patients like Derek it can sometimes help to see that this wide-open gate state as almost the default setting? The pain system has got in the habit of easily opening and staying open for long periods. (I use this little explanation when I do pain talks about this sort of thing with the patient – you'll see in little while!)

Right, so when I see this sort of thing, I might have a little questioning ponder (an amused one I add) but medically speaking, the discrepancy observation makes me quite a bit more confident that I'm not so likely to be dealing with anything nasty or there's going to be a red-flag issue here. I've watched Derek's intervertebral movement into flexion while he was sitting and despite all the grunts and jerks, it was fine, just stiff and looking unhealthy but fine, it basically moved to its gentle maximum, like most people when they sit and come forward. So the red flag which alerts us to significant loss of lumbar flexion is slipped into the 'not quite so concerned' reasoning draw (I'll re-check it a bit when he's in side lying. What we must be wary of is that sometimes very serious things can present with this exaggerated pain patterning too.)

Back to the physical exam now: Derek's just done his forward bend and not picked up on the Nice, Easy, Relaxed and Smooth movement. That needs much more work, so I'll leave it until later. As an aside, it is quite common that patients can straight away move smoothly and normally when this is sort of movement is done. The rapid turn-around from horrid jerky fearful, grunty movement to smooth and relaxed movement is usually more likely in the more acute or early stages of a problem – the key to success is doing a movement that is non-threatening.

Louis commented here: see graded exposure

I get him to sit up on the couch with legs dangling, test his calf and quads reflexes and can't get a thing. Why's that I wonder? Is it a 'hard' sign, pathologically significant and relating to nerve function? Is it my poor technique? Is he super tense and therefore inhibiting the reflexes? Is this his normal – like many others?

Louis comment: YouTube demo of sitting reflexes! Maybe somebody already has! Later he suggests the same thing for demo muscle testing!

'Go as floppy as you can Derek.' I hold his foot and gently pull it towards me, so extending his legs about five centimetres from the dangling position. I waggle the knee a bit to see if it's relaxed – nothing and tensed up to hell. I let the leg go back to dangle position and start to chat... 'Did you say you had a couple of dogs just now?' He's then off telling me how old they are, that they're his gun-dogs and so on, and all the while I'm flicking the hammer at his quads and his Achilles tendons. I get a few little contractions but not consistently. I'll come back to that later or another time.

While I'm down there I checked his foot muscle power. For two reasons, firstly I get a further handle on how 'willing' he is to be strong and low and behold, as the contractions builds up, he's suddenly going jerky and its all 'give way' and 'jerk up' again. What's sometimes called 'cog-wheel' contractions – familiar to those who deal with late stage Parkinsons disease, but it should also be very familiar to all those who deal with chronic musculoskeletal conditions. It has been labelled a 'behavioural sign' by Gordon Waddell, who sees it as strongly correlating with significant 'yellow flags' or psychosocial issues – rather than being a significant 'red' flag sign. In other words, it's something to treat and overcome rather than something that's being caused by hard pathology. Jerky backward and forward contractions like this are often labelled as being pain inhibited. Yes, too to some extent, certainly when contractions build up in the foot, there will be an increasing stabilising contraction of the trunk, hence increased forces through the super-vigilant and sensitised lumbar area and therefore a reflex letting go. Anxiety and fear about causing pain are likely big factors here too. This means the individual is so insecure about the pain coming that they let go. I see this as a semi-conscious/unconscious almost learnt issue – which can often be quickly trained out. We can analyse it to high heaven – ultimately it's a feature that goes in my shopping basket of 'things that aren't normal and that need to be checked, worked on and improved if possible'. (section GE 4 the Shopping Basket approach)

The second reason is because I want to see if his muscle strength is OK – as I've already noted that he hasn't any consistent reflexes it would be remiss of me not to at least check the major muscle groups (myotomes!). I know that 'real' neurological weakness is where the patient works as hard as they possibly can and the contraction comes but it can easily and steadily be broken. I definitely wasn't getting that here.

Light touch testing was normal. I didn't do pin-prick as I didn't think it likely to give me anything of value and it always takes a bit of time, especially if the patient gets really nerdy and focused on tiny differences. If necessary, like any good clinician, a change of opinion if new things come to light might bring me back to test it later on.

I think it's the test of a good clinician to have in mind all the physical tests they want to do and to be able to have a little prediction about what they'll be like. It shows that you're thinking in patterns, that you feel confident. What is always interesting is when what you're expecting doesn't happen!

So, what are Derek's lying down movements going to be like? Yes, movements – with most therapists it's all passive once someone lies down. For me, most of the time and especially with Derek type problems, I continue with active hands off movements. For example, lying supine I might get the patient to do crook rotation; pelvic rock; bridging; hip hitching; grab a knee; active leg lifting (SLR), mini sit-up; arms up and so forth.   Guess what they were like?   Yes, your right, all jerky and grunty and zilch good quality movement. I didn't do all those movements, just one or two, I couldn't see the point, but in some patients you often end up finding good quality movements and these can be useful to use as a first 'getting-going' phase of normal movement re-learning and confidence building. It's simple graded exposure. With Derek, 'active' SLR (can you guess) brings on the back pain at about 45 degrees and he doesn't relax at all as I try and do it passively. SLR bringing on low back pain is seen as a yellow flag – a predictor of poor outcome!

My hunch, hopefully like yours, is that lumbar area palpation is going to be incredibly tender with lots of tension, spasm and grunting.

I got Derek to turn on his side for the palpation. An aside here – is that while I do get patients to lie prone for palpation I quite often avoid it as it can make those with very poor extension (or even those that do have good extension sometimes) very painful when they go to get off. I always ask patients 'When was the last time you lay on your front?' and then if they have recently I ask how they found it. The end result is that I go very carefully with lying patients prone, especially for prolonged periods – thanks to a lot of experience of patients really struggling afterwards.

Right, Derek's lying on his right side (he chose the right as his most comfy) and I'm round the back starting to put my hands on him – gently at first a bit away from the pain area – but not too touchy feely if you know what I mean – adapt to the patient! I continue on waiting for him to start jumping but he doesn't, I carefully go deeper into the soft tissues, still OK…

'Let me know what's happening in here if you like Derek and I'm just as interested in good feelings as bad, you with me?

'Yes.'

So now I've gone deeply in all over the lateral muscular masses of erector spinae and the lateral and posterior reaching abdominals – which he doesn't mind, or says nothing and doesn't flinch. I know he would be reluctant to say that something felt good in his current state... so I'm a bit at a liberty, assuming there's possibly a bit of positive/it's ok, about what I'm doing. I now go in on the spinous processes, starting over the sacrum at about S3 and working up towards L5 and above. This more bony palpation is, as you'd expect, more discomforting to him, yet he still doesn't flinch. The main tenderness is over the S1 and L5, as in most people who have low back pain or a history of it. Push hard enough, or with nasty 'pointed' thumbs and you'll always find a tender spot!   In other words, be careful with your interpretation of what you find. The other thing here is, if you go in ham-fisted and hard (like orthopaedic consultants, some medics, 'macho' physios and the mean and uncaring do!) you're more than likely to get a huge pain response. If you're like this, you haven't understood pain processing properly. Remember the 'vulnerable organism' from section GE 02 chapter 2.3. A person in pain, who is anxious about their problem (just by seeking help with you means they are anxious and concerned) has their pain 'sensitivity' setting set at a very low threshold and therefore it will be very easy to turn it on.

The palpation examination wasn't quite what I had expected, but I was pleased; at least here was somewhere I could start some mechanical input that might bring about a bit better movement perhaps?   I felt I had the option of either, trying to get some better quality movement going or, use some simple manual therapy/physical input to see is anything would change the dire state of his movements.

I went for the hands-on option – arghh! I can hear all the 'cognitive-behavioural' – 'yellow-flaggy' – 'follow the rules of best practice' lot out there shouting... 'You'll make him dependant on manual therapy! Sorry, I won't because I take great care not to! Manual therapy here is simply an input to start a process, if it doesn't do anything I stop and I explain why to Derek. If it does help better movement then I'm getting somewhere and as time goes on my hands come off – he's got to start moving with confidence on his own and that's where the focus of future sessions have to go.

For now, I haven't got time to start explaining adequately the smooth movement issues, but manual therapy input for the last 5-10 minutes of the session is easy.

I get Derek to sit up.

'Are you comfortable to sit there for a moment or two? Look there's the good and the bit of bad about what I'm finding, ready?

'Sure.'

He looks a bit glazed but he is looking at me now.

'Before I start is there anything huge concerning or worrying you. I hear that the Drs haven't helped or been understanding, which is very common. Is there anything else?'

'Yes, big time – they're not even interested in getting a scan or x-ray. If it was me who was the Dr, right, how would I know what was wrong, if I hadn't got some handle on the inside of the back? When I mention scan and x-ray's the Dr just mutters 'They're a waste of time here... That, I'm afraid is bollocks, excuse me for swearing.'

'Got you. Does that mean you're concerned that something big and bad might be going on inside?'

'Well of course, this pain is horrendous and every three weeks or so, I just have to do a slightly odd movement, or something really simple and bang I'm stuffed and can't move for a week. They just give me painkillers and sign me off work some more. I'm pissed right off '

'Got you again! For me the situation is this: you're stuck, you don't look as if you've moved normally for all this time and that's not doing you any good and as I'm sure you know, if this goes on too long it gets harder and harder to overcome and you can end up having long term pain – what's called 'chronic pain'. We need to get you moving normally again and get your confidence back in your back. I'm only going to be able to do that if I'm confident and you're confident that there's nothing seriously wrong. So, I'm going to write to your Dr and ask for an x-ray and a scan, if you agree?'

He nods and looks relieved. I go on...

'Now, I want you to know this. When good practitioners examine backs these days there are clear guidelines that get us to ask questions and do physical tests that probe for things that indicate there might be something serious wrong. These tests are called 'red-flag' tests. Red flags are things that we find out from you that tell us there might be something serious going on. Things like broken bones, weak bones, discs pressing on and damaging nerves and also the possibility of cancer and serious disease. OK? Now, I've asked you a whole pile of these questions (I know I've not mentioned them earlier, but they get asked in every single patient) and had a detailed look at you. You don't have any 'red flags', but I still appreciate that you are concerned and would like the x-ray and scan – let me tell you that most Drs in your situation would want one too – even though they may have pondered all the red-flag information! So, you're not being abnormal. Your reflexes are tricky to find, but that's not uncommon and I'll spend a little more time having another look at them next time you come.'

He nods.

'The best thing would be for you to see one of the other Drs – is that possible?'

'Maybe, unfortunately I'm down to see Dr P tomorrow for my sick note, he's the shit one. I'll still tell him you want an x-ray.'

'Good, let me know how you get on and if there are any issues I'll write him a note.'

(Nice conflict coming up with the Dr, the patient and Dr, now the physio and Dr!

A nice yellow flag amplifier here i.e. anxiety and anger with medicine and distress related to diagnosis issues etc. Nice iatrogenesis! I'll have to work hard now to get the Dr on side with what I'm trying to achieve)

You may be thinking why didn't you give him a chance to see if he still wanted the scans and x-ray after the red-flag chat? I could have done, but I've enough experience to know that many people, perhaps most people, are totally unconvinced that listening, asking questions and observing are more revealing than a scan! It helps if you have a very good reputation, you're of a certain age and you have a whole pile of qualifications! Is it just me, or does no one believe what science and research is telling us? That may include you and of course many Drs! I want this bloke to have had the investigations and then, assuming nothing major is wrong, reassured a bit more by 'technology' we can move on with the rehabilitation process.

'Right Derek, as you've just heard, I'm not concerned about anything nasty or serious going on, but I think and x-ray and scan are a good idea to be completely sure. In the meantime the most important thing we can do is make a start with seeing if we can get you moving better. I want you to know that even if there was something serious going on what we are doing is still very safe. It is very rare that even serious back problems are required to not move at all.'

I think he is listening!

'With the time I've got left today I'm going to do a bit with my hands in your back – pleasingly it's not too sore in the muscles, but they're solid, they feel clenched and that is what they look like when you move. Appreciate for a minute that when muscles are clenched that the forces through the joints underneath the muscles are taking a huge increase in compressive forces and then, if these joints and the nerves nearby are sensitive – that increased force is going to produce more pain. Can you see why I want to get nice free relaxed movement going again?'

'Go for it!'

'I'll use my wrist as an example, see this floppy movement of my wrist, it's all relaxed...'

I move my right wrist back and forth through a large range of flexion-extension. I then tense the whole thing up by making a very firm fist, you can see the tendons tighten and muscles contract in my lower forearm. I then start moving tensely through the movement again.

'Listen to that Derek!'

There's a huge crunching, popping sound now as the joint surfaces are compressed...

'Do you see what I mean? Not the nicest thing for my wrist, if it went on and on for six months, is it?'

I'm smiling and he's nodding. I think he got the message?

So I finish the session with some nice, deep, but comfortable, muscle and back mobilisations in side lying and the muscles do let go. I also do a bit of passive flexion/extension in the same position and find that to a small extent he does let go, if I go very slowly. This is all the start of an exploration process that's trying to find some normal movement!

He gets up and I ask him to rotate, side flex and flex/extend. Result? Nope! Not one jot of difference. I smile and look at Derek...

'We've got some work to do!'

Two days later he phones,

'Saw the shit Dr and he went 'What's he want that for?' really nastily, but he still gave me the referral and I've had it done. I'll get the results by the end of the week. I'll call you again... Oh and I've made an appointment with one of the other Drs to discuss the x-ray next week.'

'Good, I'll write to him.'

Here's the letter:

Dear Dr A

Re: Derek...

Thanks for looking after Derek. I believe he has been recommended to have some physiotherapy and we have made a start! Thanks also for organising an x-ray.

My concerns are these:

1. *He has plenty of yellow flag issues and I fear he is sliding towards a chronic disability situation if not dealt with in a sensitive but positive and physically forward moving way. Yellow flags of relevance here are:*

   - *high levels of disturbing pain – he's saying the pain is 15 out of 10 – despite the Tramadol and Naproxen*

   - *the high levels of pain are associated with a high level of distress at the moment*

   - *he also has high levels of concern for the future and is starting to feel negative about the back pain ever going*

   - *he is very concerned that something more serious may be going on*

   - *he is frustrated by the lack of progress*

> • *his 'behaviour' is shifted more towards avoiding than confronting activity – due to the levels of pain with movement.*

2. *Physical examination reveals very little in the way of low back intervertebral movement and huge limitations in all directions. For example, side flexion left and right are only a few degrees before intense pain limits the movement. Rotation to the left was nil today and to the right was about three quarters, flexion was about 10 degrees and so forth. Sitting flexion however, although slow, revealed good lumbar intervertebral movement.*

3. *His reflexes are hard to get or possibly absent but I will retest again next time. There is no sensory loss. I haven't been able to do a satisfactory myotome assessment due to the pain inhibition element revealing false positives. I suspect that there is no involvement – there is certainly no referred pain suggesting lumbar or sacral nerve impingement that could lead to a neuropathy.*

4. *The SLR produced back pain at about 45 degrees with both legs. I don't think this is a true 'tension' sign and is what I'd expect due to the all round hypersensitivity presenting.*

5. *Palpation reveals marked muscle tension and tenderness around the upper sacrum and lower lumbar areas.*

My feelings at the moment are that I have to work hard on a lot of reassuring and then start a get-moving-and-get-confidence-back programme going at this late stage. I think the x-ray will help a bit in the reassuring process but I also think an MRI scan would be very worthwhile too in this respect. I hope you're in agreement here – as you know he does have private health cover.

Concern, as always in these situations, is for any red flags indicating frank spinal pathology and it would be good to rule out. My thoughts, having spent a fair bit of time examining him, is that the only pathology likely, is a central disc protrusion at around L5-S1.

Thanks for your help with Derek. I think this is going to be tricky!

Louis Gifford

Chartered Physiotherapist

Derek comes back a week later.

'I'm in bloody agony. Three days after you saw me I bent down and I then spent the whole weekend on my back. I could hardly move...'

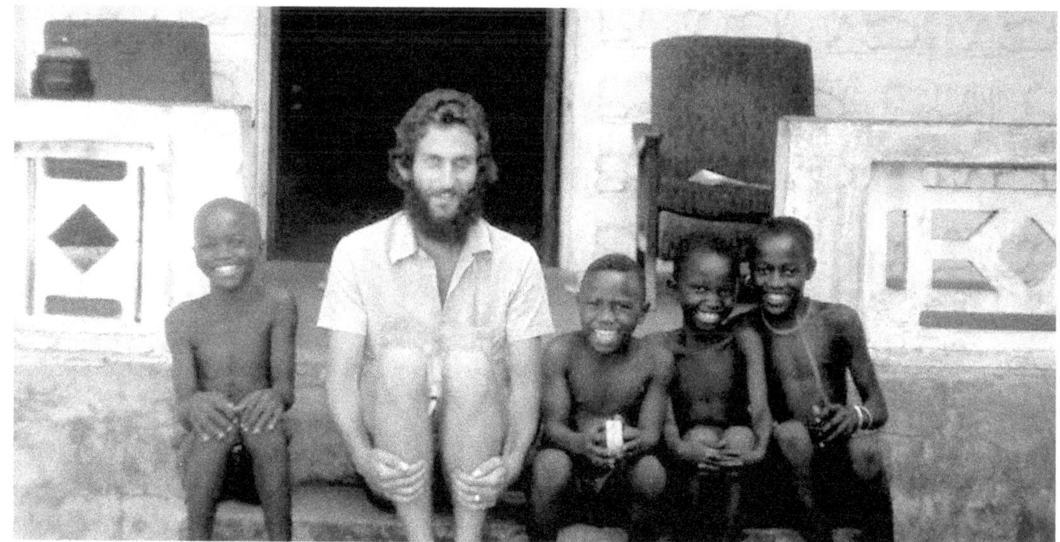

Louis with local village children Freetown, Sierra Leone 1977 - (big beards - a common thing!)

Heroes

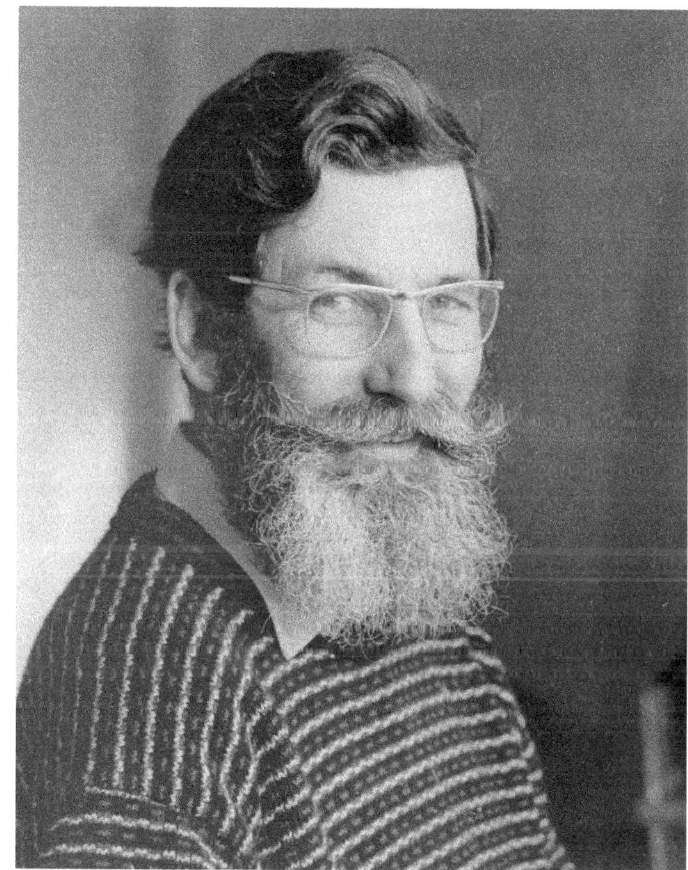

Vernon Gifford - Dad

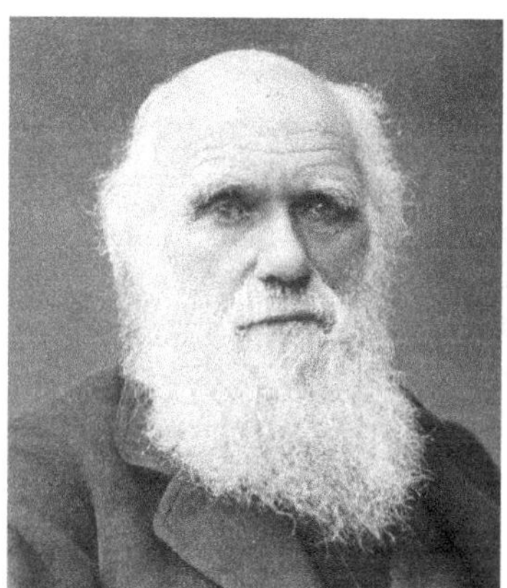

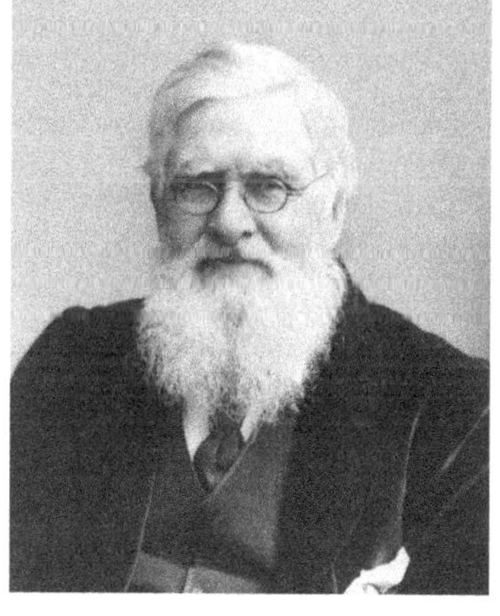

Charles Darwin (top)
Alfred Wallace (bottom)

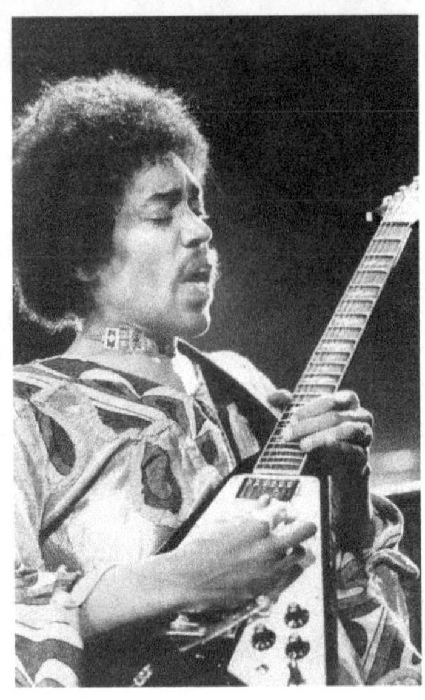

Jimi Hendrix - Isle of Wight Festival 1970

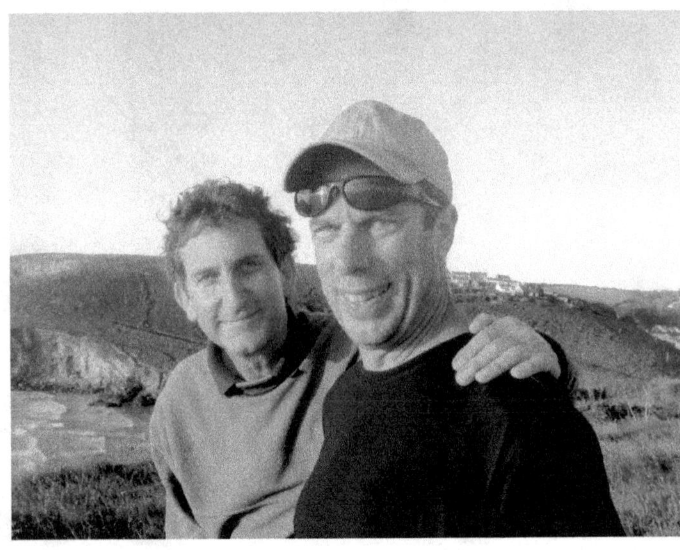

Me with Bernie Guth in North Cornwall

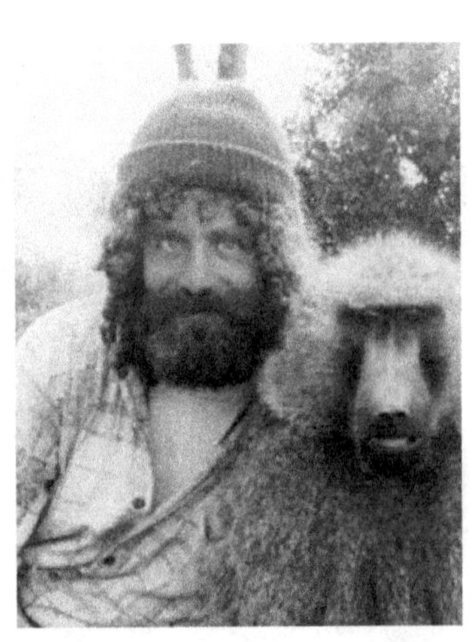

Robert Sapolsky

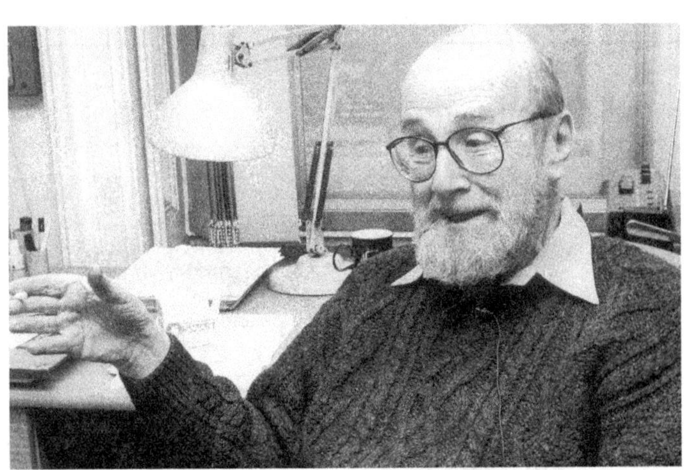

Pat Wall

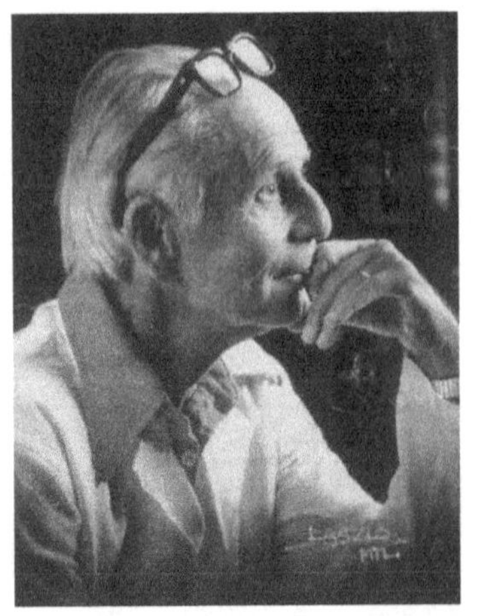

Hans Selye

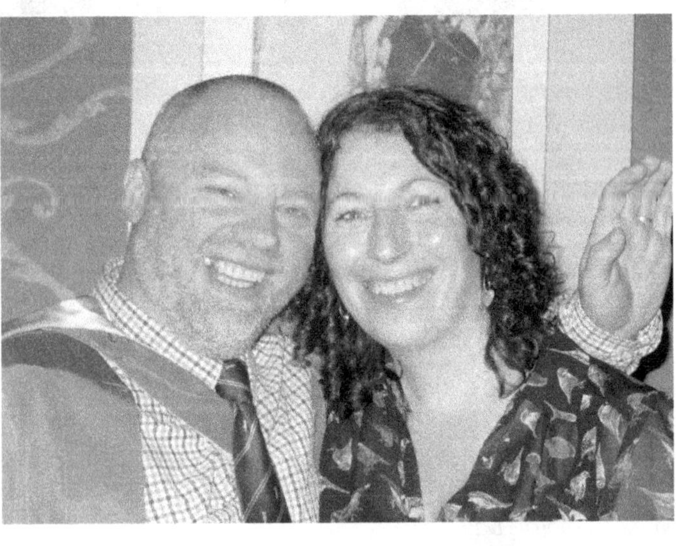

My mate Mick Thacker and his lovely wife Kath

Early Years

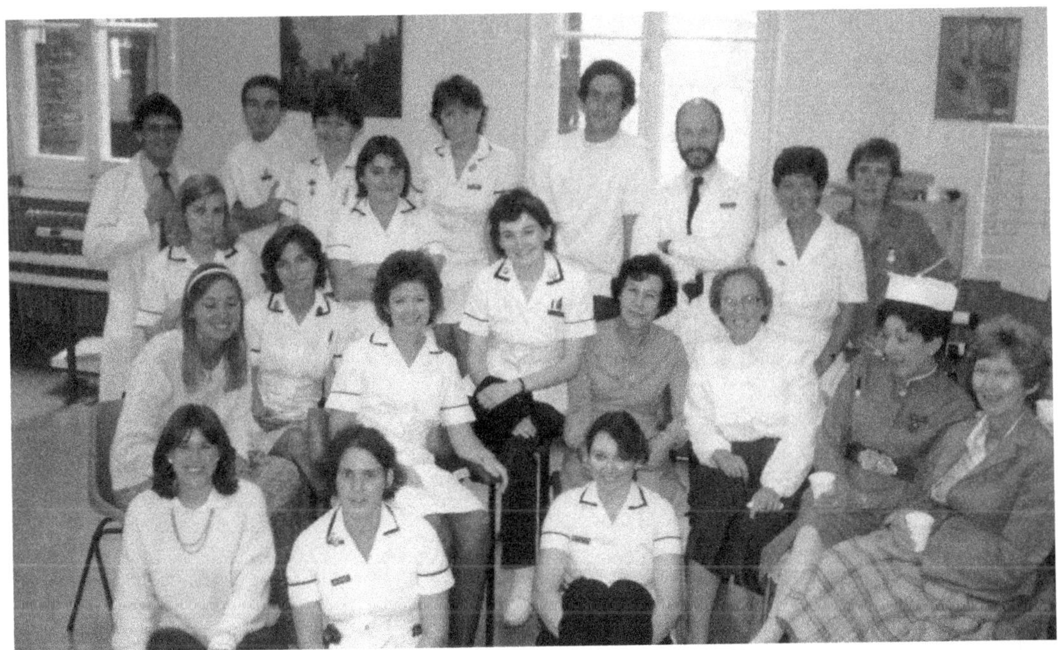

St Stephen's Physio Dept. 1984

Australia 1985-88

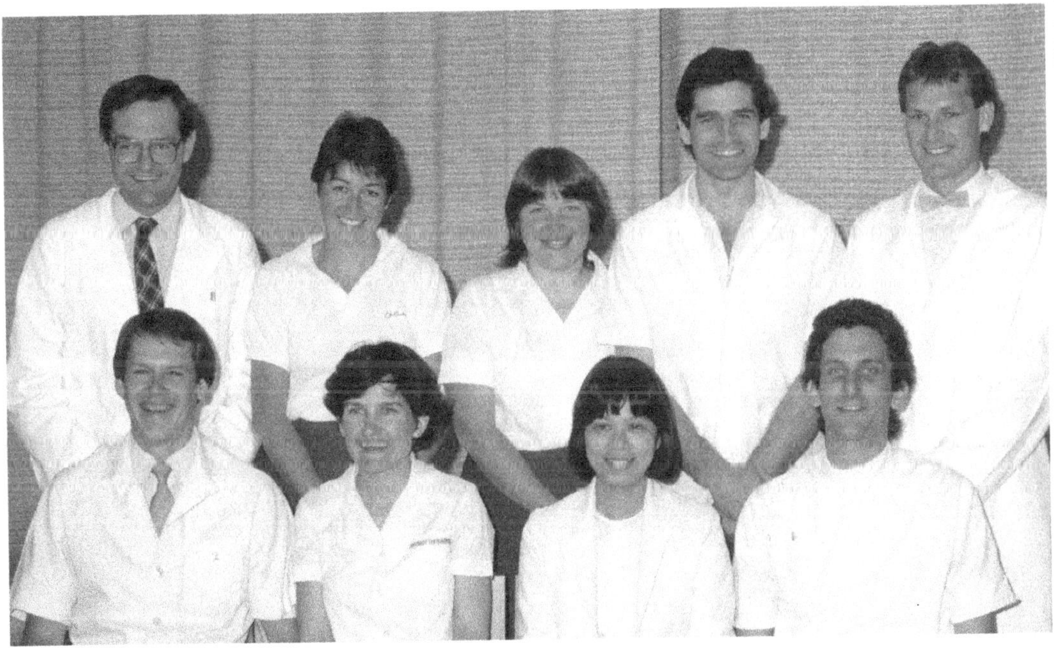

Adelaide Class of 1985 (from left to right)
Back Row: David Butler, Libby Austin (Fardy), Ellen Guth, Anton Harms, Rob Burgess
Front Row: Mark Jones, Ali Bell, Rosa Ng, Louis Gifford

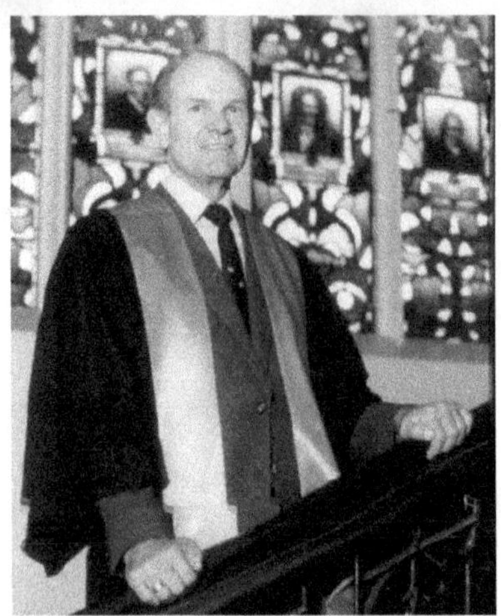

Geoff Maitland

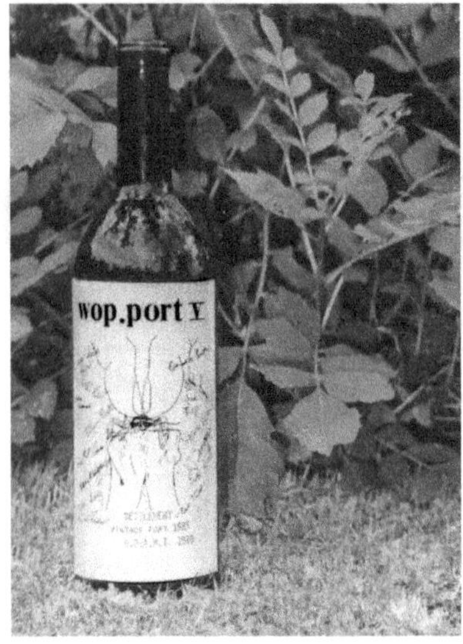

'Wop '85' Adelaide
'Bending the fly's knees'

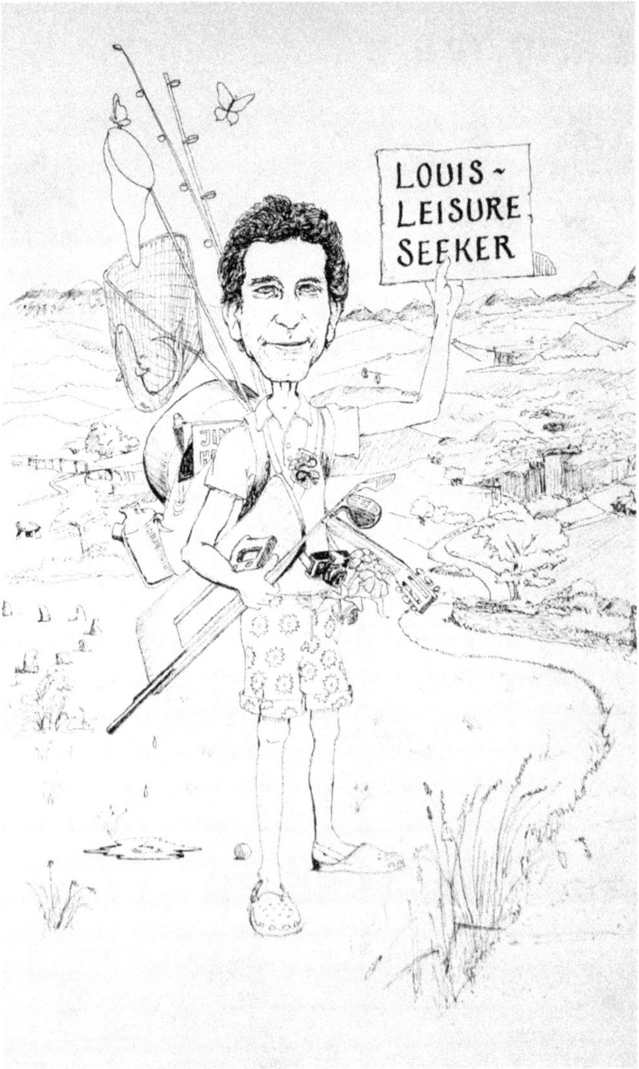

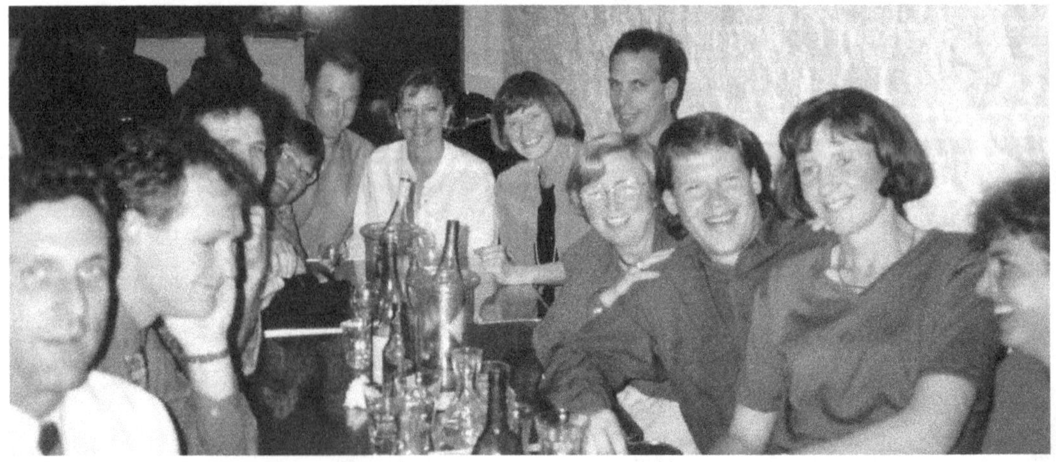

Louis 'Leisure Seeker'
Illustration by Mark Reeves

(Left to right) Louis, Rob, Anton, Ellen, Greg, Suzie, Ruth Grant,
Bernie, Pat Trott, Mark, Helen Rubenach, Tanya Harms - The Adelaide crew

Australia 1993

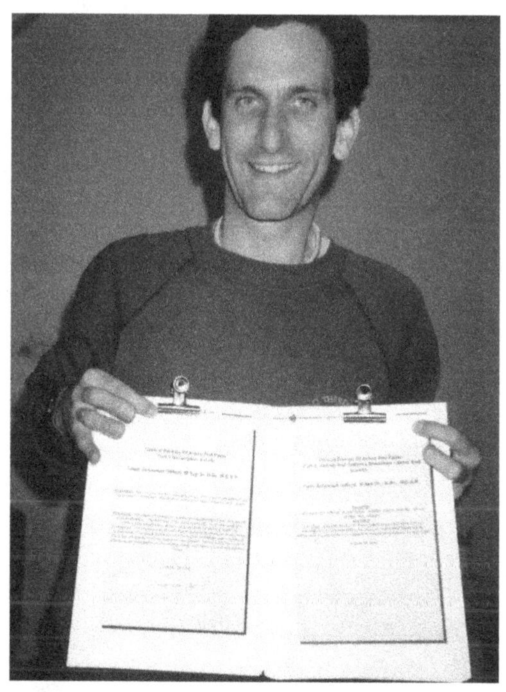

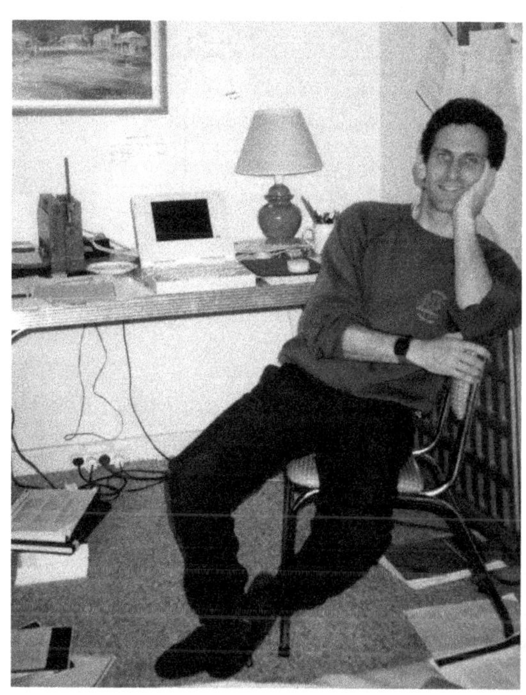

First version of the Clinical Biology of Aches and Pains workbook 1993

*1993 Adelaide - Louis' office!
Check out the computer! Louis studying for his Masters of Applied Science*

Lecturing and writing

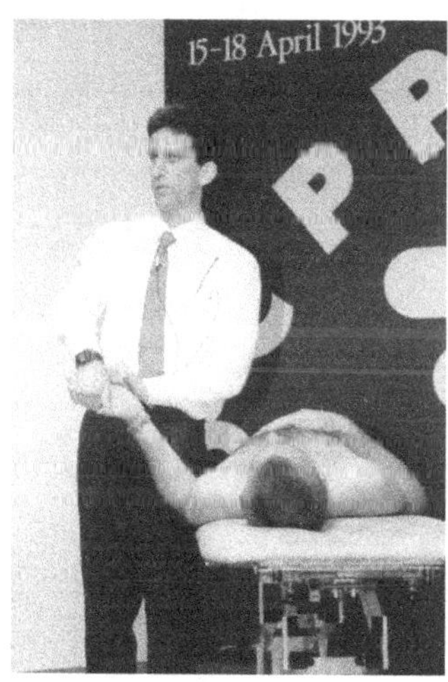

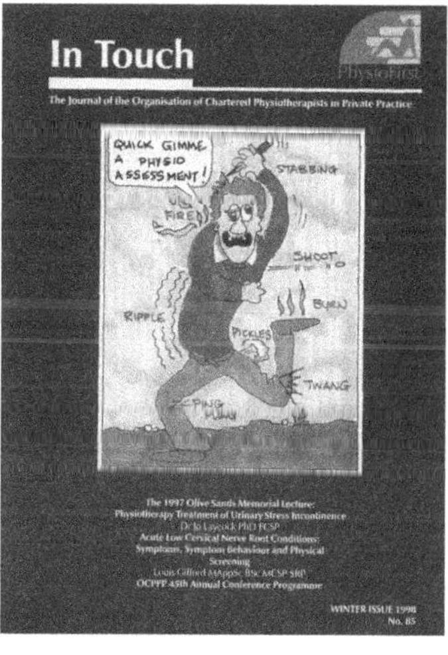

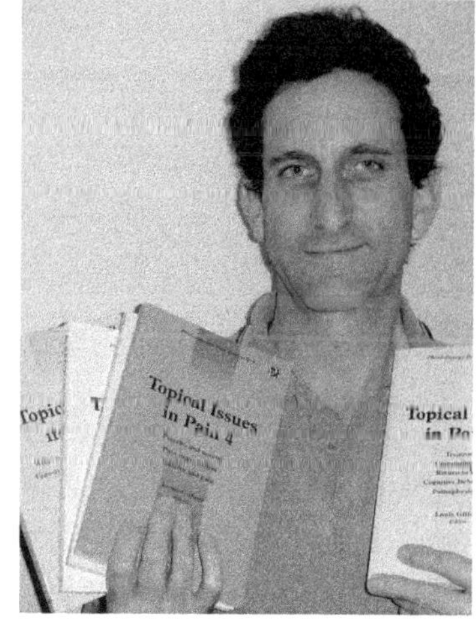

*OCPPP 1993
Olive Sands Lecture*

*'Quick Gimme a Physio Assessment!'
- The madness of pain
In Touch - Winter 1998, No.85*

TIP 1-5 1998-2006

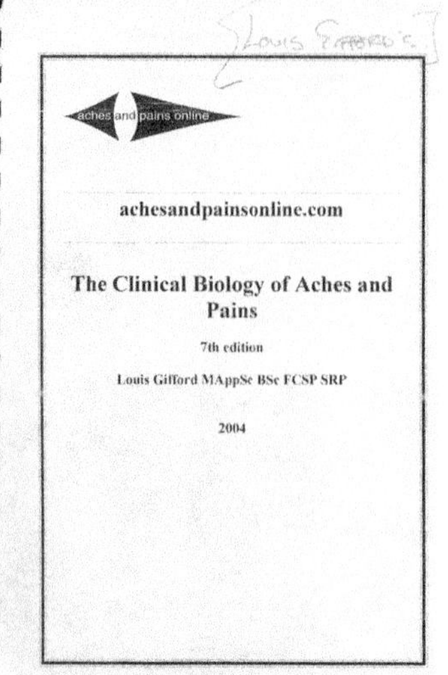

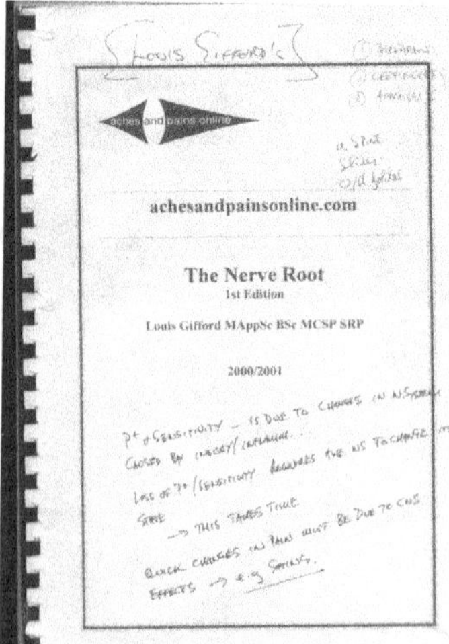

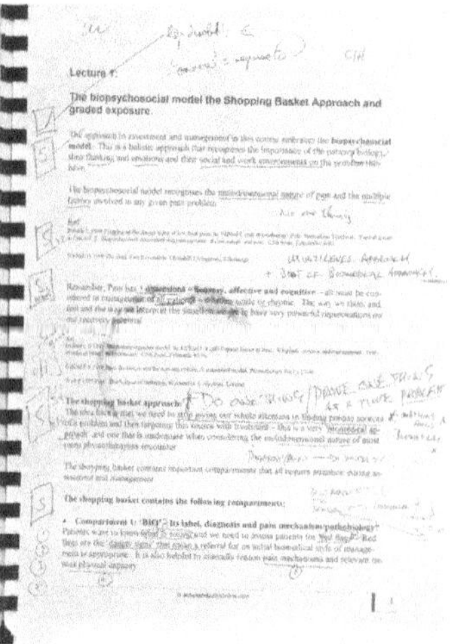

Workbooks

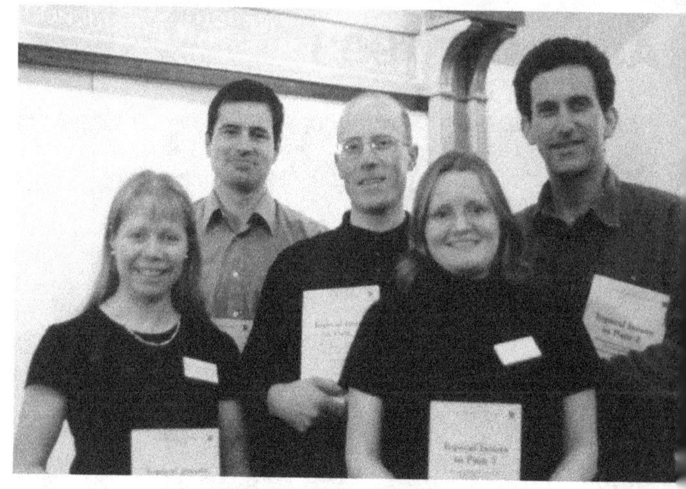

TIP 2 launch 2000 (left to right) Vicki Harding, George Peat, Paul Watson, Suzanne Brook (Shorland), Louis

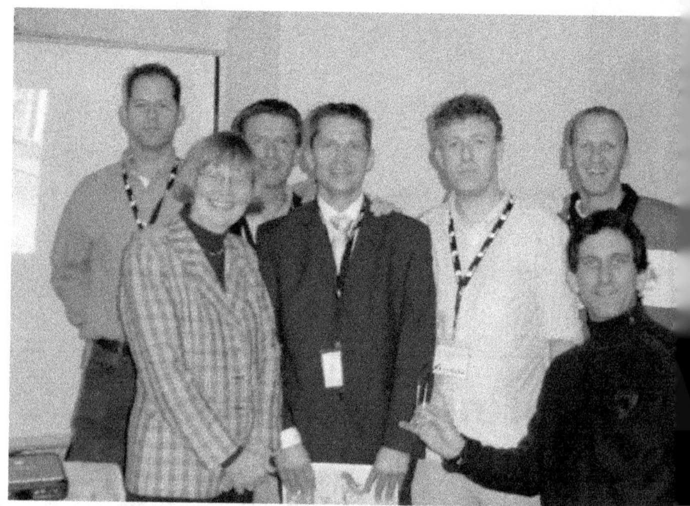

Holland 2002

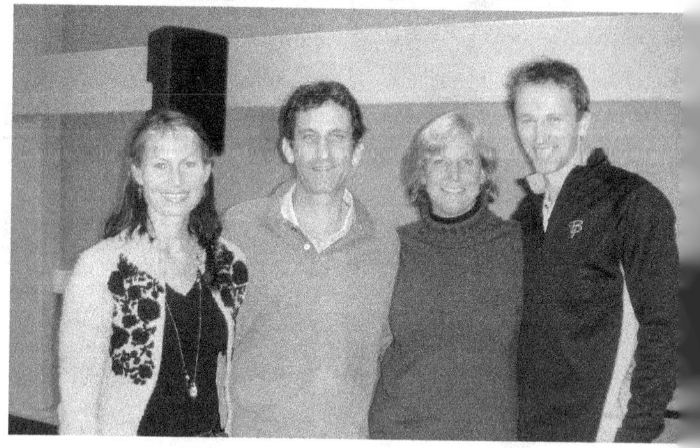

Karen Bo, Louis Gifford, Susan Mercer, Chris Drummond; Norway 2007

Some favourite teaching images

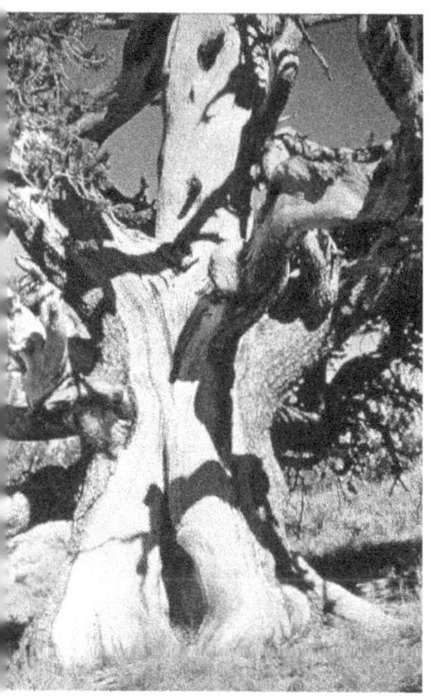

Bristlecone Pine

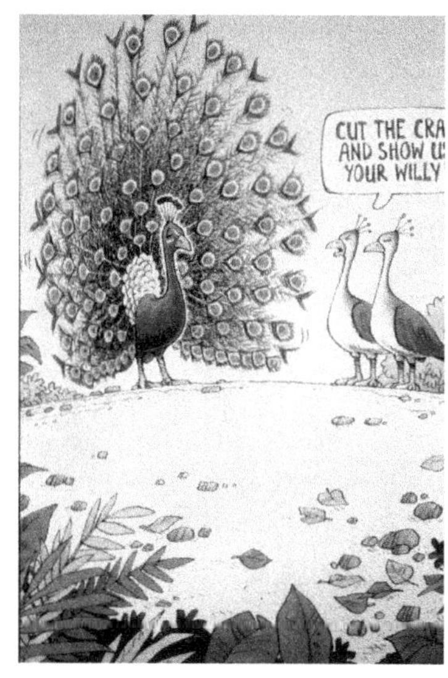

Peacocks cut the crap!

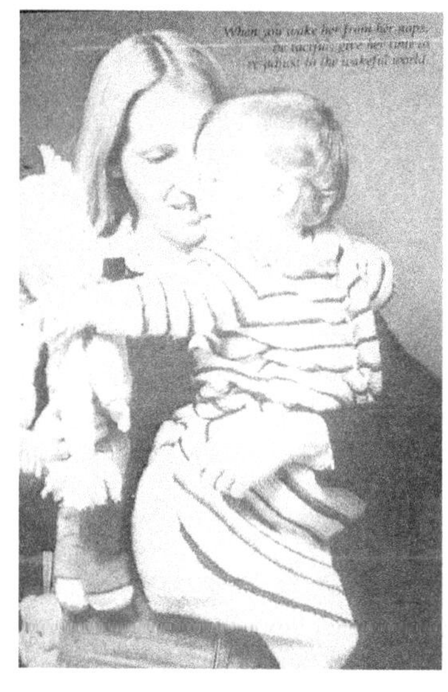

Mother and baby:
Assess, reassure, distract

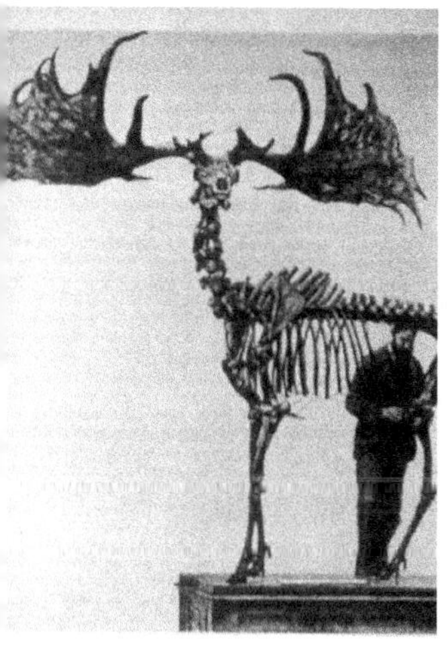

Irish Elk

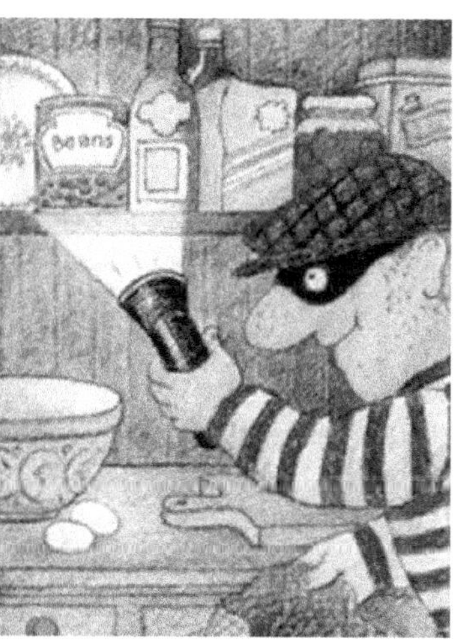

Burglar Bill

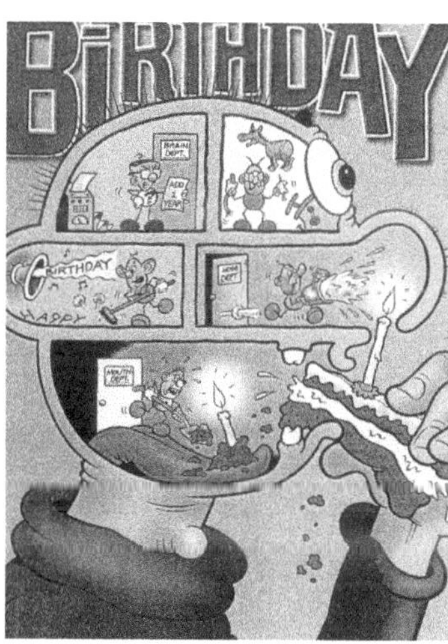

Numskulls

The 'team' at home

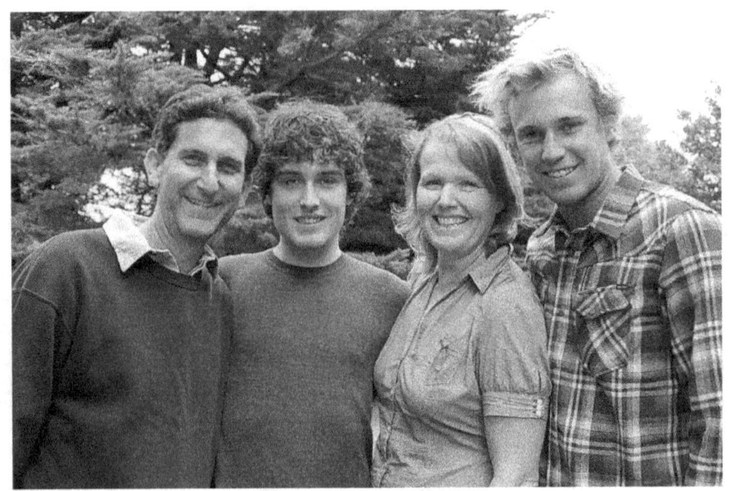

With my wife Philippa and our sons Ralph and Jake

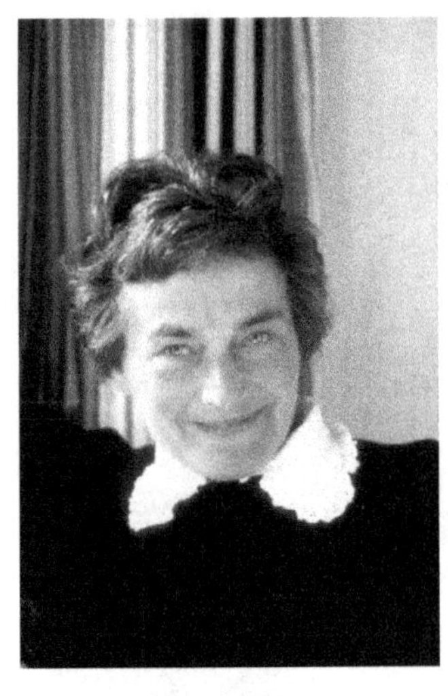

Jean Gifford - Mum

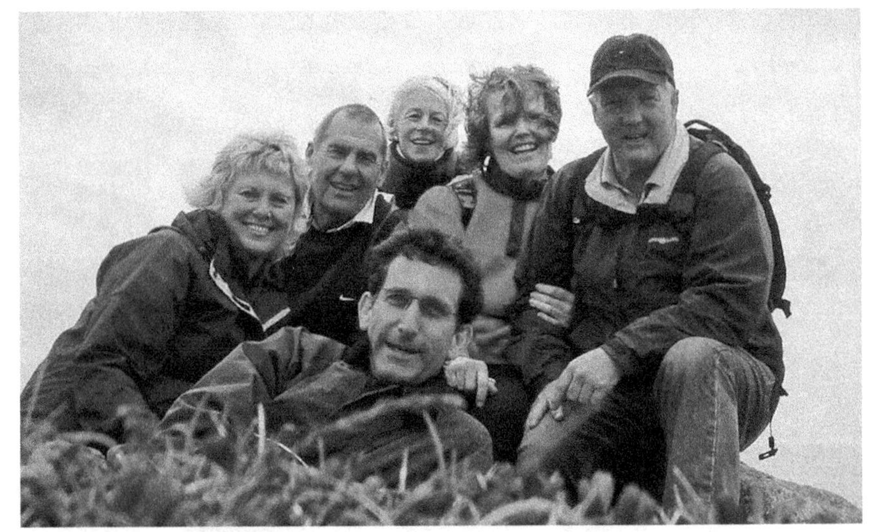

Maria, John, Jenny, Philippa, Terry and Louis

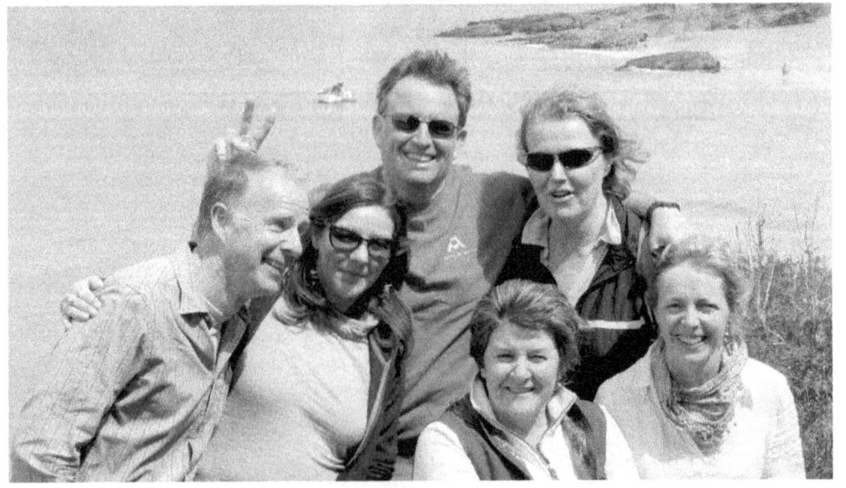

Mark, Tessa, Mike, Philippa, Julie and Jill

'How's it now?'

'Still awful, I feel it's back to where it was six months ago. The good news is that the x-ray's fine and the Drs referred me for a scan this week. I'm going to ring and sort an appointment this afternoon.'

'Did you see the Dr and was he ok with you? I assume he'd got my letter?

'Yes, all fine, he's pleased that you're trying to get me going and I'm going to meet up with him again when the scan results come through.'

I'm now thinking: great, that was all worth it. I've now got the Dr on my side and the patient's got a better relationship going here, plus we're getting helpful results from the investigations. We're starting to quell the unhelpful 'top' of 'top-down' stuff!

'Derek, I'm actually pleased that there's nothing on the x-ray, for the simple reason that x-rays are only good for showing up two things – first, really serious things like big tumours, broken bones and bad thinning of bones – osteoporosis and secondly, they show up wear and tear changes of the spine disc joints and the facet joints which are little joints that guide movement. I'll show you in a minute on the plastic spine I've got over there. I'm also quietly hoping that there isn't anything too much on your scan. I know that you're hoping it'll show what's wrong, but again, with scans they're good at showing up specific things, like the x-ray does – scans are good at showing up discs and whether the disc has bulged, or is pushing out onto a nerve, as they sometimes do. With you, because your pain is all in your back and not down your leg, you're unlikely to have any nerves being pinched, but what you could have is what's called a central disc bulge – where the disc does bulge outwards but it rarely compresses nerves unless it is a really big bulge. I'll show you what I mean.'

I get out the skeleton...

For the reader: Louis didn't finish this. I'm sure he would have edited the text. I also noted that it was started six months before he wrote the bulk of these books, therefore he would have cross-referenced it more with his later writing – if he had had the time! I decided to include it because there are some useful points that may be of interest? Louis very rarely asked for x-rays or scans for patients but as he says this guy wasn't going anywhere with rehab until these had been done. I hope the letter to the Doc highlights this? Derek's outcome: as expected, his MRI scan revealed some early disc dehydration in the lumbar spine, but no central disc protrusion at L5/S1; lower limb reflexes were there; he got going on a graded activity programme; he reported being about 99% better at his last visit! This was about four months after his first assessment; he'd been heard, activated and supported (eight sessions total – more than our average, possibly because he had the luxury of some insurance for physiotherapy input) and he was walking, cycling and working, at discharge!

Case History 4.2
Alan: an atypical nerve root problem – not to me!

In the kingdom of the fruits
The prune is snubbed by others
And they are not allowed
To mingle with the crowd
Though they're never on display
With all their highbrow brothers
They never seem to mind
To this fact they're resigned
That no matter how young a prune may be
It's always full of wrinkles
Beauty treatments always fail
They've tried all to no avail
Other fruits are envious
Because they know real well
That no matter how young a prune may be
Hot water makes 'em swell

Baby prunes look like their dad
But not wrinkled quite as bad

Song of the Prune (Extract 2)
(Crumit / DeCosta)
Frank Crumit - c. 1928

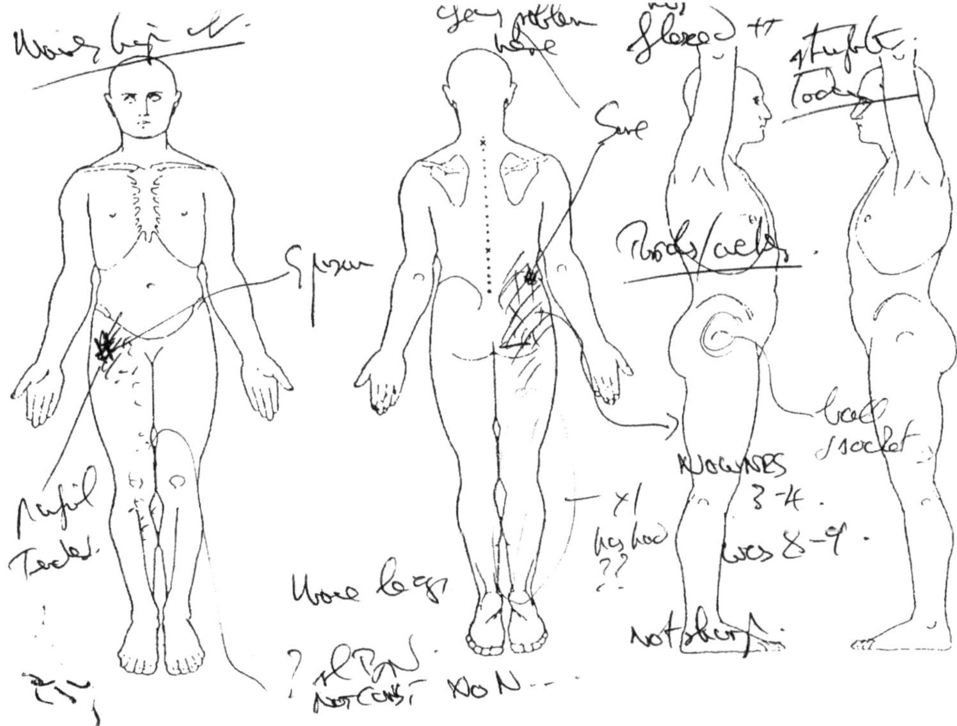

Figure CH4.1 Alan's Body Chart

Alan came to see me complaining that his main pain was in his lateral right groin, '... like a muscle spasm... it's been tweaking for several weeks with a bit going round into my backside.'

A week previously he felt it strongly, while playing tennis, he had found it hard to walk and be fully upright. Never-the-less he carried on, it felt a bit stiff and he managed to go jogging, but then it became 'agony' about five days ago. He was in Bristol at the time and saw an osteopath, who focused on the hip spasm and buttock – she diagnosed a hip muscle problem. The treatment made no difference and he had very poor sleep, the buttock pain got worse and he also described the feeling of the hip feeling 'sore' and 'inflamed'. Alan said he'd only managed about one hours sleep for the last few nights and he was constantly up and down. Lying down and trying to relax was the worst thing and he'd ended up sleeping in the chair, with his feet up and out straight. He noted that the first night when it started the only position he could get any ease was curled up on his knees on the floor.

He had been to his Dr, who agreed that he had severe muscle spasm, who gave him co-codamol and diazepam to relax the muscles and Alan was told not to drive. As he was not keen on drugs he hadn't taken any of them.

Sitting was not a problem, he could hardly walk though, due to the sharp hip pain when trying to be upright and he could really only walk in about 30 degrees or more of flexion.

Cough and sneeze were no problem, bladder and bowls were fine, his general health was really good – a retired airline pilot – into walking, tennis, gardening etc.) and he was not on any regular medication.

'Any previous problems like this?'

'I've always protected my back. I've basically had a weak back for as long as I can remember – it stiffens and is stiff every day... I'm even cautious cleaning my teeth but it's all become a normal habit...'

'Have you ever had anything like this – around the buttock and hip and so severe?'

'Not at all, just the odd few days where if I take it easy my back settles and I can carry on as normal.'

'No nerve pain down your leg, no 'sciatica' or that sort of thing?'

'Never.'

'OK, good, tell me did the Dr or osteopath check your reflexes or muscle strength?'

'No, no they didn't... '

OK, fine, anything else you want to tell me?'

'Yes, I'm on a walking holiday in five weeks, so there's a bit of pressure on!'

I smile and raise my eyes a little...

'Well, let's have a look now... '

I start the examination.

Now, this guy is in his mid 50's, nice and fit looking, is standing stooped forward and shifted off to the left. His lumbar spine is massively kyphotic and doesn't look as if it's extended for years let alone the last week or so.

He's suffering and it's building up. I get him to move and tell me what happens. He bends to the floor super flexible, he can stay there, it's relieving. His back hasn't changed, he's got good hips and very good hamstrings and sciatic length and flexibility. There's no extension as I expected – after holding upright for several seconds, the buttock and hip pain build to a very nasty level and he has to flex and hold on, while waiting for the pain to subside. Side flexion and rotation are done in flexion and the back barely moves from T9 down!

I get him to tip toe and walk on his heels and he struggles. We do calf raises and he can only just lift up on the right tip toe. The calf is clearly weak. I get him to focus on strength, not the pain and he still can't make it come up well...

I then get him to sit with his legs dangling and test his reflexes – there's absolutely nothing in both calves and nothing in his right quads. I can get his left quads reflex and he's looking at me a bit startled, so I do a bit of explaining.

'I'll tell you what I think in a minute, but it looks like you may have a disc and nerve problem – the nerves that supply these reflexes have been injured slightly and also the ones that supply the calf muscle – as you saw just now, you're a bit weaker tip-toeing on the right.'

I then check his foot dorsiflexion, eversion and toe dorsiflexors – foot dorsiflexors (main root L4) are significantly weaker as are all the toe extensors (L5 root). Eversion and quads are fine.

I check his sensation – it's fine and his slump test is fine too as I'd expected. I also get him to do some sitting hip movements – cross legs – normal and foot on knee let knee lower, hug leg etc. These are all fine. I quickly test all the static hip muscles too to see if there's any pain response or weakness – but they're all fine. I'll come back to hip ranges later if necessary.

Lying down, his SLR's are 85-90 degrees with no provocation. Right hip flexion/adduction is moderately sore, but so is the left. I don't see this as anything majorly hip but there may be something to put in the shopping basket later when he's out of this acute phase.

Thoughts:

Chris had been to an osteopath and a Dr and was given the notion that his problem was mere muscle spasm. The way I've told the story I would have thought it was obvious that this was a nerve root problem and highly likely to be 'disc' related affecting at least two levels. What's disturbing is the lack of basic objective testing – it not being at all difficult and quick to test muscle strength, skin sensibility and reflexes.

There is the 'so what?' argument though – so what if there's a disc, what are you going to do about it anyway ... it won't make any difference to my treatments... it'll get better regardless...

I don't buy that at all – most normal people want to know our fundamentals...

- What's wrong with me?

- Is it serious?

- How long will it take to get better?

- Will it recover?

- Can I do anything to help it get better...?

- Can you do anything or give me anything to help me get better...?

- Are there any other options I should consider?

... discussion of slow recovery/nerve adaptation/

Reader: Louis did not have time to complete this case history. He wanted to highlight the pain distribution on the 'body chart', with pain radiating to anterior groin/hip and also paraesthesia down the anteromedial thigh and lower leg. Louis noted that both the osteopath and Dr latched onto the 'hip muscles' as culprits, but objective tests were far more revealing. I do know that he wrote a letter to the Dr pleased that an MRI scan was arranged. Louis suggested that L4 and possibly L5 and S1 nerve roots were compromised and Alan may have significant 'stenotic effect' in his lower back (probably long standing, due to his vulnerable back history). The scan did reveal degenerative changes, some thickening affecting L4 nerve root but not impinging, not stenosis – so not too bad!

Louis went through the Toblerone recovery with Alan and all the pain reduction strategies he could – over a period of a month pain reduced considerably. Time, drugs and natural history! I don't know if Alan went on his walking holiday!

Case History 4.3

Susie: a shoulder injury what helped the most

Every day in every way
The world is getting better
We've even learned to fly
As days go passing by
But how about the poor old prune
His life is only wetter
No wonder he can't win
In the awful stew he's in
No matter how young a prune may be
He's always full of wrinkles
We may get them on our face
Prunes get 'em every place
Nothing ever worries them
Their life's an open book
But no matter how young a prune may be
It has a worried look

Prunes act very kind they say
When sickly people moan
But no matter how young a prune may be
It has a heart of stone

Song of the Prune (Extract 3)
(Crumit / DeCosta)
Frank Crumit - c. 1928'

The following is adapted from a report written by a patient about her management following a fractured shoulder:

Susie suffered a fracture of her right shoulder after falling onto her right side. This was confirmed the same day by x-ray and the arm was put into a sling. The immediate advice was that the arm would probably remain in a sling for up to eleven weeks and due to the nature of the injury, it was unlikely that any surgical procedure would be undertaken.

Two days later a second x-ray revealed that the bone had moved slightly. Susie was advised to keep her arm perfectly still and await a call regarding a 'further procedure'. She was contacted a few days later and told that a pinning/plating operation was planned. A further face to face consultation followed, but it was decided that an operation would be too complex. And that the outcome of an operation, or leaving the injury to repair naturally, would be the same. Susie's prognosis at that stage was that she may, in the long term, be able to raise her hand up to cheek or brow level, but her shoulder would probably be very stiff.

Susie…

As it turned out although this news was not the most welcome at the time, it was a blessing, because it made me determined to do my utmost to do everything in my power to improve on this prognosis!

I agreed to do as I was advised. I kept the arm in a sling at all times and very still. In these early days it was very painful but bearable. I managed some sleep, by lying on my back.

After three weeks, I attended the fracture clinic (which was run efficiently, in spite of large numbers of people waiting) but, in my eyes, I was given some slightly conflicting information. I was advised to begin to move the arm and rotate it slightly, at frequent intervals, unless it was too painful to do so.

At this point, I also noted that my elbow was extremely stiff and any movement very painful. The fracture clinic also said to, 'keep your arm in the sling' until my next appointment. Pleasingly, I was able to return to work on a five hour day basis, working from my desk. This move felt very positive and beneficial.

After five weeks I sought advice from a specialist, whose immediate response was to remove the sling and get movement going. And much to my relief an x-ray confirmed that healing had started to take place. However, after this period in the sling the shoulder was 'frozen' and the elbow was stiff. I would need a lot of physio help in order to get movement back and work the muscles to strengthen the elbow/arm/shoulder. I was very relieved to know that the fracture was repairing and that if I 'put in the work' then I should have a good, though unlikely full, return to strength.

Six weeks in and physio began! From the first moment, I felt an energy and sense of purpose. The sessions were positive, instructive and without too much discomfort. Initially, twice weekly sessions, moving on to weekly sessions quite quickly, produced rapid progress. I looked forward to them and the continued and noticeable improvement. A regime of exercises at home, with a pulley, for movement and strengthening helped a great deal. These were all practiced in the physio session, prior to the end of the session, so that both the physio and I were confident that I was carrying them out in an effective and correct manner. I became more and more determined.

At seven weeks post injury I was able to type without too much discomfort and this helped gain more movement in the elbow, which was getting easier daily.

At ten weeks I was able to drive with confidence, having had a few practice sessions, I felt that this was a great aid to strengthening the muscles and although initially very painful, soon became less so. Also, I was now working full time.

Fourteen weeks in and I was using my arm quite freely, even reaching into high cupboards.

Seventeen weeks after that fall and I was able to carry out gardening tasks, hoeing, weeding, clipping and most importantly, sweeping – all good exercise. Very little discomfort now.

Thoughts and observations:

The initial advice I received had been correct and had given the best outcome. However, it would have been of *enormous* benefit if, when attending the initial clinical appointments, I had been informed that there were signs of repair. I felt the need, not just for re-assurance, but some verbal confirmation that 'things were moving on' and that a *vital* part of regaining movement would be down to exercise and physiotherapy. And advice that a great deal of commitment in this area, would produce the best long term outcome.

Hard work and commitment by highly professional and dedicated medics is somewhat dissipated if, following an injury, there is no rehabilitation and encouragement for patients to do whatever *they* can, in order to achieve the best results. I realize that, for some people, the need to be encouraged to help themselves will be unecessary, but for many others it is not so - especially at a time when they are in pain, unsure what to do and experiencing disruption in their lives.

Being injured and incapacitated, at whatever age and by whatever problem, creates a feeling of isolation and downheartedness, one needs to see there is a 'light at the end of the tunnel'.

Since my accident I have been staggered by the number of people, of all ages, I've met who have suffered from a similar injury. This is not an uncommon result of falls in all sorts of situations. Those, who have made a good recovery, told me that physio and exercise was a vital part of it, but for a variety of reasons, for example, reduced budgets and scarcity of resources are not always readily available.

One year on –'that lightbulb moment'

It's just over a year since my injury and a visit to my physiotherapist today has confirmed that all is well and the movement good.

I have continued with the daily exercises and I continue to garden daily. I am still using the pulley and the strength has returned in equal proportions to both arms.

The occasionally ache and get the odd twinge! This positive result would not have been achieved without the expertise and encouragement of the physiotherapist, there is no doubt in my mind about that. Having had a fracture like this the most important thing is to be assured that one can CONFIDENTLY begin movement and not be afraid of so doing.

Finally and gratefully, yes, I can change a lightbulb!

Louis Gifford

Louis Gifford
Curriculum Vitae

Painkiller

Had a dream in a clean fresh Falmouth blue
Solid groundswell perfect weather.
In the middle a miracle came true
The kindest man no longer suffers

You heal people, with your head, your heart, your hand.
Painkiller.

Underneath a silver mackerel sky
You told me never to say never.
The sweetest of secrets revealed in good time
The blood between the brothers.

Ironic injustice, your muscles in agony
But even in weakness you're still thinking originally.
With your head, your heart, your hand. Painkiller

Megan Henwood from the album 'Head, heart and hand'

Louis Sebastian Gifford

DOB 07.04.1953

Aches and Pains Ltd
& Falmouth Physiotherapy Clinic
Kestrel
Swanpool
Falmouth
Cornwall, TR11 5BD
UK

T. 01326 312156
F. 01326 211149

info@achesandpainsonline.com

www.achesandpainsonline.com

www.giffordsachesandpains.com

Current Occupation:

Chartered Physiotherapist:

* Private practitioner, Director Aches and Pains Ltd and Falmouth Physiotherapy Clinic. 1988-present.
* Freelance Lecturer in England, Europe, Australia, South Africa and the USA.
* Invited author Elsevier, Butterworth Heinemann, writing and editing.
* Director CNS Press Ltd, 1998 present
* Reader/referee for *Physiotherapy* Journal, *Manual Therapy* Journal and the International Association for the Study of Pain (IASP) Journal *'Pain'*
* Retired Committee member of the Physiotherapy Pain Association (PPA)
* Retired Editor of PPA News 1995-2007
* Editor of the PPA, 'Topical Issues in Pain' book series (details below)

Academic qualifications.

- BSc Zoology University of London, 1975

- Post Graduate Certificate in Education, Bath University, 1976

- Associateship in Physiotherapy, Sheffield City Polytechnic, 1981

- Graduate Diploma in Advanced Manipulative Therapy, South Australian Institute of Technology, 1985

- Masters in Applied Science (Physiotherapy), University of South Australia, 1993

- Awarded a Fellowship of the Chartered Society of Physiotherapy – October 2001 - *The Fellowship was conferred for innovative work in the management and understanding of pain and the dissemination of the work to the profession via teaching, lecturing and writing.*

- Awarded a Fellowship of the Musculoskeletal Association of Chartered Physiotherapists – October 2011

Conference presentations - key-note and invited speaker:

Moira Packenham Walsh Memorial Lecture, London 1988: **Chasing Pain and Inventing Techniques**

World Congress of Physiotherapy, The Barbican, London 1991: **Chasing pain and inventing Techniques**

Olive Sands Memorial Lecture, OCPPP Annual Conference, Bristol 1993: **Examining and treating signs of neural tension**

Swiss National Physiotherapy Congress, Davos, Switzerland, June 1994: **Pain Mechanisms and their recognition for Physiotherapy – a new approach for the 1990's**

The Chartered Society of Physiotherapy Conference, Physiotherapy and Back Pain. London, June 1994: **Adverse Neural Tension**

Society of Orthopaedic Medicine and The British Institute of Musculoskeletal Medicine, London, December 1994: **Nerve palpation and its relevance in peripherally driven neuropathic pain syndromes**

Moving in on Pain Conference, Adelaide, Australia, April 1995: **Fluid movement may partially account for the behaviour of symptoms associated with nociception in disc injury and disease**

CSP Congress Scarborough 1995: **Central pain mechanisms and chronic pain disability**

CSP Congress Scarborough 1995: Workshop: **Central pain mechanisms and RSI**

Royal Alexandra Hospital 10th Anniversary Symposium, The Treatment of Pain. October 1996: **Pain and Physiotherapy**

IFOMT –ECE conference, Amsterdam, The Netherlands April 1997: **Recurrent and ongoing back pain – Collagen? Or the Nervous system?**

McKenzie Institute UK Conference and AGM: November 1997: **Neurobiology of Pain, consequences for diagnosis and management**

6th Nordic Congress on Manual Therapy. Oslo, March 1998: **The Mature Organism Model, the disc and the sciatic nerve**

6th Nordic Congress on Manual Therapy. Oslo, March 1998: **Case History: The shift from a passive-therapy-structure-orientated-and-focus-on-pain approach, to a self management and functional restoration approach**

OCPPP 45th Annual Conference, Balancing our Act. April 1998: **Pain, the tissues and the nervous system**

OCPPP 45th Annual Conference, Balancing our Act. April 1998. Workshop: **Integration of pain mechanisms into diagnosis, clinical reasoning and management**

Reading Shoulder Seminar, September 1998: **Neural Sensitivity – evaluation and differentiation**

Danish Sports Medicine Conference, Copenhagen, November 1998: **Pain Rehabilitation and Sports Medicine**

International Association for the Study of Pain (IASP) World Congress. Vienna, August 1999: Workshop - **Explaining Pain To Patients**

7th Nordic Congress on Manual Therapy: Low Back Pain, Clinical and Scientific Update. Copenhagen, Denmark, September 1999: **The Implication of pain science for the prevention of chronicity**

Chartered Society of Physiotherapy Annual Congress, Birmingham, October 1999: **New treatments, new assessments, new thinking: time for questions, time for change?**

Chartered Society of Physiotherapy Annual Congress, Birmingham, October 1999: **Why should the disc bother to hurt? An Introduction to Darwinian Reasoning**

Chartered Society of Physiotherapy Annual Congress, Birmingham, October 2000: **Physical Examination, pain, sensitivity, impairment and disability**

International Physiotherapists in Private Practice Association, Eastbourne. Workshops: **Nerve root**

NVMT conference, Eindhoven, Holland, 23rd March 2001- Lecture: **Impairments, disabilities and barriers – The 'shopping basket' approach**

NVMT conference, Eindhoven, Holland, 23- 24th March 2001- Workshop: **The 'shopping basket' approach: case histories, clinical reasoning and management**

Placebo study day: Treliske Hospital, Truro, 5th April 2002. **Evolutionary reasoning and the placebo**

Conference: How to explain the inexplicable: Subjective Health Complaints, Chronic Pain, Stress and other Phenomena. A one day Southwest regional meeting hosted by the Pain Management Department of the Royal Cornwall Hospitals Trust at the Alverton Manor, Truro. 14th of May 2003. **Presentation: The Vulnerable organism**

9th National Conference on Pain Management Programmes. 11-12 September 2003. John Innes Centre and University of East Anglia, Norwich. **Pain biology and clinical reasoning**

Danish Physiotherapy Congress: 'Fagfestival'. Denmark November 20-22nd 2003 **Keynote lecture: Chronic pain: If we know how it starts can it be stopped? (The vulnerable organism)**

Danish Physiotherapy Congress: 'Fagfestival'. Denmark November 20-22nd 2003 **Workshop: biopsychosocial factors – using a 'shopping basket' approach**

Norwegian Association of Sports Physiotherapy Conference 2004, Lillihammer, Feb 6-7:

   1. **Pain biology and clinical reasoning**

   2. **An introduction to pain mechanisms**

   3. **Integrating the biopsychosocial model – The 'shopping basket' approach**

   4. **The 'shopping basket' approach in practice – graded exposure**

NVMT Conference 2004, Eindhoven, Holland, March 12-13. Workshop: **Chronic pain: If we know how it starts can it be stopped? The vulnerable organism**

NVMT Conference 2004, Eindhoven, Holland, March 12-13. Keynote lecture: **The challenge of evolutionary reasoning:**

OCPPP Conference 2004, 'Turning Heads' The East Midlands Conference Centre, Nottingham 24-25th April. Workshop: **Why does acute pain sometimes become chronic pain?**

OCPPP Conference 2004, 'Turning Heads' The East Midlands Conference Centre, Nottingham 24-25 April. Workshop: **The shopping basket approach and graded exposure**

Integrated musculoskeletal trauma conference (IMTC) 2005, Waterfront Hall, Belfast. May 25-27: Complex Regional Pain Syndrome and pain management

Chartered Society of Physiotherapy Annual Congress 2005, Birmingham International Conference Centre: October 7th: **The vulnerable organism: chronic pain, if we know how it starts can it be stopped?**

Irish Society of Chartered Physiotherapy Annual Congress, The Kilkenny Ormonde Hotel, Kilkenny, Eire. **The vulnerable organism: chronic pain, if we know how it starts can it be stopped?**

Physio First Conference 2006, East Midlands Conference Centre, Nottingham University, April 1st: **Red and Yellow flags and improving treatment outcomes: or:'Top down before bottom up'**

Swiss Association of Physiotherapy Congress 2006, Lausanne, Switzerland, Saturday 22nd April: **Fear Avoidance - is therapy a part of the problem?**

Swiss Association of Physiotherapy Congress 2006, Lausanne, Switzerland, Friday 21st April: **'Meet the expert' session: Graded exposure for acute and sub-acute back pain**

Norwegian Association of Manual and Sports Physiotherapists Conference 2007: Storjfhell, Norway, February, **Chronic pain: if we know how it starts can it be stopped?**

Norwegian Association of Manual and Sports Physiotherapists Conference 2007: Storjfhell, Norway, February, **Chronic pain: permanent or curable?**

Norwegian Association of Manual and Sports Physiotherapists Conference 2007: Storjfhell, Norway, February, **Sub acute low back pain case history: 'The twisted ankle approach to low back pain'**

Physiotherapy Pain Association (PPA) Northern Branch 2007. Glasgow, February 8th 2007. Invited Speaker. Lecture day: **'I'm hoping you can cure me!'**

Rehabworks Ltd, Bury St Edmonds, Suffolk, May 13th, 2008 **'Tricking Pain'**

Oxford Physiotherapy, Wheatley, Oxford, March 20th, 2009 **'Problem pain patients assessment, treatment and management'**

Cornwall and IoS NHS Community Health Services, Pain Symposium, Truro, May 12th 2009 **'Good Pain, Bad Pain, Explain Pain'**

Additional Lectures

- Visiting Lecturer: MSc in Musculoskeletal Physiotherapy, Coventry UK, 1988-9

- Visiting Lecturer: St Georges Medical School, tutoring undergraduates in Physiotherapy 1999-2000

- Visiting Lecturer: Post Graduate Study Centre, Zurzach, Switzerland - biannual since 1991. Also teaching in Bad Ragaz, Switzerland, 1991.

- Lecturer for Neuro Orthopaedic Institute Worldwide 1994 - 2000

- Lecturer, Aches and Pains Ltd (achesandpainsonline.com) 2000 - present

Courses include:

- Mobilisation of the Nervous system

- The Clinical Biology of Aches and Pains

- Graded Exposure

- Graded Exposure - patients

- The Dynamic Nervous System

- Topical Issues in Pain Forum

- The Nerve Root

Published Material - articles, chapters and books:

Gifford L.S. (1987) Circadian variation in human flexibility and grip strength. Australian Journal of Physiotherapy, **33**, 1, 3-9.

Butler D.S. and Gifford L.S. (1989) Adverse Mechanical Tension in the Nervous System - Part 1, Testing for dural tension'. Physiotherapy 75, 622-629

Butler D.S. and Gifford L.S. (1989) Adverse Mechanical Tension in the Nervous System - Part 2, Examination and Treatment. Physiotherapy 75, 629-636

Gifford L.S. (1993) Examining and treating signs of neural tension. In Touch: The Journal of the Organisation of Chartered Physiotherapists in Private Practice, 68: 16-24

Gifford L.S. and Gifford M.J. (1994) Connective Tissue Massage. In: Pain Management in Physiotherapy 2nd Ed. Bowsher Frampton V. and Wells P. (eds). Blackwell Scientific London

Gifford L.S. (1995) The influence of circadian variation on spinal examination. In: Boyling J. and Palastanga N. (eds) Grieve'sModern Manual Therapy, Churchill Livingstone, Edinburgh

Gifford L.S. (1995) Pain mechanisms and their recognition for physiotherapy - a new approach for the late 1990's. Swiss Journal of Physiotherapy: June 1995: 4-16. **Article in German**.

Gifford L.S. (1995) Fluid movement may partially account for the behaviour of symptoms associated with nociception in disc injury and disease. In: Shacklock, M O (ed) Moving in on Pain. Butterworth-Heinemann, Australia.

Gifford L.S. (1997) Neurodynamics. In: Pitt-Brooke (ed) Rehabilitation of Movement: Theoretical bases of clinical practice Saunders, London 159-195

Gifford L.S. (1997) Pain. In: Pitt-Brooke (ed) Rehabilitation of Movement: Theoretical bases of clinical practice Saunders, London 196-232

Gifford L.S. and Butler D.S. (1997) The integration of pain sciences into clinical practice. Hand Therapy 10(2): 86-95

Gifford L.S. and Butler D.S. (1998) Integrering av smertevitenskap i klinisk praksis. Fysioterapeuten nr 9 August: 10-20 (**Norwegian translation of Gifford and Butler 1997)**

Gifford L.S. (1998) Pain, the tissues and the nervous system: A conceptual model. Physiotherapy 84(1): 27-36

Gifford L.S. (1998) Acute low cervical nerve root conditions: Symptoms, symptom behaviour and physical screening. In Touch: The Journal of the Organisation of Chartered Physiotherapists in Private Practice, Winter issue No. 85: 4-19

Gifford L.S. (1998) The mature organism model. In: Gifford L.S.(ed) Topical Issues in Pain. Whiplash - science and management. Fear-avoidance beliefs and behaviour. CNS Press, Falmouth 45 56

Gifford L.S. (1998) Central mechanisms. In: Gifford L.S.(ed) Topical Issues in Pain 1. Whiplash - science and management. Fear-avoidance beliefs and behaviour. CNS Press, Falmouth 67-80

Gifford L.S. (1998) Output mechanisms. In: Gifford L.S.(ed) Topical Issues in Pain 1. Whiplash - science and management. Fear-avoidance beliefs and behaviour. CNS Press, Falmouth 81-91

Gifford L.S. (1998) Tissue and input related mechanisms. In: Gifford L S (ed) Topical Issues in Pain 1. Whiplash - science and management. Fear-avoidance beliefs and behaviour. CNS Press, Falmouth 57-65

Gifford L. S. (1998) Pain memory. In Touch: The Journal of the Organisation of Chartered Physiotherapists in Private Practice Autumn issue.

Gifford L. S. (1999) A medico-legal report to a solicitor. Manual Therapy 4(4): 229-235

Gifford L.S. (2000) Schmerzphysiologie. In: Van den Berg, F (Ed) Angewandte Physiologie 2, Organsysteme verstehen und beeinflussen. Georg Thieme Verlag, Stuttgart 467-518 (**Chapter in German**)

Gifford L. S. (2000) The patient in front of us: from genes to environment. In: Gifford L S (ed) Topical Issues in Pain 2. Biopsychosocial assessment and management. Relationships and pain CNS Press, Falmouth

Gifford L.S. (2000) Editorial: Criticism, is it destructive or productive? Physiotherapy Pain Association News: Issue 11, May, p3-5

Gifford L.S. (2001) Editorial: A plea for descriptive research - part 1 Physiotherapy Pain Association News: Issue 12, December, p3-5

Gifford L.S. (2001) Acute low cervical nerve root conditions - symptom presentations and pathobiological reasoning. Manual Therapy 6 (2) 106-115

Gifford L.S. (2002) Editorial: Quite a pill eh? Physiotherapy Pain Association News: Issue 13, May, p3-4

Gifford L.S. (2001) Perspectives on the biopsychosocial model - part 1: Some issues that need to be accepted? In Touch: The Journal of the Organisation of Chartered Physiotherapists in Private Practice. Autumn, No 97

Gifford L.S. (2002) Perspectives on the biopsychosocial model part 2: The shopping basket approach. In Touch, The Journal of the Organisation of Chartered Physiotherapists in Private Practice Spring issue No 99: 11-22

Gifford L.S. (2002) Editorial: Therapist and patient fear of bending: Does the McKenzie approach - need a shift? Physiotherapy Pain Association News: Issue 14, May, p3-8

Gifford L.S. (2002) Memes, dreams and dualism… the flexion-extension debate and beyond. Physiotherapy Pain Association News: Issue 15, May, p14-20

Gifford L.S. (2003) Perspectives on the biopsychosocial model part 3: Patient example - using the shopping basket approach and graded exposure. In Touch, The Journal of the Organisation of Chartered Physiotherapists in Private Practice Spring issue No 102: 3-15

Jones M. A., Edwards I., Gifford L. S. (2002) Conceptual models for implementing biopsychosocial theory in Clinical Practice. Manual Therapy 7(1): 2-9

Gifford L. S. (2002) An Introduction to evolutionary reasoning: Diet, discs and the placebo. In: Gifford L S (ed) Topical Issues in Pain 4. Placebo and nocebo. Pain management. Muscles and pain. CNS Press, Falmouth

Gifford L S., Thacker M. (2002) A clinical overview of the autonomic nervous system, the supply to the gut and mind-body pathways. In: Gifford L S (ed) Topical Issues in Pain 3. Sympathetic nervous system and pain. Pain management. Clinical effectiveness CNS Press, Falmouth 21-52

Gifford L.S., Thacker M. (2002) Complex regional pain syndrome: Part 1. In: Gifford L S (ed) Topical Issues in Pain 3. Sympathetic nervous system and pain. Pain management. Clinical effectiveness CNS Press, Falmouth 53-74

Thacker M., Gifford L.S. (2002) Complex regional pain syndrome: Part 2. In: Gifford L S (ed) Topical Issues in Pain 3. Sympathetic nervous system and pain. Pain management. Clinical effectiveness CNS Press, Falmouth 75-102

Thacker M., Gifford L. S. (2002) A review of the physiotherapy management of complex regional pain syndrome. In: Gifford L S (ed) Topical Issues in Pain 3. Sympathetic nervous system and pain. Pain management. Clinical effectiveness CNS Press, Falmouth 119-142

Thacker M., Gifford L.S. (2002) Sympathetically maintained pain: myth or reality? In: Gifford L S (ed) Topical Issues in Pain 3. Sympathetic nervous system and pain. Pain management. Clinical effectiveness CNS Press, Falmouth 103-118

Gifford L.S. (2003) Behov for helhedstaenkning. Fysioterapeuten Nr 20/November/ 85.argang   (Danish translation of Gifford L S 2000 The patient in front of us: from genes to environment. In: Gifford L S (ed) Topical Issues in Pain 2. Biopsychosocial assessment and management. Relationships and pain CNS Press, Falmouth)

Gifford L.S. (2004) Unnecessary fear avoidance and physical incapacity in a 55-year-old housewife. In: Jones M & Rivett D (Eds) Clinical Reasoning for Manual Therapists. Butterworth-Heineman, Edinburgh 61-86

Gifford L S 2004 Laast sich chronischer Schmerz vergessen? Manuelletherapie. 8:181-182

Robson S., Gifford L.S. (2005) Pain and brain - a revolutionary approach to chronic injury. Peak Performance Issue 221: 1-4

Robson S., Gifford L.S. (2005) Pain And Brain - The Biopsychosocial Method Of Chronic Injury Rehabilitation. Peak Performance, Issue 222:8-11.

Gifford L.S. (2005) Schmerzphysiologie. In: Van den Berg, F (Ed) Angewandte Physiologie 2, Organsysteme verstehen (2nd edn). Georg Thieme Verlag, Stuttgart 481-535 (**Chapter in German**)

Gifford L.S., Thacker M. and Jones M. (2006) Physiotherapy and pain. In: McMahon S, Koltzenburg M. Wall and Melzack's Textbook of Pain, 5th Edn pp:603-617

Robson S., Gifford L.S. (2006) Manual Therapy in the 21st Century. In: Gifford L S (Ed), Topical Issues in Pain vol 5, CNS Press, Falmouth 3-34

Gifford L.S. (2006) Red and yellow flags and improving treatment outcomes or: 'Top down before bottom up!' In Touch, Summer 2006 issue no: 115:18-24

Robson S., Gifford L.S. (2008) Manual medicine. In: Breivik H, Campbell WI, Nicholas MK (Eds): Clinical Pain Management (2nd Edn) : Practice and Procedures. Hodder Arnold, London 230-239.

Edited Books:

Gifford L.S. (ed) (1998) Topical Issues in Pain 1. Whiplash - science and management. Fear-avoidance beliefs and behaviour. CNS Press, Falmouth

Gifford L.S. (ed) (2000) Topical Issues in Pain 2. Biopsychosocial assessment. Relationships and pain. CNS Press, Falmouth

Gifford L.S. (ed) (2002) Topical Issues in Pain 3. Sympathetic nervous system and pain. Pain management. Clinical effectiveness. CNS Press, Falmouth

Gifford L S (ed) (2002) Topical Issues in Pain 4. Placebo and nocebo. Pain management. Muscles and pain. CNS Press, Falmouth

Gifford L.S. (ed) (2006) Topical Issues in Pain 5. Treatment. Communication. Return to Work. Cognitive-behavioural. Pathophysiology. CNS Press, Falmouth

Current writing projects:

Gifford L.S. (1978-2009-2014) Louis Gifford Aches and Pains. Pain explanations: Management foundations. CNS Press/Aches and Pains, Falmouth Physiotherapy Clinic.

A practical and easy to read book that contains patient narratives, pain explanations and management foundations. Intended for physiotherapists treating and managing acute and chronic musculoskeletal pain states.

Member of the following professional organisations:

- Member of the Chartered Society of Physiotherapy (MCSP)
- Member of the International Association for the Study of Pain (IASP)

- Member of the Manipulation Association of Chartered Physiotherapists (MACP)
- Member of the Organisation of Chartered Physiotherapists in Private Practice (OCPPP)
- Member of the Health Professions Council (HPC)
- Honorary Life Member of the Physiotherapy Pain Association (PPA) and executive committee member. Formerly Education chair.
- Member of the Pain Society

Previous Employment

Lecturer:

- Department of Biology, Milton Margai Teachers College, Freetown, Sierra Leone, West Africa. 1976-1978.   Biology lecturer.
- Department of Health Sciences, South Australian Institute of Technology, Adelaide. 1986-87. Part time lecturer on the post graduate diploma in advanced manipulative therapy.

Physiotherapist:

- Walton Hospital, Liverpool: 1981-1982
- St Stephens Hospital, Fulham, London: 1982-1984
- G D Maitland and partners, Adelaide, South Australia: 1986-1987

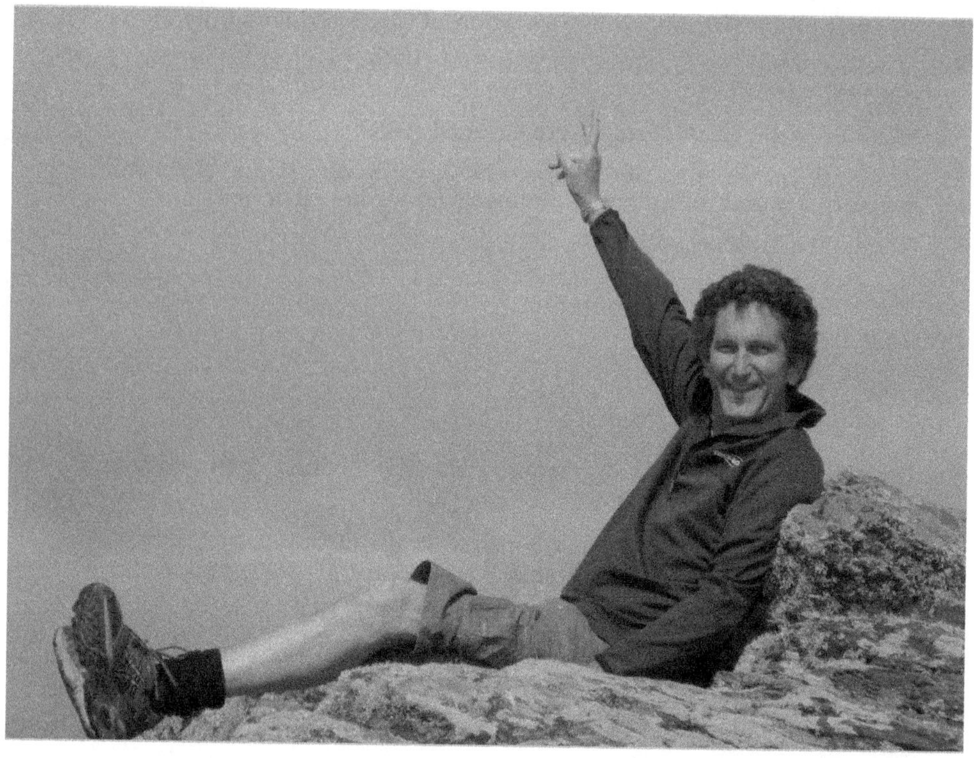

'Louis was a true inspiration and advocate for living life to the full and I have many fond memories of his infectious positivity. I will never forget him telling me not to screw my face up in pain "because it really is unattractive!" He explained pain to me and that wisdom helped me through the first of a double hip replacement. I will stay faithful to his expertise and remember him always.'

Emma Teague
- a message from one of Louis' patients February 2014 (with permission)

Printed in the USA
CPSIA information can be obtained
at www.ICGtesting.com
CBHW061633110224
4273CB00033B/484